Virtuous Liaisons

Virtuous Liaisons

Care, Love, Sex, and Virtue Ethics

RAJA HALWANI

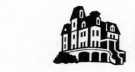

OPEN COURT
Chicago and La Salle, Illinois

To order books from Open Court, call 1-800-815-2280 or visit www.opencourtbooks.com.

Cover painting by Christopher Koch, "Infinity," 2001, oil on linen, 2'4" × 2'4". Reproduced with permission.

Open Court Publishing Company is a division of Carus Publishing Company.

Library of Congress Cataloging-in-Publication Data

Halwani, Raja.
    Virtuous liaisons : care, love, sex, and virtue ethics / Raja Halwani.

        p. cm.
Includes bibliographical references and index.
        ISBN 0-8126-9543-7 (trade pbk. : alk. paper)
    1. Virtue. 2. Ethics. 3. Caring. 4. Love. 5. Sexual ethics.   I. Title.
        BJ1531 .H25 2003
        179'.9—dc22

                                                                2003018107

To my brothers Firas, Omar, and Makram.
For their goodness.

Contents

Contents   ix

Acknowledgments

A number of individuals have been invaluable to the writing of this book. Claudia Card, Rosalind Hursthouse, Mary Jeanne Larrabee, Catherine Lord, Margaret McLaren, and Richard Mohr have all read parts of an early draft. Their comments were extremely helpful. My thanks go to them.

John Corvino, Marianne Janack, Steve Jones, and Christopher Koch have read an early draft of this book and have supplied me with valuable insights and comments, and often saved me from contradicting myself. My gratitude and thanks are immense.

Special thanks go to Alan Soble who has read a penultimate draft of this book. His comments and suggestions, often laced with humor, helped make the book what it is in its final form.

Much of my thinking about sex and love has matured due to the work of Alan Soble. Much of my thinking about virtue ethics has matured due to the work of Rosalind Hursthouse. My intellectual debt to them is infinite.

Both Kerri Mommer and Cindy Pineo from Open Court have made wonderful editorial suggestions to the manuscript, both substantive and stylistic. Their editing has put a final stop—and thank goodness for that—to my verbosity and tendency for wordiness (just witness this last sentence). I thank them.

It is surely much more than thanks and gratitude that are owed to those who make our lives meaningful and worth living. Whatever its nature, it is this debt that I owe to Steven William Jones.

Parts of chapter 1 were published as "Care Ethics and Virtue Ethics" in the journal *Hypatia* (vol. 18, no. 3, summer 2003). I am grateful for Indiana University Press and *Hypatia*'s permission to reprint the material.

Introduction

Care, love, and sex. These are three phenomena considered central to our lives, but they are also rife with moral issues.

It is not an exaggeration to state that most people are, have been, and will be part of a close, caring relationship. Our parents, hopefully, cared for us when we were young—at least those of us who had parents. Many of us have and/or will care for our own children. Moreover, many of us are in other types of caring relationships: we are a friend to someone, a lover to another, a sibling to yet another. That we are in caring relationships is, for many reasons, an important fact about our lives, and it is one that merits close attention. Consider the following examples. Lovers sometimes spend large amounts of money on their beloveds, lavishing on them expensive gifts. Parents sometimes buy their children toys upon toys upon toys, sometimes to be discarded by their children after a few days. Siblings sometimes lie on behalf of each other. Lovers sometimes stay with each other, stick by each other, no matter what. Parents often defend their children no matter what their children have done. Because all of this occurs, one can argue, at the moral expense of others, there seems to be something morally suspicious about such actions. Why? Perhaps because one of the parties to these caring relationships is simply undeserving. He is, say, a bad person, period. Or, if he is not a bad person, there are other people that require our moral attention. Why should someone buy her daughter bags full of dolls when there are children in the world who are starving? Why should someone spend hours cooking yet another elaborate meal for his beloved, when he could have spent his time doing something else much more morally worthy? Why should a sister hide her brother from the law when she knows very well that her brother is a criminal?

The answer usually given is, "Because we love them. Because we care for them." Caring, as I said, is a pervasive activity in our lives. Without caring, no one really knows what we—human beings—would be or what we would "look like." In this respect, caring is not just pervasive to our lives. It is also important. But caring is also often used to shield morally dubious activities from scrutiny. This cannot be right. There is a need to be able to critically examine care and caring activities from a moral and philosophical perspective and to put care in its proper place. But it is difficult to discern what this proper place is. Presumably, it would give care the importance it deserves, without, at the same time, allowing it to trample on and to occupy other aspects of our moral lives.

Turn next to romantic love. Being in a romantic relationship with someone is one example of being in a caring relationship, and so the general issues surrounding morality and care apply to romantic love. But there is more. Judging from what one sees and hears in popular culture, love seems to be considered an ideal that we should all aspire to. This is, moreover, not a phenomenon confined to the Western world. Much of popular culture elsewhere in the world seems to reflect a similar view of love. Compared to friendship, for example, love receives a lot more attention. Philosophers, psychologists, novelists, and other people working in the humanities and social sciences do not generally depart from this view, either. But surely this view, if not wrong, merits some close attention. Are people who are not in love—better yet, who do not want to be in love— objects of pity? Is there something wrong with them? If yes, why? What is it about romantic love that deserves the emphasis put on it? And what proper place should love have in our lives? Even more important, perhaps, are issues regarding the connections between love and morality. We often hear it said, for example, that love makes people better. But what does this mean exactly? And is it true? If yes, how does love make people better— morally better, that is? If the answer is no, then why not?

Sex is yet another area that raises numerous issues. Though cultural norms are changing, most people still believe that certain types of sexual activities are wrong. Let me give a few examples. Many people still consider homosexual sex to be wrong, not only people who, because of their religious views, consider gay sex wrong (though that is not true of all religious people, of course), but also many seemingly ordinary people on the street. Consider promiscuity. Promiscuous people are still judged to a large extent to be defective in some way. At worst, they are considered immoral people and their actions are also considered to be wrong. At best, they are viewed as somehow lacking in something, as psychologically off, as being compelled to be promiscuous perhaps because of some trauma or other. Indeed, and to link these two examples together, often times the reason given—even by some philosophers—as to why homosexuality is wrong is because gay people are thought to be promiscuous. Consider next sex work, a line of work in which one earns one's living through sex, be it prostitution, phone sex, stripping, or acting in pornographic movies. Many people in society look down upon sex workers for doing something shameful or beneath them. At best, sex workers are objects of pity to those who view such workers as somehow forced into that line of work. This attitude is found not only among lay people, but also among quite a few philosophers, including a few feminists. Consider, lastly, open marriages, which are relationships in which the spouses agree to have sex with people other than their spouses. People who are in open relationships are looked upon as being weird and others often question why they would be in a marriage to begin with. Gay men, some of whom are in such relationships, are often accused of not being in "real" love relationships precisely because of this.

Such issues deserve close attention. We cannot rest content with the fact that today many people accept premarital sex as okay, with the fact that they accept masturbation as healthy, and with the fact that they have reconciled themselves to the idea that some couples live together without being legally married. But why stop there? Why not go on to question other views about sexual practices? What exactly is supposed to be wrong with promiscuity, open marriages, and sex work? However, before going into the issue of how virtue ethics is relevant to these phenomena, a few more words about them are in order.

1. Care, Love, and Sex

The main reason for choosing care, romantic love, and sex as my areas of focus is that these comprise three domains thought to be essential to a well-lived life. Caution, however, must be exercised in fleshing out what is meant by "essential." Consider care first. It is undeniable that without care few human beings could grow up to be well-adjusted, well-functioning individuals. Without proper nurturing, attention, education, and general guidance, it is hard for people to lead healthy lives. Moreover, even after human beings have reached adulthood and are on their way to taking charge of their own individual lives, they still need care. They need the support of their friends and their family so that they can pursue and engage in their projects; they need intimate relationships in which and through which they can share their joys, sorrows, worries, good news, important moments, and their time with friends, siblings, lovers, and/or children. Furthermore, and as Aristotle recognized (e.g., 1985, 1128a), leisure and relaxation are important elements in a well-lived life. For usually periods of relaxation and leisure are shared with intimate others, precisely because the having of such intimate others constitutes what it means to enjoy such periods of relaxation, rather than just simply the idea that many people would rather not spend their leisure time alone.

Moreover, intimate relationships (to which care is essential) often confer meaning on people's lives. Though it is usual, of course, that people have multiple goals in life, most people also desire to have other people in their lives in intimate ways. In this regard, such intimate relationships confer meaning on life—in the simple sense that one would find minimal reason to continue one's pursuits without the presence of such intimate others. The loss of a good friend, for example, can render one's life inane and empty of purpose (even if only temporarily), and individuals who lose intimate others have to struggle in order to maintain what before was a normal life. All of this should strongly indicate that in adulthood one not only needs care from others, but one also needs to give care to others, the care that comes simply with the territory of being in an intimate relationship.

Care, then, is essential to a well-lived life because without it we are hard-pressed to see how individuals can lead healthy and normal lives. We need care as infants and as children in order to grow up to be healthy, and we need to receive and give care in adulthood as part of the much needed element of having intimate relationships as part of a well-lived life. This is not to say that care cannot be mismanaged, that it cannot go wrong, that it cannot be given to the wrong people, and I will address these points in the first chapter. But the issue is our recognition of the claim that care is needed for a good life. And in this respect, care is a crucial area of investigation for a neo-Aristotelian virtue ethicist (more on this below) insofar as her concern is the idea of a flourishing life, that is, a well-lived, moral life, and what goes into this life.

Let us consider next romantic love. Romantic love is one example of a type of intimate relationship, and, to this extent at least, embodies care as an essential dimension of it. Moreover, one often encounters, mostly in popular opinion and writings, the idea that romantic love is essential for a happy life, and that a person who goes through life without love is a person fit for pity. In the chapter on love, I will challenge this idea, but I will not challenge one possible reason behind it, namely, that it is because love involves intimacy to a high degree that love is thought to be essential to flourishing. One cannot challenge this idea without also challenging the general one that intimate relationships are important for a well-lived life, and this idea, it seems to me, is one that is foolish to challenge. There is, then, an important reason behind the claim that love is needed for flourishing, and in this respect it is necessary to address it. In this regard, neo-Aristotelian virtue ethics cannot afford to neglect the topic of romantic love.

Because we recognize care as obviously necessary for human flourishing, we also recognize that care is a universal phenomenon. No one has questioned the idea that all human societies have practiced care in one form or another. However, we cannot say the same about romantic love. It has recently become somewhat fashionable to claim that romantic love is not a universal human trait, that it has its origins in the European phenomenon of courtly love, and is thus to that extent a culturally-bound phenomenon.[1] This claim cannot withstand much scrutiny. It requires only a bit of perusing of the literature, philosophy, mythology, and poetry of cultures and societies which predate or lie outside of twelfth-century Europe to realize that the phenomenon of romantic love is more pervasive. To give just two examples from Arabic literature, pre-Islamic Arabic poetry (sixth century C.E. and before) has as one of its central concerns romantic love, and Ibn Hazm, the Andalusian writer, devoted an entire book to romantic love (written sometime early in the first half of eleventh century). As would be expected, the phenomenon of romantic love was understood, explicated, discussed, treated, and regulated differently by different cultures. But one cannot conclude from this that before twelfth-century Europe there was no such thing as romantic love (the best defense we can make on behalf of such claims is that perhaps only in the modern age has romantic love become a dominant cultural theme). The point of this excursion is that if one is tempted to dismiss the topic of romantic love on the basis that it is not a universal phenomenon and so not a fit subject for a book concerned with the virtues and flourishing, then one should definitely reconsider this claim.

Sex, too, is thought of as an area important to consider when it comes to deliberating about how to lead a well-lived life. As human beings we need to consider seriously the place that sex should have in our lives and we need to think hard about what form it should take. In this regard, most, if not all, of the ancient Greek philosophers recognized the importance of this question, and they all sought, in their own ways, to regulate it and give it its proper place. Aristotle (and others) believed that the virtue of temperance is the correct way of manifesting and feeling the sexual urges. Just as we recognize the importance of care and intimate relationships, we also recognize the importance of sex, and the question, which has historically been more prominent in regard to sexual activity than it has been in regard to care and romantic love, is how to regulate it and what importance to give it. While most philosophers agree that the topic of sex is important, they also agree that sex is not one of those areas in life that one ought to place in high priority, that is, that one ought not to organize one's life around it. And while I will not challenge these claims, I will challenge some of the ways in which such claims have manifested themselves, such as the claims that certain forms of sexual behavior have no place in a well-lived life (such as promiscuity, open relationships, and sex work).

There is, however, a second reason why care, romantic love, and sex are the focus of this book in addition to their being centrally connected to the issue of a well-lived life: each can be a virtue. At the very least, each corresponds to a virtue appropriate to the ways in which each can be felt and acted upon. In this respect, they would be natural domains of investigation in a book inspired by virtue ethics. For instance, it has not escaped the notice of some philosophers that care can be thought of as a virtue (see the first chapter), and so the questions surrounding this idea become pressing: How is care a virtue? What would some of the corresponding vices be? And why should we think of it as a virtue? With respect to romantic love, some contemporary philosophers (for example, R. Solomon [1991]) claim that it is virtue, while others deny this (for example, Pettit [1997]). Aristotle seems to be of two minds about this issue. In laying the ground for his definition of "virtue," he claims that feelings are not virtues, and he gives love as an example of a feeling (1985, 1105b20–1106a5). But in his discussion of friendship, he claims that love is the virtue of friends (1985, 1159a35). And so again the question of whether romantic love is a virtue and why (or why not) becomes pressing. Temperance has traditionally been thought of as the virtue concerned with sexual activity. It becomes important to ask some crucial questions: What is temperance, exactly? Is it even possible to have temperance with respect to sex, or is continence (self-control) the best we can hope for? What forms of sexual behavior does temperance rule out and what forms does it allow? Is it true that some maligned sexual practices can only be vices (intemperate forms of behavior) or can they be accommodated by temperance? It is these questions, among others, that the three following chapters seek to address.

But it is not only the fact that these three topics are importantly connected to the notions of flourishing and virtue that constitutes the reasons for addressing them. These three topics, in addition, exhibit some strong internal connections, and this makes them obvious candidates for discussion, because they go together. Despite the fact that some think romantic love is nothing but a form of egoism (an objection I will address in the second chapter), it nevertheless seems to be an important example of a type of caring relationship. But romantic love is also often characterized by sexual activity. Indeed, many philosophers consider sex to be *the* aspect of romantic love that sets it apart from other types of intimate relationships. While this cannot constitute a necessary aspect that sets romantic love apart from other intimate relationships (not all romantic love relationships include sex, and some friendships include sexual activity), it does correctly display a general characteristic that does indeed mark the distinction between these relationships. So romantic love is internally connected to both care and sex.

But whatever other internal connections may exist, there is one *characteristic* thread that runs through all of these three—intimacy. Intimacy is marked by the close and deep knowledge of two people of each other. It is also marked by privacy: privacy in the sense that intimate relationships require some amount of sheltering to flourish, and in the sense that they require, again, sheltering to establish trust—another marker of privacy—by way of the person-affecting information that intimates have of each other. There is no denying that both care and romantic love, as concepts, make reference, implicitly or explicitly, to intimacy. Furthermore, and while *some* forms of sexual promiscuity do not involve any intimacy (and I will discuss the importance of this in the third chapter), almost all other forms of sexual behavior involve some degree of intimacy. Even casual sex, often found in one-night stands, involves some intimacy, though it differs importantly from that found in affairs (another issue I will address in the third chapter). Care, romantic love, and sex are domains that necessarily bring other human beings into intimate relationships with the agent. To that extent, they naturally belong together (this is not to say, of course, that intimacy does not occur in other types of relationships). Add to this the idea that intimacy, in one form or another, is humanly important, and we can see why intimacy as a thread through care, romantic love, and sex forms one justification for discussing these three phenomena.

There is one more obvious reason why I discuss these three areas: virtue ethics, the virtues, and flourishing aside, they are all domains of life that are important, period. In this respect, any ethical theory worthy of consideration will have to address them.

2. General Problems Raised by Care, Love, and Sex

Historically, philosophers have not discussed care as such.[2] Usually, when one comes across a discussion of care, one does so in one of the guises that care can take. For example, one can find discussions of care as found in friendships. Aristotle, for instance, devotes two chapters of his major ethical work, *Nicomachean Ethics,* to the issue of friendship. Discussion of care as such only became prominent with 1982's *In a Different Voice,* in which Carol Gilligan, a developmental psychologist, argues that women in general reason morally by relying on the notion of care, as opposed to men, who reason morally by relying on the notion of justice. Gilligan's work ushered in a flurry of philosophical debate. On the one hand, many philosophers agreed that she was on to something important. But many other philosophers also thought that her work re-emphasized traditional feminine values that contemporary women and society at large were advised to handle with care. Because traditionally women have been thought of as caring and nurturing, many philosophers viewed such re-emphasis on care as a threat to the feminist struggle against sexism.

This issue of reaffirming feminine values became more pressing when Nel Noddings published a book on care in 1984 in which she argued that caring can serve as the foundation of moral theory. One problem with Noddings's view is not only that such a conception of moral theory might undermine feminist claims, but also that Noddings seems to put too much moral emphasis on care at the expense of other moral concepts, such as justice and integrity. So the situation that many philosophers came to be faced with was this: on the one hand, caring seems to comprise an important moral dimension of our lives, a dimension not explicitly addressed by most past philosophers. There is a need to accommodate it in our moral thinking and theory-building. On the other hand, care does not seem to be able to theoretically support the emphasis that has been put on it by people such as Gilligan and Noddings. So the issue boils down to the following question: What are we to do with care, philosophically and morally?

Historically, philosophers have not been as negligent of romantic love as they have been of care. One finds interesting discussions of it in, for example, Plato, the Stoics, St. Augustine, Arthur Schopenhauer, and Søren Kierkegaard. But what one often finds lacking in them are explicit, plausible, and/or nonreligious discussions of the connections between love, on the one hand, and morality and living a flourishing life, on the other. The Stoics' discussion, for example, is implausible insofar as it is part of their general project of ridding us of emotions. Kierkegaard's discussion, to give another example, is shot through and through with Christian themes, and Kierkegaard thought that personal (romantic) love had no moral value (my assumption here is that it is desirable to fasten upon accounts that can be agreeable also to the nonreligious mind). Contemporary philosophers have addressed these issues, especially the one regarding the connections between romantic love and morality. But what one sometimes finds are claims that, on the face of them at least, seem to be false. So, for example, one finds claims to the effect that romantic love and morality have nothing to do with one another (indeed, that they are even antagonistic), or that romantic love is one of the most important values to our lives. What is also often missing is a sustained discussion of the question of how exactly love is important to a well-lived life.

The problems that romantic love raises can be encapsulated in two main questions. First, what are the connections between romantic love and morality? Second, to what extent, and why, is romantic love important to a well-lived or flourishing life?

Sex has been an issue of interest to philosophers, especially to the ancients and the medievalists. But after the medieval period, few philosophers addressed sex at any length. One often finds scattered remarks here and there about it, and what one finds is not very uplifting. Immanuel Kant, for example, condemned to the realm of the immoral all sexual activity outside of a marriage context—a position that a few contemporary philosophers still accept. But this has not been the generally accepted view among other contemporary philosophers, who have recently begun paying attention to sexual issues, be they moral or conceptual. Most contemporary philosophers have accepted a general liberal position in regard to sexual activities, a position that can be summed up in the statement that sexual activities are morally acceptable as long as certain conditions are met, such as not harming others and having the consent of both (or more) parties to the sexual act. Indeed, even when philosophers discuss the issue of sexual perversion, many of them are quick to point out that perverted sex is not necessarily immoral sex. So the dominant view about sex is, generally, a liberal one.

However, this does not mean that there are no problems raised by sex. For one thing, even though the ancients and the medievalists did address issues of sex, there is scant attention to particular forms of it that are of interest to us, such as promiscuity, sex work, and open relationships. For another thing, many feminist philosophers are not content with the contemporary liberal position about sex, arguing that in the context of sexism, liberalism fails because there is no genuine equality between the sexes. Indeed, much of the ire of these feminists is directed at sex work and sex workers, on the grounds that women sex workers are in a highly morally precarious position when it comes to our sexist societies and that their lives leave much to be desired, morally speaking. For yet another thing, even if the liberal position is correct, it leaves out some questions unanswered. In its focus on sexual *acts*, it generally neglects the broader issue of what place particular sexual activities are to have in well-lived lives. For example, one can argue that even if particular sexual acts of promiscuity are morally permissible, there is still the further question of what place promiscuity can have in the life of a decent human being: Can a good, virtuous person nevertheless be promiscuous?

So the main problem that sex raises, in light of what I have said, can be summed up in the following question: Can one be a decent, morally good human being, lead a flourishing life, and yet also be promiscuous, be in an open relationship, or be a sex worker? To put the question in a stronger way: Is there anything about promiscuity, sex work, and open relationships that would endanger one's moral decency?

It is my contention that a neo-Aristotelian virtue ethics can adequately address these problems. With respect to care, a virtue ethics approach advises that we think of care as a virtue and house it among the other virtues. With respect to love, virtue ethics advises that we claim that love is an emotion (not a virtue), even though love, as a concept, is an essentially moral one. It also advises that romantic love is important to a flourishing life only because of those features that it shares with other intimate relationships. With respect to sex, it states not only that one can be morally decent and yet be promiscuous, a sex worker, or in an open marriage, but also that there is nothing about these—with one exception regarding certain forms of open relationships—that raises the likelihood that one's virtuous character would be put at risk by adopting such ways of life. This is not to deny that other moral approaches can offer similar answers, but only to assert that virtue ethics can also do this. Now it is time to say a few things about virtue ethics.

3. Neo-Aristotelian Virtue Ethics

It is often customary to begin a work on virtue ethics by stating that, in comparison to other moral theories such as utilitarianism and Kantian ethics, virtue ethics is still in its infancy. To some extent, this claim is no longer true because much has been written recently on virtue ethics, though the volume of literature is still somewhat small in comparison with what has been written on some other theories.[3] In the present book, I do not attempt to contribute to the body of work on virtue ethics as a theory, nor to add to the endeavor of applying virtue ethics to social problems. Rather, I assume a particular version of virtue ethics and use this version as the basis for an investigation into what virtue ethics might have to "say" on three crucial areas of our lives: care, love, and sex.

3.1. The Foundations of Virtue Ethics

Starting around the 1950s, some philosophers became discontent with the two dominant moral theories, Kantian ethics and consequentialism. Whether correctly or not, they thought that these two theories left out important questions about ethics. They thought that these theories were too focused on issues having to do with the rightness and wrongness of *action*, and not focused enough on the issue of what it means to be a good *person* and on what it means to live a flourishing, decent life. So they began to look for an alternative view. Since the ancient Greeks had made these two latter questions the center of their moral views, these contemporary philosophers thought that perhaps the new theory should be a revival—with some necessary adjustments—of ancient Greek theories. Virtue ethics was "born."

Generally speaking, contemporary virtue ethics is an ethical approach to moral theory and problems that importantly uses and relies upon the notion of virtue or the virtues, such as justice, courage, temperance, wisdom, generosity, kindness, and benevolence. Put in this way, virtue ethics would *not* necessarily be a moral theory on a par with other moral theories such as consequentialism, Kantian ethics, and care ethics. The reason is simple: most, if not all, moral theories can admit of versions in which reliance on the virtues is crucial. Consider, for example, consequentialism, the theory that—roughly stated—claims that an action is right if it brings about the best consequences. One could formulate a version of consequentialism in which one makes central the proposition that the cultivation of virtue is the best means of securing good states of affairs (see, for example, Adams [1976]). In this respect, this version of consequentialism would indeed crucially rely on the virtues, and so would rely on the concept of virtue in essential ways. Similar claims can be made about possible versions of Kantian ethics, care ethics, or contractarian moral theories. If we are to claim that virtue ethics is indeed an independent moral theory, we must offer more on its behalf than merely saying that it relies importantly on the notion of virtue.[4]

In this respect, Gary Watson, in "On the Primacy of Character" (1997), identifies one important way to carve out an ethics of virtue that not only relies essentially on the virtues, but also does so in a way which prevents it from collapsing into a type of consequentialism or deontology. He does so by claiming that at the very foundations of the theory, there is no appeal to the notion of the good, but rather to the notion of a "characteristically human life." Once we have the idea of living a characteristically human life in our grasp, we can *then* go on to say that whoever exemplifies this life is a *good* human being. According to this view, the virtues are traits needed to live a characteristically human life. It is an Aristotelian view in the sense that it fits in with Aristotle's claim that a good human life is a life lived in accordance with virtuous activity, and because it fits in well with Aristotle's ethical naturalism, which is, roughly, the view that ethics should be based on human nature. Recently, both Rosalind Hursthouse (1999b, part 3) and Philippa Foot (2001) have explicitly attempted to defend such a view.

It is important to emphasize one point. On Watson's construal, which is accepted in its basics by both Hursthouse and Foot, what sets virtue ethics apart as a theory from other moral theories is found at the very foundations of the theory, and not necessarily in what virtue ethics tells us, say, about how one should act given a particular circumstance, or about the importance of emotions in action. Both a Kantian and a virtue ethicist, for example, could agree that in many cases euthanasia is wrong because it is unjust, and both could agree that justice is a virtue. (This, by the way, goes far to show that the "rivalry" between virtue ethics and other moral theories is somewhat exaggerated.) What they would disagree on is *why* justice is a virtue, and they would disagree on *that* issue because they disagree about what the foundations of morality are. The reader must exercise some caution in reacting to the conclusions of this book. The reader might, for example, exclaim, "But a consequentialist could—as long as she accepts the role and importance of the virtues in the ethical life—argue that care is a virtue (chapter 1) or that promiscuity is compatible with temperance (chapter 3). We don't need to marshal a new theory—virtue ethics—to reach these conclusions. All we need is the notion of virtue(s)!" In a sense, this would be correct. But in another sense, it would miss an important dimension of my claims. For an essential aspect of my position is not only that we can reach these conclusions if we use the notion of virtue, but also that we can reach these conclusions if we use the notion of virtue as housed in and understood by a particular version of virtue ethics, namely, a neo-Aristotelian one. My aim is not only to exhibit the fruitfulness of virtue in regard to these issues of care, love, and sex, but also to exhibit the fruitfulness of neo-Aristotelian virtue ethics in this regard.

I have mentioned that according to this version of virtue ethics, a virtue is a trait that one needs to flourish, to lead a good human life *qua* being human. But what does flourishing mean? This is a complicated question. But, to put it roughly, to flourish is to lead a well-lived life, and an essential, large part of this is to have and exercise the virtues. According to neo-Aristotelian ethics, having and exercising the virtues is constitutive of living a good life, because we as human beings can lead *good* lives only if we do so in the way that is good for us (as opposed to, say, what is good for anteaters). And what is good for us is the possession and exercise of the virtues. However, to flourish is to also be happy and content with one's life. Thus, to Aristotle, it is important that the person in question also have the requisite amount of external goods, such as money and friends, and to not have serious misfortunes affecting the person. Otherwise, we are hard put to claim that a person whose family died in an accident is flourishing. (Requiring the presence of external goods and the lack of misfortunes in one's life is one claim that set Aristotle's views on the good life apart from the views of other ancient Greek philosophers, such as the Stoics.) However, how much and what kind of external goods are needed in order for one to flourish, and how serious a misfortune must be so that the one hit by it does not flourish, are debatable issues. But the general point about what it is to flourish, though vague, is nevertheless plausible.

In each of the following chapters, I briefly discuss why and how care and temperance are virtues in this sense, and why romantic love is not (chapters 1, 3, and 2, respectively). My main aim is not to *show* that these traits are virtues, but to strongly indicate that they are (or as in the case of love, are not) virtues. What I do is to briefly argue how such traits are indeed plausible candidates for being virtues, and I do so by arguing how care and temperance are crucial for a human being to flourish *qua* being human, and how they benefit their possessor, while arguing that romantic love is not crucial for flourishing and that it does not benefit its possessor in the *basic* ways that the virtues usually do. Thus, care and temperance, but not romantic love, satisfy the two important criteria for a trait being a virtue. Since a general discussion of what and why particular traits are virtues can be, and is, much more complex and much richer than my treatment of it in this book is, and since Rosalind Hursthouse and Philippa Foot have successfully broached this complexity and richness, the reader is strongly advised to refer to their work (Hursthouse 1999b, part 3; Foot 2001), work on which my own is ultimately based.[5]

3.2. Neo-Aristotelianism

I would like to highlight, in this section, what it is exactly about the version of virtue ethics that I accept that is Aristotelian. But before I do this, let me describe the two main reasons I have relied on neo-Aristotelian virtue ethics. The first and more important one is that neo-Aristotelian virtue ethics, as a theory, seems to be on the right track. It captures the important aspects of morality that a moral theory should capture. To anticipate my remarks below, its emphasis on character, on the question of what a good life is, on the role of emotion and wisdom in action and on their importance in a moral life, and on moral education, to name a few aspects of virtue ethics, are highly appealing and promising. Moreover, its ethical naturalism is one strike in its favor, for the reason that, if true, it allows virtue ethics to be a moral theory that is *fit* for us human beings. No doubt, other moral theories have their appealing aspects also. For example, Kant's insistence on the idea that the right moral theory must be in principle applicable to all rational creatures, and not just human beings, seems to capture something important about our intuitions regarding moral theories (and I am not here denying that virtue ethics can be extended to other rational creatures; I am simply shelving the issue). But the fact that other moral theories have their own appealing and plausible aspects does not deny the claim that virtue ethics is also an appealing moral theory.

The second reason I rely on neo-Aristotelian virtue ethics is that such a theory is the only *plausible* one that has been defended and explicated at length. For example, Hume's virtue theory is not very convincing. Also, some contemporary forms of virtue ethics, like the version formulated by Michael Slote (2001), still require more defense by way of explication and warding off their seeming implausibility.[6]

To return to the goal of this section, what is so Aristotelian about neo-Aristotelian virtue ethics? The phrase "neo" in "neo-Aristotelianism" is meant to capture two general ideas. First, not all elements of virtue ethics are Aristotelian. It is a theory which is strongly inspired by Aristotle's thought, though it does not accept everything, or even many, of the things Aristotle himself accepted. In other words, it may very well depart from Aristotle in certain areas. Second, "neo" captures the idea that one can extend Aristotle's thought to areas that Aristotle himself did not discuss. Again, much of the work on these two points has already been accomplished by Hursthouse and others, and so I will be brief in my treatment of them in this introduction. However, there are two points worth keeping in mind. First, and despite its debt to Aristotle, the issue as to whether those Aristotelian elements in virtue ethics have also been accepted by other ancient philosophers and by the medievalists is left open. What is crucial is that these *are collectively* found in Aristotle, and that they are contrasted with what is often found in some *contemporary* moral theories. Second, despite the contrast with contemporary moral theories, no claim is made in this book that these latter theories are in principle inhospitable to revision, thus narrowing the gap between them and virtue ethics. There is no reason, for example, to think that Kantian ethics cannot adopt a position on the emotions similar to that of Aristotle's, despite the current contrast between the two views.

It is an extremely tricky issue to identify the elements that make virtue ethics an Aristotelian-inspired theory. However, six elements readily come to mind (and it is crucial to note that these six elements are assumed rather than argued for in this book, since it is not on or about virtue ethics as such). First, virtue ethics takes seriously the question of what a well-lived or flourishing life is. In this respect, virtue ethics is not narrowly act-centered. Moreover, its understanding of flourishing is not confined to subjective reports from the agents themselves as to whether they think they are leading a well-lived life (though it does not neglect these). Second, it accepts the idea that the virtues are needed if one is to flourish: for an agent to live a good life, the agent's best option is to have and to exercise the virtues. Third, it accepts the second claim because it accepts the further claim that how we flourish is anchored in our nature as human beings (and not in one aspect of our existence, such as our rationality or our capacity for feeling pleasure). Fourth, it gives emotions—which it construes as not only affective but as also cognitive—an essential place in having a moral character and in acting morally correctly. Fifth, it emphasizes the importance of the moral training of our emotions, thought, and values from early on in our childhood. In accepting this claim, neo-Aristotelian virtue ethics accepts also the claims that the better one's political and social environment is, the better one's moral upbringing will be, and that the emotions can be trained and so subjected to the regulation of wisdom and reason. Sixth, virtue ethics rejects any claims to the effect that (i) what is the morally right thing to do can be simply read off from a principle or rule or algorithm, and/or that (ii) there is one ultimate principle by which the rightness of actions is justified (for instance, that the action maximizes pleasure).[7] It is important to note, in connection with (i), that virtue ethics does not deny the importance of moral rules. Rather, it cautions against the mechanical or blind application of these rules. It is also important to note, in regard to (ii), that virtue ethics' emphasis on character and the virtues entail neither the claim that actions are justified by reference to the flourishing of the agent nor the claim that the issue of rightness of actions is secondary in importance, as some writers on virtue ethics claim (for example, Statman 1997, introduction). Aristotle's views, it seems to me, contain the insight that, given the absence of a set of principles by which we can decide what is the morally right thing to do in a given situation, we need to rely on moral wisdom and the other virtues. And this claim naturally leads to the idea that it is the person with the virtues, including that of wisdom, who knows and emotionally reacts to what is rightly to be done. Hence, the virtuous person can be used as a standard by which we decide what the right actions are in particular circumstances. But none of these claims entails that the issue of rightness of actions should take a philosophical back seat. At best, it takes a back seat only methodologically, in the sense that we arrive at it via an analysis of the virtues and what a virtuous person would do in the particular situation.[8]

It is also important to note that the claim that one needs the virtues in order to flourish yields a *criterion* for what a virtue is, namely, that a virtue is a trait or a disposition that one needs to flourish. What virtue ethics does not assert in this regard is that this is a *definition* of what a virtue is. The claim simply asserts a functional criterion. In this regard, it is a mistake to accuse advocates of virtue ethics, as Peter Simpson (1992) does, of being un-Aristotelian in defining "virtue" in this way because not all advocates of neo-Aristotelian virtue ethics make this mistake nor are they logically compelled to do so. Now, and as far as the definition of virtue is concerned, it is an open issue. There are competing definitions, and it requires much care and thought to decide what is the best definition. In this regard, however, one can, without too much worry, adopt Aristotle's own definition of virtue: "Virtue . . . is a state that decides, consisting in a mean, the mean relative to us, which is defined by reference to reason, i.e., to the reason by reference to which the intelligent person would define it" (1985, 1107a). Caution must be taken in explaining and plausibly fleshing out certain central notions in this definition, such as those of "state that decides" and the mean (and it is the contentiousness of these issues which supplies us with one reason why I leave the issue of defining "virtue" an open one).

Alternatively, one might, depending on the definition, adopt a more contemporary one, without much loss of the Aristotelian spirit. Consider a modified version of a definition offered originally by Linda Zagzebski (1996): "a virtue is a deep and acquired excellence of a person, involving a characteristic motivation to produce a desired end" of a worthwhile type, "reliable success in bringing about that end," and a characteristic disposition to react emotionally to one's situation.[9] This definition is much closer to Aristotle's than it first appears: it emphasizes the idea that virtue is a state, and a good one at that, that it is acquired, and that it involves the ability to achieve a particular end (and this must assume some notion of decision). In its notion of motivation, it brings in the idea of emotional involvement, an idea which Aristotle emphasized and which is found implicitly in his own definition (in the notion of the mean as exhibiting the right emotion). I am, of course, simplifying here. But my point is that as long as we are able to preserve certain ideas central to the notion of virtue (an acquired excellence, the role of decision, the notion of hitting upon the right end and action, and the role of emotion) we can choose from a number of competing definitions of "virtue," all of which are good. And whether one of these is the best is an issue that we need not settle now and that we can leave open.

Neo-Aristotelian virtue ethics departs from Aristotle in important ways. There are, to my mind, four important issues that advocates of virtue ethics either do not accept from Aristotle or, at the very least, are subject to give and take.[10] First, neo-Aristotelian virtue ethics is not committed to Aristotle's own list of the virtues. Aristotle listed as moral virtues those of bravery, temperance, generosity, magnificence, magnanimity, the virtue concerned with small honors, mildness, friendliness, truthfulness, wit, and justice (1985). Neo-Aristotelian virtue ethics is not committed to this list in two ways: we can add virtues to the list (e.g., care, kindness, and integrity), and we can drop virtues from it (e.g., the headache-inducing one of magnificence). In this respect, advocates of virtue ethics are not logically required to stick with Aristotle's own list, though some virtues from his list *must* be present, or one's position would, simply, not be Aristotelian. One criterion that can be used to decide which virtues should be retained and which should not is the importance of the trait in question to a flourishing life. Courage and generosity, one can argue, *are* needed for flourishing, whereas magnificence is not. It requires much thinking as to how we go about deciding whether a trait is indeed needed for flourishing, but my emphasis is on the very idea found in this criterion.

Second, even if one were to accept many or all of Aristotle's virtues, there is room for disagreement as to how the virtues are to be fleshed out. For example, we can agree with Aristotle that bravery is the virtue of facing important dangers, and that death is one of these, but we might disagree with him that only death in war is the right type of death to face, as he seems to suggest (1985, 1115a30).[11] Third, even if we agree with some interpreters of Aristotle (such as Kraut 1989 and 1999) that the life of *theoria*, roughly defined as the life of intellectual contemplation, is *the* life of perfect happiness, and that the life of virtuous activity is a happy life but in a secondary way (and this is a matter of some serious scholarly dispute), we might depart from Aristotle on this score. We might simply reject the idea that the former life does indeed constitute the happiest life. I say "might" because it seems to me that an advocate of virtue ethics might also accept this interpretation of Aristotle and yet not be bothered by it, on some such grounds as that even if it is true it does not, morally, matter. Or that in today's world precious few people can or are willing to practice it, and so it is of little consequence. Be that as it may, this third point of departure—like the first two—is one that allows for some give and take.

The fourth issue, however, does not allow for give and take. There is unanimous agreement—and rightly so—among advocates of neo-Aristotelian virtue ethics that Aristotle's views on women, slavery, and elitism ought to be rejected. Whether we can remain Aristotelians while rejecting Aristotle's views that—roughly stated—women are intellectually inferior to men, that some people are slaves by nature, and that the practice of virtue requires a certain amount of leisure in one's life (and so the manual labor has to be done by others who will not be able to be as actively virtuous) has been denied by some philosophers (for instance, Susan Okin with respect to Aristotle's views on women [1996] and Peter Simpson with respect to Aristotle's views on elitism [1992]). I believe that we can do so. Virtue is not necessarily the domain of men, or of men of a certain class and political stature. Aristotle's list of virtues, though in his time mostly practiced by men, is not necessarily confined to men. Moreover, we can add to his list of virtues ones traditionally thought of as feminine (such as care) and not confine these to women. In addition, the view that some people are slaves by nature is simply ludicrous. The above points containing the elements of virtue ethics that render it Aristotelian are perfectly compatible with the denial of these pernicious claims by Aristotle.[12]

The list just offered of the areas in which neo-Aristotelians agree with Aristotle and in which they part company with him is not meant to be exhaustive, of course, as there might be elements that other philosophers deem important enough to be included in it. However, it does contain the crucial ones that have been discussed in the literature. Moreover, my emphasis on *neo*-Aristotelianism should tell the reader that this book is not one on *history*. Though I take Aristotle to be an important, if not the main, source for the ideas in this book, it is not an exegesis of his ideas. I depart from Aristotle in important ways. For example, Aristotle did not discuss care as such, and my conclusion that care should be thought of as an Aristotelian virtue is an extension of Aristotle's views. Nor did Aristotle discuss romantic love as such. Again, my own discussion of romantic love is inspired by Aristotle and virtue ethics's views on the virtues and on flourishing, but what I end up concluding is an extension of Aristotle's thought. Similar remarks apply to my conclusions regarding promiscuity, open relationships, and sex work.[13]

4. A Preview of the Chapters

In this section I highlight the main arguments and conclusions of each of the three chapters to come. The reader may skip it and go directly to the chapters themselves.

The concept of care that I focus on in the first chapter is confined to the sense of "care" applicable to caring activities that occur in intimate relationships, such as those between lovers, friends, siblings, and parents and their children. Thus, it is not the broader concept of care that applies to caring about causes, ideals, and strangers. Moreover, in chapter 1, I do not attempt to offer an exhaustive analysis of the concept of care. Rather, this issue is dealt with only in order to support my thesis that care is best construed as a virtue, along Aristotelian lines. In this regard, I offer an argument to the effect that care is a virtue because it fits the criteria for a trait being a virtue and because it fits the definition of "virtue." And it is the thesis that care is a virtue that I take to be the answer to the problem of what theoretical place the concept of care has in our moral thinking and theorizing. This is an issue that has arisen over the past few years from the debates—occurring mostly within feminist ethics—regarding the importance of care as an ethical concept and behavior, especially in comparison with issues about justice and the way some traditional moral theories have been propounded. It is, then, my view that situating the notion of care within the theoretical framework of virtue ethics allows us to sidestep the important objections given against using care as the sole foundation, or basic concept, of a moral theory rivaling other theories.

It is also my view that by situating care within virtue ethics, we are able to preserve the required balance between partiality and impartiality, and that we are able to preserve the most important aspects of caring—those aspects thought to be missing in moral theories such as consequentialism, Kantian ethics, and others—and which are thought to give care ethics its appeal, such as the importance of intimate relationships to our lives, and the importance of emotions and affectivity in moral action. In short, by subsuming care ethics within virtue ethics, we can keep what is important and desirable about it, while also being able to reject what is objectionable about it.

My focus in the second chapter is on romantic love, as opposed to, for example, agapic love or the love that occurs between friends and between siblings. Moreover, in chapter 2, my aim—again—is not so much to analyze the concept of romantic love, or to investigate the connections between the concept of love and other surrounding ones, such as those of exclusivity, constancy, sexual fidelity, and marriage. Rather, my aims are to trace the connections between romantic love and virtue, and to investigate the issue of what place and importance romantic love has in a flourishing life. Given these ends, I *do* engage in some analysis of the concept of romantic love, but that is because this is necessary in order to offer a philosophically plausible defense of the idea that romantic love is a moral concept, in the sense that it cannot be understood without reference to concepts that are moral in nature. In this regard, I first discuss a number of positions offered in the literature on the connections between romantic love and morality, and then I discuss positions on the connections between romantic love and virtue. I argue that the concept of romantic love is essentially a moral concept, in the sense that it necessarily refers to moral terms, but that it is not a virtue. I do this by arguing against positions that claim that there are no connections between romantic love and morality and that romantic love is morally neutral, against positions that claim that romantic love is not an emotion, and against positions that claim that romantic love is a virtue. In doing this, I am able to preserve the popular, though crucial, belief that romantic love is an emotion. If it is an emotion, then, and given that virtues are not emotions, it follows that romantic love is not a virtue. I also argue directly for the claim that romantic love is not a virtue by arguing that it fits neither the criteria for a trait being a virtue nor the definition of "virtue."

Claiming that romantic love is an emotion and not a virtue allows me to clear the way for the next investigation, namely, what connections there are between romantic love and virtue. My position is that the virtues enable romantic love in the sense that the best—meaning "moral"—romantic love is the one that issues forth from a virtuous person, and defend this view in light of two possible and powerful objections. Finally, I turn to the issue of the role of romantic love in a well-lived life, and I argue that romantic love is not necessary for a flourishing life, as long as the person living this life has other deep and intimate relationships. In other words, what is important about romantic love as far as flourishing is concerned are those aspects of it having to do with care, intimacy, trust, and the sharing of a life, elements which are conceptually found also in other, nonromantic types of relationships. In this regard, the claim is an Aristotelian one, given Aristotle's own emphasis on friendship and his subsuming love under it. However, what this claim implies is that in those social and cultural configurations that allow for only one deep and intimate relationship for each person at a time, romantic love might indeed be necessary for flourishing, since in such configurations friendships and other such relationships would not contain the depth and intimacy found in romantic love.

The last chapter is concerned with three areas of sexual activity, or, to put it more specifically, three ways in which one can lead one's sexual life: promiscuity, open relationships, and sex work. My aim in this chapter is not to offer any novel conclusions about the moral permissibility of these ways of life, but rather to argue that their moral permissibility can be argued for on Aristotelian grounds, rather than just on liberal ones, as some philosophers' discussions might (unintentionally) mislead us to think. This I achieve by first discussing the virtue of temperance and by arguing that there are two concepts of temperance, one which revolves around the rational and psychic health of the agent, and one which revolves around the good of others. Moreover, I argue that both of these concepts of temperance are virtues, in the Aristotelian sense that each contributes to making a human being better *qua* being human and that each benefits its possessor. Second, I argue that none of these three ways of sexual life necessarily contravene the two aspects of temperance or other relevant virtues. Thus, they are not at odds with flourishing and can, indeed, be part of a well-lived life. Indeed, not only *can* they be part of such a life, they are perfectly compatible with it. Thus, I am out not just to defend a weak claim of logical and psychological compatibility, but a stronger one, namely, that there is nothing about promiscuity, open relationships, or sex work that would, as such, detract from or endanger one's virtuousness. Conversely put, there is nothing about virtue as such that ought to lead an agent to avoid promiscuity, open relationships, or sex work. The one exception I take to this claim is in regards to certain forms of open relationships and their likelihood of putting romantic love between the two spouses in danger. If this is so, then such relationships threaten an external good needed for the two agents' flourishing. But this is the only exception to my general conclusions. Promiscuity, for example, is compatible with a life governed by reason, as long as the agent does not allow his sexual activities to take priorities over other things in his life. Promiscuity need not, as it is often portrayed, denote unbridled and all-consuming lust, and to this extent may be practiced without undermining the agent's rational ability to pursue goals more worthwhile than sexual activity. Similar reasoning applies to open relationships and to sex work. In the cases of promiscuity and open relationships, I use the lives of some gay men as examples of leading a rational life that involves promiscuity or being a party in an open relationship. I use the lives of gay men not because these lives are representative of the rest of the population, be it gay or straight, but because they provide actual and obvious (insofar as such gay couples are known by the general populace to exist) models with which my position can arm itself. With respect to sex work, I draw on, for help and support, the lives of actual sex workers and what these workers had to say about their jobs and their lives.

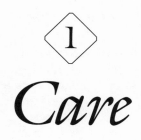

Care

What is the status of care ethics in moral theory? If, as has been argued, care ethics cannot constitute a comprehensive moral theory, and if care cannot be the sole foundation of such a theory, the question of the status of care ethics becomes a pressing one, especially given the plausibility of the idea that caring does constitute an essential component of moral thinking, attitude, and behavior. Furthermore, the answers given to solve this issue are inadequate. For instance, the suggestion that care ethics has its own moral domain, such as friendship, in which to operate, while, say, an ethics of justice has another domain (such as public policy), seems to encounter difficulties when we realize that, as Susan Okin has argued, in the former domain justice is necessary.

I want to suggest that care ethics be part of a more comprehensive moral framework, namely, virtue ethics. Doing so allows us to achieve two general desirable goals. First, by incorporating care within virtue ethics, we will be able to accommodate the criticism that such an ethics cannot stand on its own because it allows for morally corrupt relationships and because it neglects justice. I will argue that reason has an important regulative role to play in intimate relationships, and that a virtuous person is equipped, given that she has the intellectual virtue of practical wisdom, to evaluate intimate relationships as being morally desirable or not. I will also argue that virtue ethics has a principled way of adjudicating between the claims of partiality and impartiality and is thus able to make the needed room for justice.

The second desirable goal achieved by incorporating care ethics into virtue ethics is that we can preserve the most valuable elements of care ethics. These elements are: its appeal to partiality as a legitimate moral concern, its application to individuals intimate to the agent, its emotive component, and its relevance to areas in moral life that have been neglected by some traditional moral theories.

23

I will first explain the type of care ethics that I focus on and review two important objections to it. Next, I will highlight those elements of virtue ethics relevant to its adequacy as a framework for care ethics. I will then explain how subsuming care ethics under virtue ethics helps us achieve the desired goals mentioned above. I then discuss a few considerations having to do with the status of care as a *virtue*, and an important one at that, such as its role in *eudaimonia* and its connection to emotions. In the penultimate section, I consider the question why Nel Noddings—whose views on care are the focus of this chapter—rejects the suggestion (and the thesis of this chapter) that care is a virtue. A discussion of this issue is important since it helps focus my claims and enrich the discussion. I also explain and criticize Michael Slote's attempt to make care *the* basic virtue in virtue ethics. In other words, I discuss and reject two attempts—by Noddings and by Slote—which try to give care a more foundational role than my account does. Finally, I explain briefly how my approach towards care ethics avoids the pitfalls of previous ones regarding the connections between care ethics and justice morality and discuss one possible objection.

However, to avoid confusions, I will first say a few words about what this chapter is *not* concerned with, namely, three aspects of the debate that are essentially about gender issues. Since Carol Gilligan's work in moral psychology, much has been written on the gendered nature of moral thinking. Gilligan's arguments contain two compatible claims. First, that women's moral reasoning, in general, differs from men's; specifically, the former tends to center around the notion of care, while the latter around justice. Second, that care reasoning and justice reasoning are separate and incompatible ways of moral thinking (this second claim should not be confused with the claim, which Gilligan accepts, that a comprehensive moral theory should emphasize both care and justice concepts).[1] Gilligan's research has been subjected to some powerful criticisms that target both the conceptual and empirical aspects of her work. For example, both her interpretation of the interviewees' responses and her choice of what moral problems to focus on have been contested, and other empirical studies have yielded the result that men and women do not reason differently.[2]

It is not true, however, that a discussion of care ethics *must* raise the gender issue. For *suppose* that women do *not* reason differently than men, and, moreover, that they reason by focusing on the notion of justice. This would not show that the philosophical questions about care ethics are moot. Care ethics would remain an important an important issue for moral theory because, among other reasons, moral theory does not adequately address areas that concern care ethics, and care is important to moral thinking, emotion, and behavior. On the other hand, *suppose* that *all* women reason differently than men, and, moreover, that they reason by focusing on the notion of care. But suppose also that women reason in this way because of cultural influence. In other words, suppose that due to sexism, women have been strongly influenced by certain values and social beliefs, such as that they should be nurturing, loving, and caring, and that these values are a result of a sexist system that relegated women to certain spheres of life.[3] This would still not show that the philosophical questions about care ethics can be set aside, for, again, the issue of the importance of caring, acting from care, and the disposition to care, for moral theory would remain. In short, the question of the status of care ethics in morality is conceptually independent from the gender one, and this is the first gender aspect of the debate that is not a focus of this chapter.[4]

Another aspect of the gender issue I am not concerned with is the issue whether, even if virtue ethics can successfully incorporate care ethics, this would still have the implication of marginalizing women. That is, another issue I will not address is the possibility that virtue ethics could consistently include care ethics, but that philosophers who write on virtue ethics would nevertheless continue not to address issues of specific concern to women.[5] While this is also an important issue, it concerns the political practice of philosophers and so falls outside the scope of this chapter. A third aspect of the gender issue that I will not attend to *as such* is whether incorporating care ethics within virtue ethics would meet the needs of feminist ethics, that is, whether this would yield certain desiderata for ethics that feminists have been arguing for.[6] Again, I will not address this issue since it is conceptually different from the one I am concerned with, namely, the status of care ethics in moral theory. However, much of what I say will, *ipso facto*, address such feminist concerns insofar as these have coincided with what has been thought important about care ethics. Ultimately, however, whether virtue ethics—the theory that I propose should be the host of care ethics—does meet feminist concerns is a complex topic that can be only fully addressed in a separate work that can give it the attention it requires.

1. Noddings's Care Ethics

What is caring? What is involved in the very concept—or idea—of care? What are the characteristics of caring actions and caring relationships? And how can caring be morally risky or dangerous? It is these questions that this section addresses.

An influential attempt to build a comprehensive moral approach on the concept of care is Nel Noddings's (1984). It is important to look at

Noddings's attempt since this allows us to see what is lacking in her approach and to pin down more precisely what care, as a concept, is.[7] Starting with the claim that relations between human beings are *ontologically* basic, Noddings construes caring relations as *ethically* basic.[8] In order to be moral, according to her, one must maintain one's self as caring. She calls this view of oneself the "ethical ideal": "We want to be *moral* in order to remain in the caring relationship and to enhance the ideal of ourselves as one-caring. It is this ethical ideal . . . that guides us as we strive to meet the other morally."[9] This ethical ideal comes from the two sentiments of natural and ethical caring (104). The former is the natural sympathy we feel for others; it is the sentiment expressed when we *want* and *desire* to attend to those we care for, such as a mother's caring for her child (79). The latter occurs "in response to a remembrance of the first" (79), and it forms the basis of ethical obligation: it is the "I must" that we adhere to when we want to maintain our ethical ideal as ones-caring (82). So even in situations when I find it difficult to engage in caring action, I am under an obligation to do so if I want to be moral, that is, to maintain myself as one-caring (82).

What, however, is involved in caring relations? Noddings claims that for caring to be genuine it has to be for persons in definite relations with the one-caring.[10] Though she makes room for the idea that one can expand one's circle of those cared-for, she insists that genuine caring is not "caring about," namely, the caring for abstract ideas or causes (112). Caring targets the well-being of the cared-for. But more specifically, genuine caring involves what Noddings calls "engrossment and motivational displacement." In engrossment, the one-caring attends to the cared-for without judgment and evaluation, and she allows herself to be transformed by the other, while in motivational displacement the one-caring adopts the goals of the cared-for and helps the latter to promote them, directly or indirectly (see especially pp. 15–20, 33–34). This account has the result, which Noddings emphasizes, that caring has its limits. If genuine caring is not to be corrupted, the one-caring simply cannot care for everyone (18, 86). This, moreover, is not simply a practical consequence but a conceptual one: given Noddings's requirements of engrossment and displacement, it is impossible for any one person to engage a large number of people, let alone the whole world, in such caring relations.

Before moving to criticisms of Noddings's views, it is worthwhile to note that Milton Mayeroff, in *On Caring* (1971), offers an account of caring that is very similar to Noddings's. For example, Mayeroff emphasizes the idea that caring is essentially helping the cared-for to grow on the latter's own terms, by allowing the cared-for's "direction" of growth to lead the one-caring's efforts in responding and attending to the cared-for. The claims contained in these assertions are extremely similar to Noddings's engrossment and motivational displacement. The latter has a similar-sounding claim in Mayeroff's belief that caring is helping another to grow, while the former has its counterpart in Mayeroff's idea that helping another grow should be done by responding to the cared-for's own needs and direction of growth.[11] I do not wish to claim that Noddings and Mayeroff's positions are identical. My point, rather, is that Noddings's view of caring as involving engrossment and displacement is not entirely new, not because Noddings is not an original thinker, but because it is difficult to offer a plausible account of caring without arguing that caring involves *something* along the lines of engrossment and displacement. I will, however, return to this issue briefly when I explicitly evaluate Noddings's views.

Noddings's views have been subjected to severe criticism.[12] Two of these are crucial to bringing out what is essentially missing in a moral view that is built solely on the notion of care. Claudia Card (1990) takes as her starting point the fact that on Noddings's view caring cannot be extended to everyone. If so, Card asks, how are we to think of our moral obligation to the people that we are not in caring relations with? We seem to need another moral concept that would ground our moral obligations to those non-cared-for, and Card opts for justice: "in a densely populated world life is not apt to be worth living without justice from a great many people, including many whom we will never know" (107).

Victoria Davion's (1993) criticism of Noddings has as its starting point the moral dangers attending engrossment and motivational displacement. If one cares for someone who is evil, then the one-caring might himself become evil. For if engrossment and displacement are, respectively, allowing oneself to be transformed by the cared-for and adopting the goals of the cared-for, then in caring for someone who is evil the one-caring allows himself to be transformed by the cared for and to adopt immoral goals, and such a person, the one-caring, simply cannot be viewed as a moral paradigm. Hence, something is needed to regulate care and to ward off the possibility of such moral corruption. Davion opts for integrity, and her argument is that integrity is necessary to one's ethical ideal, since "seeing oneself as a being with moral integrity is part of seeing oneself as one's best self" (175). Since caring is sometimes incompatible with maintaining integrity, caring simply cannot be the only absolute moral value, as Noddings would have us believe.

Both of these criticisms by Card and Davion can be made more vivid when put in the context of Noddings's notorious discussion of Ms. A, a fictitious woman who opts to fight on the side of her racist father and aunt rather than on the side of Jim, a black man who "spoke eloquently of the prevailing injustice and inhumanity against blacks" (Noddings 1984, 109–11). Ms. A would fight on the side of her racist relatives, but if she were to see Jim on the other side, she would point her gun at some "other target." The reason is that on Noddings's view, caring for her relatives constitutes the supreme moral imperative, given that caring is the only absolute moral value that Noddings accepts. Ms. A cannot decide to start caring for Jim and fight against her family, because she already has a relationship established with her aunt and father, whereas her relationship with Jim is potential. And on Noddings's view, actual relationships take priority over potential ones. The problem here is that in not fighting on Jim's side, Ms. A not only neglects considerations of justice, but is also willing to violate her integrity, given that she believes that Jim is morally correct in his demands. She allows herself to degenerate into someone whose tribal loyalty trumps any other morally correct action.

The two objections point to an important conclusion: *any* ethics that attempts to build itself simply on the concept of care is bound to face some severe difficulties. Though my discussion relies only on Noddings's account, the conclusion is nevertheless plausible. For it seems simply wrong to believe that caring is the only basic component that goes into an ethical life: if one understands "care" along the lines of Noddings's understanding of it, it is clear that in being one-caring one can nevertheless be acting morally wrongly. The trick here is to balance two things: first, to offer a plausible concept of care without, at the same time, packing too much into it so that it loses its substance (a mistake which Slote succumbs to; see last section). Second, we must be careful not to be too ambitious in what theoretical ethical work we want our concept of care to perform. We should not, for instance, claim that our concept of care can be the sole basis of a good moral theory. In this regard, Gilligan's views are more plausible than Noddings's. Though Gilligan and Noddings agree on a number of claims about morality (for example, they share the views that moral agents are particularized and not abstract agents, that moral action requires a deep knowledge of the moral patient, that the self is relational, and that moral action has essential emotive components), Gilligan is not committed to the idea that an ethics built solely on care would yield a comprehensive moral theory. Indeed, Gilligan (1982) often claims that a care approach needs to be combined with other approaches. However, it is precisely this issue that makes the problem of the status of care ethics within moral theory pressing, for it is not clear how this combination is to be articulated. Before we turn to it, however, we need to try to understand whether Noddings's analysis of the concept of care is acceptable. Doing so allows us to trace in a more accurate way the contours of the concept, and this offers us a good entry into the status of care ethics in moral theory.

Should we accept Noddings's characterization of care? Is it true that caring involves engrossment and motivational displacement? Is it true that genuine caring is personal? It is important to note that accepting an affirmative answer to these questions does not commit one to the claim that the *only* features that go into the concept of care are those of engrossment and displacement. After all, in caring for another one tends to the cared-for's well-being in general, not just his goals. Still, the issue is whether these two features are two of the essential ones to the concept of care, and it is difficult to see how we can escape such an account of caring if we are also to maintain its intuitive appeal. After all, much of the interest in care ethics stems from the fact that it attends to those areas in life, such as friendship, parenting, love, and marriage, that have been neglected by some traditional moral theory. In all of these areas there is an essential element of attention to particular individuals. Moreover, in all such areas there is an essential element of motivational displacement. Surely it is correct to state that friends support and promote each other's goals, that parents do the same for their children, and that lovers do so for each other. This, we should keep in mind, need not always be done directly but can also be done indirectly. For example, since friendship involves the friends' intimate knowledge of each other, including their goals and aspirations, then when friends provide support, comfort, and care for each other they are indirectly promoting each other's goals.[13] Furthermore, the fact that the one-caring can support the cared-for's goals indirectly should indicate that the promotion and support of these goals need not—and hopefully in many cases does not—come at the expense of the goals of the one-caring. In other words, the notion of motivational displacement—and despite its possibly misleading phrasing—does not entail that if x promotes and supports y's goals, then x does so at the expense of x's own goals. Even in cases in which the support is direct, x need not sacrifice her own goals. For instance, it might be the case that x shares the goals of y, or it might be the case that x has time and energy to promote both her and y's goals.

However, it might *seem* to be hasty to consider motivational displacement as essential to caring. For consider the following objection: it is indeed plausible to claim that much that goes under the activity of caring involves the support and promotion of the goals and life plans of the cared-for. But this seems to deny the truth of describing some relationships as caring even though such relationships do not involve the elements insisted upon by Noddings. To give an example my students are especially fond of, it is plausible to claim that two siblings or two friends care for each other even though they have been geographically and temporally distant from each other. Since such relationships are caring and yet do not involve engrossment and displacement, it would seem that Noddings's account is at best incomplete; it would have emphasized some central elements of the concept of care but would not have given an exhaustive analysis of it.

I think, however, that such objections involve underdescribed examples and cases. Noddings, for instance, can respond by asking for more detail. Consider the siblings' case. The fact that they have not seen each other for a long time need not entail that there is no support and promotion of each other's goals. After all, they could have been corresponding with each other consistently, emotionally, and substantively. Furthermore, if the two siblings are not only geographically and temporally out of reach of each other, but also psychologically and emotionally, then there would be no plausibility to the claim that they are in a caring relationship with each other. The fact that they are siblings should not pressure us into thinking that they must have an intimate and close relationship; they could be, simply, emotionally and psychologically distant from each other. And if so, there ought to be no temptation at all to describe their relationship as being one of caring.

Still, let us reconsider the example of the two siblings who live far apart from each other, who have not seen each other for a while, and yet who correspond intimately and continuously with each other. There is one thing that is nevertheless missing and which should make us hesitate before describing this case as one of caring, namely, the intimate knowledge required for full-fledged caring. The idea is that no matter how frequently and in how much detail the siblings correspond with each other, the fact that they are far apart weakens their ability to know each other. They do not, for instance, see each other's facial expressions, hear each other's voices, or have day-to-day encounters, and these are sources indispensable to robust, intimate knowledge of others. And if knowledge is essential for genuine caring, then we ought to think twice before calling such relationships "caring ones" à la Noddings.[14]

This point is plausible, but its force should not be exaggerated. For it only forces us to acknowledge that when discussing *actual* relationships, we need to discuss them along a spectrum ranging from "uncaring" to "full-fledged caring," with a number of cases in between (such as the case discussed in the paragraph before this one). But the *conceptual* point behind Noddings's claims is the centrality of relationships. If there is no relationship between two people, or if the relationship is too superficial or maintained out of obligation, then we should not acknowledge it as a caring one, even if the two parties in question are biologically related and even if they have *had* a close relationship (e.g., as kids growing up in the same household). So the example of the psychologically close but geographically distant siblings *is* one of caring, yet it cannot be one of full-fledged caring precisely because of the lack of some sources needed for a robust and intimate knowledge of the other.

There is still one important question which remains for Noddings's account: Is it sufficient that the goals of the cared-for be believed by her (the cared-for) to be good in order for her friend, the one-caring, to promote them? Or should the goals be genuinely good? Suppose a friend of mine—Lois—is in a love relationship which, though it began well, has turned sour.[15] My friend's spouse, Clark, has started abusing her, say, verbally and psychologically. Lois, given her love for Clark and her closeness to the situation, cannot perceive that the situation is hopeless and clings to the goal of preserving the relationship. I, on the other hand, having the advantage of being an external observer, am able to grasp the basic fact: Clark is a man who does not love and respect my friend. The question that this case gives rise to is whether it is a requirement that the goals of the cared-for *be* good in order for the one-caring to support them, or whether it is enough that the former *believes* that they are good. In the above case, my friend believes that her goal of preserving the relationship is a good one, while I believe—and know—that it is not only futile, but quite bad.

There is a straightforward answer to this question: the goal should not be supported. Since my friend's well-being is primary, and since supporting her goal would help further damage her well-being, then I should not support it. What I should do is talk to her, try to understand her point of view, and, if upon finding that she is being deluded, try to reason with her and try to show her why the relationship is not worth pursuing. This much, perhaps, is uncontroversial.[16] However, there is a tougher question: Is it morally permissible that I act in such ways so as to *frustrate* Lois's goal? Should I, directly or indirectly, bring it about that her efforts to achieve her goal are defeated? I want to leave the answer to this question open for three reasons. First, the answer to it depends on the case (how fragile she is, how damaging the abuse is, how clingy she is to Clark, and so forth). Second, and related to the first, positively interfering to thwart my friend's goal seems to be an interference with her autonomy, and this is a thorny issue, at least in the sense that interfering with one's autonomy affects one's well-being. So if care is directed generally at promoting the well-being of the cared-for, thwarting the latter's goals seems to adversely affect the cared-for's well-being via interfering with her autonomy. And perhaps it might not even yield a unitary answer but one that depends on the case: Would not interfering at this point thwart her future autonomy by allowing my friend to degenerate into a hopeless state? So it is a thorny issue.

But, third, in distinguishing between goals that are genuinely good and goals merely believed to be good, we have all that we need by way of a theoretical restriction on the notion of motivational displacement. Genuine friends support those goals that are not only believed, by their friends, to be good for them, but that are also genuinely good. This fact also reminds us how motivational displacement can work in cases of parents supporting the goals of their infant children. For even though infant children do not, and cannot, entertain goals of their own, parents can nevertheless support goals objectively true of them, namely and minimally, of growing in a healthy way to lead a healthy life.

The case of Lois and Clark, moreover, brings out an important point. If Noddings views caring as the basic moral value—as she indeed does— then her account will be crippled by such a case: if the one-caring refuses to support and promote the goals of the cared-for, then the one-caring would be acting under a diminished ethical ideal on Noddings's account. Since this is an implausible result, we have clearly laid out before us the need for an ethical scrutiny of caring relationships, so that one does not end up caring for another no matter what the other's goals are. To summarize, then, the discussion up to this point: it is plausible to claim that the parties in intimate relationships adopt and support each other's goals, and that for this motivational displacement to be ethical, the goals adopted must be genuinely good for the cared-for.

Considerations similar to those about motivational displacement apply also to engrossment. While uncritical acceptance of another is morally undesirable, no friendship or marriage can last if each party subjects the other to continual evaluation. After an initial screening, so to speak, one can rest content that his friend is not an immoral person, so that befriending him presents no danger for the former's moral integrity. Also, this need not foreclose on change. If one's friend begins to show signs of corruption, one could start a process of reevaluation and of slow detachment to prevent further engrossment (and future pain should the friendship be severed). Incidentally, the idea of an initial screening lends further support to the idea that there is a need for some moral concept (e.g., integrity) and/or some concept tied to moral ones (e.g., reason), other than care, to do the work alongside care, since we cannot get this type of evaluative posture out of care alone.

We can conclude that caring, for it to retain the moral appeal and importance that many have attached to it, has certain aspects that are deemed by its advocates as crucial. Care, first, is aimed at particular people that the moral agent is in relation with (without denying the possibility that the agent might expand such relations to include new people). Second, it must involve the element of motivational displacement, especially in an indirect form, and it must involve a certain critical amount of engrossment. Third, since care relationships typically involve caring for our loved ones, for those who are dear to us, we can add the further element that care has an important emotive dimension, such that when one cares for x one also expresses emotion, by, for example, being happy to care for x, being pleased to do so, and desiring to.

In addition, we can highlight some salient features found in *acting* from care.[17] First, the agent acts with respect to another that the agent knows and is in relation with, such as friend, lover, and offspring (Mayeroff 1971; Noddings 1984; Benhabib 1987; Friedman 1987, 1995; Blum 1993; Jaggar 1995). This distinguishes care from other altruistic motives that typically target strangers and perhaps acquaintances, such as sympathy, pity, and compassion. This need not deny that caring can involve sympathy and compassion (pity is controversial since it might be an innocuous form of contempt and superiority), but it does distinguish care from these in terms of their objects. Second, what is involved in caring is the intimate knowledge of the person cared-for (Mayeroff 1971; Gilligan 1982; Friedman 1987, 1995; Benhabib 1987; Blum 1993). In acting from care, one utilizes one's knowledge of the cared-for to tailor one's action to suit the needs of the cared-for.

Third, acting from care does not typically involve the use of moral principles (Gilligan 1982; Noddings 1984; Benhabib 1987; Blum 1993; Held 1995). Indeed, this is one crucial element of care ethics that has been emphasized so as to distinguish it from justice reasoning. In justice reasoning, it is claimed, an agent uses some moral principle or other and applies it impartially to the issue at hand to act correctly. By contrast, in acting from care one can act directly without the mediation of principles. However, acting without the mediation of principles should not tempt us to understand caring action as thoughtless and impulsive. Indeed, in using one's knowledge of the cared-for, one takes account of relevant features that help determine one's action, and this is not usually found in cases of acting impulsively.[18] (Closely related to the issue of emotion, one can also find in the literature on care—in Blum, for example—the claim that caring action can often be spontaneous, though with the emphasis that spontaneity need not render the action thoughtless.)

Fourth, in acting from care one typically acts emotively and affectively (Mayeroff 1971; Noddings 1984; Blum 1993; Friedman 1995; Jaggar

1995). The one-caring has an attachment to the cared-for and is concerned for her well-being. The one-caring is concerned for the needs of the cared-for, takes pleasure in her happiness, and is sad when she is not faring well. When one cares, then, it seems that one would also enjoy, and take pleasure in, one's caring actions. In cases when caring is done to alleviate suffering and ease pain, an emotive component is also present: one shares the pain of the cared-for. However, in either case, the one-caring gladly acts out of care, much as the brave person à la Aristotle gladly acts courageously even though facing fear and danger is unpleasant.[19]

The word "typically" in the first sentence of the above paragraph is important. For there might very well be cases of caring actions that carry with them no affective components. Cases of this sort are easy to envisage. Consider, for example, actions such as cleaning, cooking, and doing the laundry. These might be done for another *because* the one-caring cares for another, that is, they stem from the commitment of the former to care for the latter, yet they need not involve any pleasure in being carried out, nor do they need to be motivated by a desire to do them. This is not to say that they involve pain (although they certainly could), and it is not to say that they never involve pleasure or motivating desires, but simply to say that such emotional components are not a necessary requirement for such types of action. If this is required, then many actions that are caring—and they are so precisely because they are the actions of an individual who cares for another—would turn out to be not so. This, however, is a high price to pay because it simply goes against the way we describe and think about such actions in our daily lives.

These characteristics of care and of acting from care yield four desiderata of care ethics, all of which are emphasized in the literature: the concern with people embedded in contextual relations; attention to areas of life, neglected by some traditional moral philosophy, such as friendship and the family (indeed, the above contextual relationships are usually found among friends and family members); the emphasis on the affective component in ethical engagement; and partiality. But with partiality, the issue is more complicated. While many advocates of care ethics claim that it allows us to be both partial and moral, we will see that what care ethics demands of us need not conflict with impartiality (or universalizability, for that matter). For now, the question is whether virtue ethics can incorporate care ethics within its framework while at the same time (i) preserving the elements of care ethics thought to be valuable, (ii) answering the objections to care ethics, (iii) explaining how caring action need not conflict with certain traditional moral constraints (impartiality and universalizability), and (iv) giving us a unitary moral framework for both care and justice reasoning. But before we delve into these issues, there is a basic question that—though its answer might be obvious—needs to be briefly dealt with, namely, whether care is a plausible candidate for being an *excellence* in a person. If care cannot be a candidate for a trait of excellence, and if virtues are traits of excellence, then care simply cannot be a virtue and so the thesis of this chapter would not even take off the ground.

2. The Goodness of Care

We can perhaps all agree that there is something good—morally good—about care. But it might not be as easy to say what this general goodness amounts to, and so the issue that needs to be dealt with in this brief section is whether care can be plausibly thought of as a moral good, an excellence. This is a difficult question due to one important consideration: if the objections we have considered against care ethics have any merit, they should tell us that caring can be corrupted and can put the one-caring in morally dangerous situations, in which the one-caring ends up supporting the goals of an immoral person. And we have, in effect, recognized the need for a method by which caring relationships can be evaluated. But if this is correct, then we cannot simply state that care is a virtuous disposition. Much like daring and risk-taking, caring can become corrupt.

The issue here, I should note, is not the one—over which a good amount of energy and ink has been spent—that asks whether courage in a villain is a virtue or whether courage in a villain is even courage to begin with. This latter issue has to do with identifying conditions under which a particular trait of character is a virtue. And it seems to me that the answer to this question can be settled—in a classical and neo-Aristotelian sense—by claiming that a trait is a virtue that a person needs to flourish and that makes the person good *qua* being human. I will address this issue in regard to care below. However, the question that I am concerned with in this section is the far more basic one of whether care is *generally* a good trait to have, despite the fact that it can become corrupt. It is like asking whether risk-taking is a generally worthwhile disposition to have, despite the fact that risk-taking can be part of immoral ends. This question is more basic than the former one because if the trait in question were not generally worthwhile, we would not bother with raising the above question about it. No one bothers, for example, with trying to see under what conditions paranoia is a virtue, or under what conditions putting on one's left shoe before putting on the right one is a virtue, or under what conditions eating with one's hands is a virtue, or under what conditions making a sculpture out of marble is a virtue, or under what conditions greeting someone by asking, "What's up?" is a virtue. Some of these are traits that might be classified as habits; others as skills; and others as personality quirks. But each is either positively bad (such as the first one) or simply an issue of indifference to us as human beings. And my quest here is to see whether care belongs on that list. If not, then we can meaningfully go on to ask under what conditions it would be a virtue.

Furthermore, that a trait or an object can become corrupt does not entail that it is not a generally good trait to have. Knives can be used to kill, but this does not show that knives are not good to have. Caution can become excessive and lead to forms of catatonia, but this does not show that caution is not a good trait. To claim that a trait *can* be bad does not settle the issue of whether it is a generally good one to have.

Now it seems obvious that care *is* a generally good trait to have. We must, as philosophers, keep in mind the pervasive fact that all human beings come into this world as infants, and that without proper attention we cannot grow up to be mature and functioning entities, let alone survive. And much that goes under the rubric of "proper attention" is caring activity on the part of our parents and family members. A number of studies have shown that infants who receive improper attention tend to face many difficulties in life in terms of their ability to relate to and cooperate with others. Moreover, infants who grow in badly tended orphanages tend to develop psychological illnesses and to require much special attention and toil on the part of their future adoptive parents.[20]

But care is not just practiced by parents. Friends, siblings, and lovers are also paradigmatic examples of people whose relationships are characterized by care. Indeed, we would readily withhold the descriptions of friendship and love from relationships that do not (or only minimally) include caring activities or in which the parties involved have no desire to care for each other. A husband, for example, who claims to love his wife but who does not care for her in the ways emphasized in this chapter cannot be plausibly described as loving her, not unless some special explanation is offered, such as that he suffers from depression or some psychological trauma or other. Nor would anyone seriously consider that these relationships are not generally good to have. We know that love can go sour, that love-stricken individuals can do all sorts of crazy or immoral things, and that love has often been described as an illness. Nevertheless, we persist in believing that love is a good thing to have, and this is not just because people in love also often exhibit tendencies that are good (and thus opposite to the ones just mentioned), but because love—especially in its earlier stages of passion—allows the lover to experience joy, elation, and an openness to the world of a type rarely felt in other experiences.

Or consider friendship: Aristotle claimed that friendship is a virtue because without friends we cannot practice many of the virtues, such as generosity and beneficence (1985, 1155a5–12). As one recent philosopher puts it, "Friends help friends to be virtuous, by enabling them to be happy in their efforts to achieve moral excellence" (Jacquette 2001, 380). If, moreover, moral excellence is part of, or constitutive of, a flourishing life, as Aristotle insists, then friendship, and *philia* in general, would be part of such a life. Aristotle, moreover, offers, in the same passage, other reasons why friendship is important. Without friends we cannot—or it is difficult— to guard and protect our prosperity. And without friends we have no one to turn to when misfortune hits. If we keep in mind that *philia* covered not only what we today consider friendships but also the love between siblings, lovers, and parents and children, Aristotle would be giving us very powerful reasons for the importance of these relationships, and hence also for the importance of care, which characterizes such relationships.

Yet another important role for care in human life is the fact that caring can give meaning to our lives. Caring for someone we love, be it a parent, an offspring, a sibling, a friend, or a lover, can give meaning to our lives by providing us with a focus, a goal, or a center around which our lives can revolve. Of course, we need not have just one goal or focus. But the fact remains that having such goals allows us to separate what is worthy from what is not worthy of pursuit, and this gives us something to live for—a meaning. The point is not that we care for others *in order to* have meaningful lives, but, rather, that *in* caring for others, our lives have meaning.

A number of contemporary philosophers have recognized this point. For example, James Rachels, while attempting to see whether there is any justification for our partiality towards loved ones, accepts the position that personal relationships are integral to a rich and fulfilling life. In answering the question, "Why are personal relationships a great good?" he offers the following answer (among others): "Bonds of affection are more than just instrumentally good. . . . There is, at a deep level, a connection between love and the meaning of life. . . . Loving relationships provide individuals with things to value, and so give their lives this kind of meaning" (1989, 54–55). Milton Mayeroff states something similar: "When a man who has been unable to care or had no one or nothing to care for comes to care for some other, many matters previously felt to be important fade in significance, and those related to caring take on new importance" (1971, 51).

The issue of caring and the meaning of life should not tempt us to believe that only caring for intimate others can give life meaning.

Obviously, caring for animals, causes, strangers, activities (e.g., writing, painting, and playing soccer professionally) can also give life meaning. Nevertheless, the fact that caring for nonintimate others or activities can give life meaning does not detract from the truth that caring for intimate others does also give life meaning, and this is all we need to make the point. Consider, as an illustration, the novel *Silas Marner* by George Eliot. Silas, disillusioned with humanity, moves from his town, Lantern Yard, at a young age and takes up residence in the town of Raveloe, leading a reclusive life as a weaver. With time, one thing comes to take paramount importance in his life: hoarding the money and gold he made from weaving. Later in his life, a young child, whose mother had just died out in the cold, wanders into Silas's cottage, and Silas decides to take care of her (he calls her "Eppie"). Here is Eliot's description of the effect Eppie had on Silas's life:

> Unlike the gold which needed nothing, and must be worshipped in close-locked solitude—which was hidden away from the daylight, was deaf to the song of birds, and started to no human tones—Eppie was a creature of endless claims and ever-growing desires, seeking and loving sunshine, and living sounds, and living moments; making trial of everything, with trust in new joy, and stirring the human kindness in all eyes that looked on her. The gold had kept his thoughts in an ever-repeated circle, leading to nothing beyond itself; but Eppie was an object compacted of changes and hopes that forced his thoughts onward, and carried them far away from the old eager pacing towards the same blank limit—carried them away to the new things that would come with the coming years, when Eppie would have learned to understand how her father Silas cared for her; and made him look for images of that time in the ties and charities that bound together the families of his neighbours. The gold had asked that he should sit weaving longer and longer, deafened and blinded more and more to all things except the monotony of his loom and the repetition of his web; but Eppie called him away from his weaving, and made him think all its pauses a holiday, reawakening his senses with her fresh life, even to the old winter-flies that came crawling forth in the early spring sunshine, and warming him into joy because *she* had joy. (2001, 144)

With Eppie in his life, Silas came to realize that hoarding gold was an inane and pointless activity. He was able to see what was worthy about life.

Much about life that is worthwhile would be lost without intimate and close relationships. If we emphasize flourishing, and not just living or surviving, then without *philia* we would not flourish; intimate relationships are part of a flourishing life. And if caring is essential to *philia*, then its importance would stare us squarely in the face. Therefore, caring would surely be a generally good trait to have and to cultivate.

3. Care Ethics as Part of Virtue Ethics

3.1. Reason, Emotion, and Caring Actions

Caring actions are often thought to be spontaneous, impulsive, and done out of emotion, such as love, for the cared-for. This might tempt some to think that there is some tension between acting from care, on the one hand, and having such action be moral and suffused with reason, on the other. This section shows that this temptation can be easily resisted.

My overall suggestion in this chapter is to think of care as a virtue, as one virtue among those that go into constituting a flourishing life.[21] As a virtue, care would not simply be a natural impulse, but, to use Noddings's terminology, also ethical. In Aristotelian terms, it would not be a natural virtue, but one harnessed by reason. This allows us to maintain what is most desirable about care ethics. First, consider its insistence on the idea that human beings are not abstract individuals who morally relate to each other following principles such as justice and nonviolation of autonomy. One of virtue ethics' main claims is that we are social and political animals that need to constantly negotiate the ways we are to deal and live with each other.[22] With this general claim about our sociality, virtue ethics also claims that without certain types of relationships we do not usually flourish. Without friends and family members, human beings typically lead impoverished lives, being unable to partake in the pleasures of associating with people whom they can trust and share their joys, sorrows, and activities with. Virtue ethics, then, gives pride of place to care ethics' insistence on the sociality of human life and to its emphasis on the importance of certain types of relations such as those of friendship and family ties.[23] The point, I take it, is obvious enough and requires no further elaboration.

However, there might be a potential difficulty as far as virtue ethics' ability to accommodate care ethics well in this area: care ethics often takes human relationships to be ontologically basic, but virtue ethics does not. It seems to take instead the individual as ontologically basic and the individual's flourishing as ethically basic. If so, then virtue ethics does not take caring for others as ethically basic, and if it does not do this, then it does not incorporate care ethics' claims *well*. If virtue ethics is to do justice to care ethics, then it must be able to set aside its claim that flourishing is the ethically basic concept in its repertoire. This is, I think, a serious issue, and much depends on what we take these terms of contention to mean.

It is true that virtue ethics takes the concept of flourishing to be ethically basic in important respects. First, virtue ethics focuses not only on the issue of what makes acts right and wrong, but also on what the well-lived life is. Second, virtue ethics, as a neo-Aristotelian theory, claims that it is *rational* to be virtuous because being virtuous is one's most reliable way to flourish (Hursthouse 1999b, part 3). But from these claims it does not follow that flourishing is ethically basic *in the sense* that it gives agents moral license to violate the claims of others, be these strangers or intimates, when the agent's flourishing is at stake. Being virtuous is not a tactic, a policy, one adopts and one drops when it suits one. When one is virtuous, one has, among other things, the right attitudes, values, thought, and emotions with respect to, generally, what is good and bad, right and wrong, worthwhile and not worthwhile. This implies that being virtuous is compatible with, and often requires, sacrifices, sometimes of one's own very self. One cannot coherently claim, for example, to be courageous but also claim that even though such-and-such a good is absolutely worth fighting for, one will not because one's life is at risk.

Thus, given the thesis that care is a virtue, a virtuous, caring agent would act in a caring manner and would feel the requisite emotions when the situation calls for care (unless, of course, defeating conditions were present). In this respect, virtue ethics does accommodate care ethics' emphasis on caring, and it does so well by giving care an important status among the virtues (but more on this in the penultimate section). What virtue ethics does not accommodate is care ethics' claim that human *relationships* are ontologically basic. It does not do so not because it accepts the claim that the individual human being is ontologically basic (I am certain that virtue ethics is not committed to such a claim). It does not do so because it has no reason to be committed to such a controversial claim: what is important for virtue ethics to accommodate are care ethics' *ethical* claims, not its ontological ones. Furthermore, care ethics' claim that caring relationships are ethically basic does not entail the claim that human relationships are ontologically basic, and so virtue ethics is not logically committed to accept the latter, ontological claim. This is, by the way, a good thing, because the ontological claim seems to face a severe difficulty: a human relationship cannot be ontologically basic if it conceptually *requires* human beings to be the nodes of the relationship.

Let us turn next to the issue of emotion. As we saw, under care ethics acting typically involves acting emotively, being prompted to act by one's care for the cared-for, and this implies the desire (conscious or not) to promote the cared-for's goals and to allow oneself to be transformed by the cared-for. (For the sake of this discussion, I am setting aside those humdrum cases of caring which do not involve emotive components.) Furthermore, and under virtue ethics, when a virtuous person acts, she will also, characteristically, have the requisite emotion, both as an impulse to act and as a reaction.[24] This claim is part of the Aristotelian view—and most contemporary views on the emotions—that the emotions partake in reason. Virtue ethics then accommodates care ethics' concern about emotion quite easily: when a virtuous person acts in a caring manner towards another, he also feels the tender emotions associated with caring action. Moreover, he is also prompted to act out of the desire and love for the cared-for. This is a desirable view to have since we do not want caring actions to be unthinking and devoid of reason.

That the emotiveness of caring action and reason can be in harmony with each other is nicely demonstrated through Aristotle's conditions for virtuous action and a discussion of some possible worries found therein. Aristotle states that "first [the agent] must know that he is doing virtuous actions; second, he must decide on them, and decide on them for themselves; and, third, he must also do them from a firm and unchanging state" (1985, 1105a30–1105b). Consider the first condition. Aristotle here requires that if one, for example, tells the truth, that one also *know* that one is telling the truth. However, there is more to this than meets the eye. For as is well known, one can tell the truth, know that one is telling the truth, and yet not know that telling *this* truth in *these* circumstances is the good or virtuous or right or correct thing to do. And Aristotle seems to be requiring that the agent *also* know the latter, that is, that the agent know that her action of telling the truth in this situation is the right thing to do. This requirement is crucial: without it, it would be hard to see how his conditions are conditions for virtuous action, rather than actions that are right accidentally, so to speak. The requirement, moreover, does not entail that emotion cannot be present: having the requisite emotional motivation can go hand in hand with such thoughts as "I must do this," or "I should take the knife away from her before she harms herself," or "This is the right thing to do."

The reason for having the requirement found in the first condition is the sensible one that without it, it is difficult to set the virtuous apart from the vicious and the happy-go-lucky. It is the former, *because* they are virtuous, who engage in their actions with knowledge rather than accidentally and by morally stumbling through their daily lives. The idea is that virtuous agents are the ones who are able to tell the difference between actions that are good and right and those that are not, and this is part and parcel of Aristotle's requirement that decent agents be morally wise. And, as far as caring actions are concerned, this is surely a plausible demand: no matter how emotional and spontaneous we desire caring actions to be, we do, and should, also want them to issue from reflective and morally committed agents. Otherwise, we will all be in danger of being like Ms. A

(Noddings's woman who is willing to fight on the side of her racist family, discussed in section 1 above).

Turning to Aristotle's second condition, we find that it requires the virtuous agent to act *because* the action is just, or honest, or courageous, or, to stick to our topic, caring.[25] The harmony between reason and emotion should again be evident: a caring person can act caringly with all the needed and felt emotion while also acting for the right, virtuous reasons. But this might seem to pose a problem. For it might be thought—plausibly enough—that it is too demanding to require of caring agents that they say to themselves, "I am doing this *because* it is caring" (see on this Broadie 1991, 86–87). Indeed, as far as care ethics is concerned, such a requirement would run directly contrary to care ethics' emphasis on the *spontaneity*—though not the unthinkingness—of many caring actions.

This is a tricky issue. It is difficult to see how agents can act and yet not act for reasons, or even have their reasons for action present in their minds. It is, for example, difficult to see how a brother can act and take away the knife that his baby sister has in her hand without having some relevant reason to motivate him, such as "Knives are dangerous," or "She could hurt herself," or "She is my baby sister." Spontaneity, in short, does not preclude acting for reasons. The difficulty with Aristotle's condition might be not so much that it is too demanding to require that reasons be compatible with spontaneous caring action, but that the sort of terms that agents construct their reasons out of are too sophisticated. For example, the objection might be that it is too demanding that agents use such terms as "just" or "benevolent" or even "virtuous" to articulate their reasons. This would be too demanding because not all caring, virtuous agents will be philosophers, or will have taken Ethics 101.

This is a perfectly plausible objection. It is fully correct in claiming that such requirements are too demanding and, more importantly perhaps, unrealistic. But Aristotle's second condition need not be interpreted in this way. There are arrays of terms that agents can, and do, use, that do not require philosophical training, and that reflect perfectly the virtuous reasons for action. Hursthouse gives a very clear presentation of such terms:

> What are reasons 'typical of' a virtue? They will be the sorts of reasons for which someone with a particular virtue, V, will do a V act. So, thinking of the sorts of reasons a courageous agent might have for performing a courageous act, we can come up with such things as 'I could probably save him if I climbed up there,' 'Someone had to volunteer,' 'One can't give in to tyrants,' 'It's worth the risk.' Thinking of the range of reasons a temperate agent might have for a temperate act, we can come up with 'This is an adequate sufficiency,' 'I'm driving,' 'I'd like you to have some,' 'You need it more than I do,' 'She said

"No".' With respect to the liberal or generous, 'He needed help,' 'He asked me for it,' 'It was his twenty-first birthday,' 'She'll be so pleased.' With respect to the agent with the virtue of being a good friend, 'He's my friend,' 'He's expecting me to,' 'I can't let him down.' For honesty we get such things as 'It was the truth,' 'He asked me,' 'It's best to get such things out into the open straight away.' And for justice we get such things as 'It's his,' 'I owe it to her,' 'She has the right to decide,' 'I promised.' And so on and so forth. (1999b, 128)

Notice the reasons Hursthouse offers for the virtue of being a good friend. These are perfectly adequate as reasons given for caring actions in the context of a friendship. We can also generate a large number of others as we move from caring within friendships to caring within other types of relationships such as those between lovers, siblings, and parents and children. So a brother can say, "She's my sister." A wife: "He's my husband." A father: "They need me." A lover, "He's my one and only." Another lover, "She's my world." The examples can easily be multiplied.

Alternatively, the difficulty with Aristotle's second condition might be that the condition is taken to require of agents to *deliberate* prior to their actions, and *this* surely is in tension with spontaneity. But this difficulty can only come if we adopt an uncharitable interpretation of Aristotle. For we know, and so did Aristotle (1985, 1117a22, for instance), that not every action on the part of the virtuous person requires deliberation. Deliberation is a time-consuming process that requires the agent to weigh reasons for and against one or more courses of action. In addition to the fact that there are numerous situations in which agents simply do not have the luxury of time that deliberation requires, not all actions require deliberation for the obvious reason that on many occasions what ought to be done is perfectly clear. In caring relationships, moreover, a virtuous agent would not need to deliberate every time he acts in a caring manner towards his cared-for. The agent need not, prior to assisting her friend in correcting the latter's architecture plans, deliberate about whether she should do so, whether *morally* she may help her friend. For if her friend is *good*, and if her friend's projects are also good (and so do not, say, include, designing propaganda buildings for some fascist regime), then there is simply no need for the virtuous agent to scrutinize her actions towards that friend on every occasion. And similar reasoning applies to all other caring relationships.

It is the third condition, namely, that the agent act from a "firm and unchanging state," that will allow us to successfully complete the discussion of the harmony of emotion and reason. The firm and unchanging state of which Aristotle speaks is, roughly, the agent's character. A virtuous agent is *reliable*: because of her moral education, training, and upbringing, she can be relied upon to do what is virtuous. Part of what this helps us see is that the reliability in question is not just that of thought and action, but also that of emotional reaction and motivation. For an essential part of the virtuous agent's moral training is that of her emotions, and so when she acts from a stable state she does the right thing but she also has the right emotional reaction and motivation. (Of course, all of this assumes that the agent is not acting out of character, or is being coerced, etc.) Thus, we can now put the point of this discussion about caring action, emotion, and reason as follows: caring, virtuous action is typically emotive. Its emotiveness goes hand in hand with the agent's knowledge that her actions are virtuous and with the agent's acting for virtuous reasons. Indeed, caring action that is *virtuous* is virtuous precisely because of the presence of the correct rational and emotional response. Virtue ethics accommodates care ethics in this respect with a vengeance.

The discussion thus far has been on the compatibility within virtue ethics of the emotiveness of caring action with reason. It has not yet addressed the different issue—with which Davion's worry is mainly concerned—as to whether the caring relationship *itself* is moral or not. Thus, the discussion thus far has been concerned with caring actions *within* caring relationships. Our next issue is the ethical standing of the relationships themselves.

3.2. Caring Relationships, Reason, and Davion's Criticism

No doubt, being in a caring relationship can be, and generally is, a good thing. But caring relationships can be morally bad. There is the need, then, to give a general account of the conditions under which a caring relationship is deemed by the virtuous person to be good to begin with. This is the task of this section. I will begin by looking at some remarks Aristotle gave on friendship, since these offer a good segue into my account.

Aristotle claims that the virtuous person's friend is another self: "The excellent person is related to his friend in the same way he is related to himself, since a friend is another himself. Therefore, just as his own being is choiceworthy for him, his friend's being is choiceworthy for him in the same or a similar way" (1985, 1170b6–7). In the *Eudemian Ethics*, Aristotle states, "For friendship seems something stable, and this alone is stable. For a formed decision is stable, and where we do not act quickly or easily, we get the decision right. There is no stable friendship without confidence, but confidence needs time. One must then make trial. . . . Nor is a friend made except through time" (1984, 1237b10–17). Though

Aristotle does not explicitly speak of choosing our friends, his remarks indicate that there is a choice involved in friendships, a choice to the effect that we choose our friends given certain standards, such as having a morally desirable character. His remarks commit him to the idea of choosing our friends because without such an idea his points about building confidence and making trial would not be plausible: Why test the character of our potential friends if we do not have the option to choose not to be their friends? The choice need not be about *initiating* friendships, though this is true in many cases, but is about opting to continue or to quit them. Furthermore, the choice takes time and needs to be tested until a certain amount of confidence and trust is established. In addition, the friend, who is "another self," will share "a sense of our commitments and ends, and a sense of what we take to be ultimately 'good and pleasant' in living" (Sherman 1989, 131).

It is crucial to note that the notion of choice is important not just for its own sake, but for what it also indicates, namely, that with choice comes rational deliberation, and this implies that we can use reason to evaluate and regulate friendships. (Indeed, the notion of choice provides a poor basis for intimate relationships that do not involve much choice for their parties in *initiating* the relationships, such as siblings and, in parental ones, children.) Reason, then, plays a crucial role in our choice of friends. In choosing Richard for a friend, I need to make sure that he has a character compatible with mine, that his goals and activities are morally in the clear, and that I can even share them and be willing to (indirectly, at least) promote them. Such a choice, of course, requires the time needed to evaluate my friend's character, actions, and goals. With time, my choice of Richard as a friend is either cemented or shaken. If the former, then, in caring for him, I need not always deliberate about whether my action is right. In caring for Richard by, say, helping him to achieve a certain goal, I need not deliberate about whether doing so is ethically correct, for this has already been established. He would not have been my friend if his goals were deemed unworthy. We have to remember that friendships involve a good amount of trust between the friends. If I come to know that my friend is a morally decent person, and given my intimate knowledge of his character and his life (he is, after all, my friend), then I can trust that his goals would be morally in the clear, especially in those cases when he adopts new goals. Unless a special case arises (for example, caring for him conflicts with another moral requirement, or I have reason to believe that he is changing and so realize the importance of not automatically trusting a new goal of his), I need not deliberate about whether my action is morally permissible.

To be clear, my claim is neither that a friend does not deliberate about the goals of his friend, nor is it that he should not deliberate about these goals. There are situations within friendship when deliberation is called for, and these are not confined to ones in which caring for a friend conflicts with another moral requirement. It might be that, for example, Richard undertakes a project that I think could be, for one reason or another, unsuitable for him, and so have to deliberate as to whether I will support him. However, I also do not want to make the weak claim that deliberation is always appropriate within friendship or the strong claim that it is always necessary. These extreme positions, I believe, would make the conceptual claim that friends trust each other shaky, and would, if acted upon, causally endanger the trust that friends do have for each other.

This account need not deny the possibility that a friend's character changes. If this were to occur, we use reason to reevaluate our actions towards him. Aristotle recognizes that friends sometimes change (1985, 1165b12–36), and if a friend changes to the point where he is no longer the same person, the grounds of the friendship dissolve. The point is that reason, or wisdom, plays a crucial regulative role: it assesses the goals and the general character of a friend, and in doing so, it offers a generally reliable mechanism through which we can check whether the friendship is morally in the clear, so to speak.[26]

The preceding account applies as well to married couples and lovers, insofar as these relations involve an amount of choice, and to other relations that do not involve as much choice in initiating the relationship, such as child-parent ones, but which also essentially involve caring. The regulative role of reason would allow the one-caring, be it the offspring or the parent, to decide whether to continue to be in such a relationship and so to continue to be caring or not. And surely this is a result that ought to be welcome. For insofar as care ethics has been criticized on the grounds that it does not leave room for a mechanism by which the caring relationship is evaluated as good or not, such an account of the role of reason would, in principle, supply such a mechanism. Furthermore, we can here see a role, though a limited one, for choice: if the emphasis is placed not so much on the choice to *enter* a relationship but on the ability to leave it, or at least to withhold care, then the one-caring would have some choice in the decision to minimize care, to cease caring altogether, or to even suspend the relationship entirely. I do not mean to deny, of course, that sometimes a wife is unable to leave her husband, that a son who realizes that his father is corrupt cannot just pack his bags and go. But this is an issue that has to do with specific and contingent obstacles to actual relationships.

However, one might find the idea that a parent or a child can opt to leave a parent-child relationship to be highly unrealistic or implausible. It might be thought unrealistic not because it is sometimes difficult to leave such a relationship due to factors specific to the case, but because, in addition to social pressures, few parents or children can just simply decide to leave such a relationship, even after much deliberation. For aside from the rare case in which the child or parent is thoroughly evil, children and parents find themselves to be, for good or ill, emotionally attached to their parents and children, respectively, in ways that spouses—perhaps—do not. Furthermore, opting to leave such relationships might be thought implausible because children-parent relationships have special obligations. Even if my mother, say, is self-centered and rarely shows concern for me, it is still my obligation to tend to and care for her.

The above reflections are plausible. However, they do not threaten the idea that reason has, and should have, a regulative role to perform in intimate relationships. In those cases of parent-child relationships in which one (or both) of the parties shows signs of moral corruption, and if opting to leave is an implausible solution, then reason will have to play a more direct role, much like it would have to in cases of friendship that exhibit signs of going awry. Wisdom would have to play a role in how best to care for the other party in the relationship in order to make sure, for example, that the moral integrity of the one-caring is not compromised, or that the one-caring does not open himself up to corruption. So a son might decide to do the minimum that is required in terms of his duties to his father but maintain his emotional distance from him as much as possible. And a mother might lie to her son about how much money she has so that he won't forcefully take it and spend it on alcohol and gambling, even though she continues to perform her household activities, including those that tend to her son's domestic life (e.g., his laundry). I mention these suggestions not because I believe that, say, a mother *should* continue to care for her son, no matter what he is and does. Indeed, there are clear cases in which mothers, and parents in general, should cease to care for their children, period. Rather, I mention these to indicate that my account is not silent about tough, realistic cases in which the ones-caring *cannot*, for whatever reason, simply opt out of a relationship.

The account of the regulative role of reason is able to supply us with an adequate way of accommodating Davion's criticism of Noddings's ethics of care, namely, that one can care for someone who is evil and so open oneself up to moral corruption. We can see this in terms of the concept of integrity, the concept that Davion herself uses. It should be clear that a virtuous person is one who has integrity, and it is hard to see how one can be virtuous and yet lack integrity. A virtuous person is one who has and exercises the virtues, and to exercise a virtue is to act rightly from a *stable* character. But this means that when one acts virtuously one acts *reliably* because one is committed to acting rightly, and to doing so *because* it is morally correct. A virtuous person, for example, tells the truth *because* doing so is honest. Someone who tells the truth because it secures an advantage for him (for example, becoming his boss's favorite employee) is the paradigm picture of someone who is *not* virtuous. No person can be virtuous and yet lack moral integrity. To think otherwise is to think of someone who has what Aristotle calls "natural virtue," someone who acts rightly and desires to act the way he does, yet does and is so accidentally, so to speak. To be virtuous one must subject one's conduct and desires to the scrutiny, and shaping, of reason. If so, then if a virtuous person finds herself in a relationship such that the one cared-for is turning evil, and if she fails to reverse or at least prevent such a change from being completed, then her concern for her own character would call for severing such a relationship.

We can even go a bit further. Davion (1993, 179) recognizes that the role of integrity in her account is one of necessity and not of sufficiency. In other words, while integrity is necessary to maintain a morally good relationship, it is not sufficient, because two evil people can have integrity (so long as their actions, say, cohere with their values) and so maintain a strong relationship. Whether Davion is correct in thinking that having integrity is compatible with being evil is an issue we need not go into, because we do not need to settle it in order to see that a *virtuous* person cannot have integrity and be evil. For under virtue ethics integrity comes after certain conditions have been met. Simply put, a virtuous person is someone who is *virtuous* (excuse the banality). Her integrity will, ipso facto, be that of a person who is good, not evil, because whatever commitments and principles she abides by and give her agency a sense of coherence, these commitments and principles are to what is morally right and good. So the sufficiency condition is met.

As a side note, this discussion of integrity and virtue might, however, usher in the troubling thought that when it comes to virtuous people, integrity is a superfluous trait. What role does it possibly play in the behavior of the virtuous person? One can see its role in the behavior of a continent agent: if integrity is plausibly, though partially, understood as resisting temptation, and if the continent agent is one who struggles against his desires, then we can see a role for integrity in such a person's life. But what role would it play in the life of the virtuous agent? In reply, we should keep in mind that virtuous people are not immune to temptation. A virtuous person might, because of financial difficulties, very much desire a promotion or a raise, and so he might be tempted to "sleep his way to the top," but his integrity would prevent him from succumbing to the temptation or to even giving it much thought. Hopefully, we can begin to see a role for integrity in the lives of the virtuous.

There is one more serious issue that I will attend to before turning to partiality. I have emphasized the idea that it is important that friendships and intimate relationships in general be subject to the regulation of reason, understood in the Aristotelian sense as oriented towards the good. This claim entails that for an intimate relationship to continue and to flourish, both (or more) parties of the relationship must share a good amount of basic values and commitments to moral ends. However, this seems to run counter to a claim, made by Marilyn Friedman (1993) and recently accepted by Richard White (2001), to the effect that one crucial value of friendships is that the parties to it, *because of their friendship*, can morally grow and change in *deep* and *radical* ways. However, given my account, sharing some deep values might preclude this growth, since without difference in these values it is difficult to see how one friend can influence another to such deep change. If so, then my account would end up denying—if Friedman and White are correct—an important value of friendship, namely, its ability to effect deep and radical changes in the friends. A brief treatment of this issue will enrich the discussion so far and allow us to arrive at some interesting insights about friendship. Since Friedman goes into this issue in more depth than does White, I will focus on her claims.

Friedman claims that "to suppose that the abstract commitments to values and principles that we happen to hold at a particular time should always prevail in any conflict with our commitments to loved ones would be to cut ourselves off from an invaluable source of inspiration for critical moral thinking" (1993, 140). This seems to go directly against some of my own claims. Friedman is claiming that one's values should not always win in a conflict between these and one's belief that one ought to support one's friend in a certain circumstance. One reason why Friedman puts her claim in such a way is because she thinks that a commitment to a friend or an intimate other has as its object the friend herself in her particularity, and acting on behalf of such a commitment is motivated by the friend as an individual, not some abstract principle: "One's behavior toward the friend takes its appropriateness, at least in part, from her goals and aspirations, her needs, her character. . . . Partiality for a friend involves being motivated by the friend as an individual, by who she is and not by the principled commitments of one's own which her circumstances happen to instantiate" (1993, 191–92). This is contrasted with commitments to abstract moral guidelines, such as moral rules, values, and principles. Moral guidelines "structure modes of reasoning from which one derives specific judgments governing the situations and choices faced in daily life. Abstract moral guidelines are general and make no reference to particular persons or occasions" (190).

Friedman states that the conflict often arises when a friend, x, is prompted to act out of her friendship for y but x's principles do not support such a purported course of action (192). It is here that one important value of friendship can be clearly seen, according to Friedman: given the conflict, and given that we take our friends seriously, there is an opportunity for moral growth. For now x is in a position where she is able to rethink and possibly revise the principles and guidelines she has hitherto been committed to. In this respect, our commitments to particular intimate others act as a counterbalance to our commitment to principles, and in those cases in which they take precedence over the latter, we see how x can grow due to her friendship and due to her friend y (195).

Friedman argues that:

> friendship is a close relationship in which trust, intimacy, and disclosure open up for us whole standpoints other than our own. . . . Because we know, in minute and intimate detail, so much of what is happening to a good friend, those experiences live for us with narrative specificity and richness. Because a friend is other than oneself . . . a friend will differ from oneself in some ways. Usually she conceptualizes experience and comprehends its significance in terms that are at least somewhat different from one's own. Because of those differences, the narratives and judgments she shares will implicitly reveal a moral perspective that is, to at least some extent, unlike one's own. (198–99)

It is because of these differences and the interaction between the friends that a "profound" moral growth and change can occur: "Friendship can open up the very possibility of growth in our *deepest moral values, rules, and principles and not simply their fuller articulation.* . . . What a friend may provide for us is a viewpoint informed by an *alternative set of principled moral commitments*" (201; my emphasis).

One craves, at this point in Friedman's discussion, some examples. The reason I say this is because of a worry I have: Friedman's account is plausible because it is set at a somewhat high level of abstraction. But once we try to think of it in more concrete and applied terms, it turns out to be conceptually too ambitious: friends, I want to argue, *cannot* effect such a *radical* moral change in each other. But to see this, consider first what Friedman has to say about x's and y's effect on each other when x and y are like each other to begin with. According to Friedman, the more friends are alike, the less likely they are to bring about such deep changes in each other. This, she emphasizes, does not deny that in such friendships there is moral growth and change, but it does deny that the growth and change amounts to "radical transformation of deep-level, abstract moral commitments and more likely to amount to a fuller articulation of the moral values both friends already have in common" (203).

This is exactly correct. But what Friedman does not see is that similarity between the values which friends have is a necessary condition for two people to be friends to begin with. And once this is granted, the possibility that friends can effect deep and radical moral changes in each other becomes much less obvious. To elaborate: Friedman, given her discussion, obviously does not have in mind friendships of mere utility or of pleasure; she has in mind friendships that are pervaded by intimacy, deep trust, and other crucial notions. But for trust and intimacy to ground such friendships, they require an important dimension of commonality between friends, a dimension that has as one essential constituent the sharing of deep and basic values. It is hard to think of Simona and Salma as being *friends* were Simona and Salma to differ in their regard to the value of human life, or in their regard to human equality, to give a couple of obvious examples. In this respect, if Simona and Salma are friends, the kind of effect they would have on each other is less of the radical kind and more of the kind that allows the friends to articulate their values better—as Friedman states—and of seeing how their values and principles apply to situations whose relevance they have not hitherto seen. For example, Simona, a staunch defender of the state of Israel and its foreign policies, might be committed to the value and equality of human life in the abstract and to the value of a people's right to live on their land in dignity and freedom. But Simona might have been also blind to the fact that Palestinians are as deserving of these rights and values as are Israelis. It might take Salma, a Palestinian friend, to open up her eyes in this respect and on this issue.

Without a shared amount of deep values and principles, Simona and Salma cannot be friends in the sense that Friedman and I have in mind. For without such shared deep values, they cannot attain the level of trust and intimacy requisite for such friendships. But if this is correct, then friends cannot affect each other in the ways that Friedman suggests. (Perhaps Friedman has something specific in mind when she mentions "radical" and "deep" changes. If so, she does not tell us.) Her account applies better to relationships between colleagues and acquaintances, although here we must tread carefully. For to the extent that such deep changes are indeed a function of trust and intimacy, then they might not be able to occur between colleagues and acquaintances either. Of course, in *actual* cases, we have a lot more room for give and take. For example, Shay and Justin might be coworkers who have radically different values. But in the process of getting to know each other, Shay may be able to change Justin's deep values about certain things, as they get to be friends. In other words, the change might occur as their intimacy and trust grows and develops.

Of course, actual cases also show us one way in which Friedman is correct. If two friends can share *some*, but not all, of their basic and deep values, then they might—depending on the case—have enough common grounds for them to effect the kind of changes Friedman has in mind. Moreover, it seems to me that such cases are entirely possible and coherent. However, and as I have been arguing, we should not make the mistake of thinking that such changes can occur if the friends have no common grounds of basic and deep values.

I should add that these points, though made with regard to friendships, apply with equal force to other intimate relationships. Indeed, it is often the case that lovers stick together—and are friends—precisely because they share deep values and beliefs. This also applies to siblings and to parents and their children. What accounts for much of this is the fact that children, siblings, and parents all usually grow up in the same household and are thus educated and raised under the same rubric of values and beliefs. And often, when siblings break the relationship between them, for example, they do so precisely because they do not see eye to eye on certain deep matters and values.

Thus, the difference between Friedman's account and mine is not limited to scope of application in that mine is confined to friends who are virtuous while hers is not. There is another genuine difference: her account does not preserve the truthful insight that for *x* and *y* to be friends they must have an overlap of deep values and basic moral principles and commitments. In the context of caring, a relationship cannot be a caring one in a morally healthy way unless both parties' deep moral commitments and values are shared to a good extent. In this way the goals, projects, and aspirations of both parties would be based on healthy moral values.

To summarize the conclusions of this subsection, virtue ethics requires that caring relationships be subject to the regulative role of wisdom to ensure their moral desirability. Virtue ethics' emphasis on moral wisdom and on the virtues supplies us with an in-principle mechanism with which to morally scrutinize such intimate relationships. This, moreover, should be a welcome result given the need to supply care with a method of self-evaluation.[27] I should also emphasize that this account is not a temporal one, that is, it is not an account stating that *first* reason must evaluate a potential friendship or relationship, and *then* the virtuous person can rest assured that her caring actions are morally okay. This would be implausible because evaluating relationships cannot realistically be done in this way, since the evaluation typically goes temporally hand in hand with the development of the relationship. As Diane Jeske, in a slightly different context, puts it, "Coming to know other people . . . is a complex and difficult process, because persons are not transparent. . . . it is likely that we may form friendships before we know all of the faults of our potential friends" (1997, 71).[28] Rather, my account is a conceptual one: it makes room for the role of reason in the evaluation of relationships by giving reason a regulative role to play. I turn next to partiality.

3.3. Card's Criticism, Partiality, and Universalizability

It is sometimes thought that caring somehow precludes one from being also fair and just towards those with whom one is not in a caring relationship, because caring requires one to be partial towards those one cares for. This section's task is to show how a virtuous agent can be both caring—and thus partial towards her cared-fors—and yet also just—and thus impartial.

Card's objection to care ethics is that it does not give us a way to ground our obligations to nonintimate others, especially strangers, who, as far as the one-caring is concerned, comprise the bulk of humanity. However, once care ethics is incorporated into virtue ethics, Card's worry would be adequately addressed: justice is a crucial virtue for virtue ethics, since virtue ethics insists that it is a virtue that a virtuous person possesses. The reason is not simply that all virtue ethicists have said so, but that justice is a necessary virtue when it comes to some aspects of our dealings with strangers (how to distribute resources, how to ensure compliance with noninterference between people, etc.), and so no person can claim to have an ethical character if he, say, violates people's rights. Thus, while virtue ethics is able to account for our caring relations to others, it does not neglect justice.[29] It is furthermore within a discussion of justice that the issue of partiality arises in full force, for it is here that we see the need to find a way to justifiably adjudicate between the claims of partiality and impartiality.

Now advocates of care ethics usually construe the demand of impartiality as the claim that all persons should be treated on equal footing and that displaying favoritism in one's moral actions is morally prohibited. They then claim that such a demand is not plausible when it comes to our actions towards family members and friends. The idea is that it is not only morally permissible but also praiseworthy that we attend to our cared-fors, and that in (at least) some cases of *conflict* between partiality and the demands of impartiality, being partial is ethically acceptable, if not even laudable. In other words, the idea is not simply that people, as a matter of fact, feel the pull of partiality, but that they *ought to* feel it.[30]

Furthermore, there are at least three important aspects to partiality that connect quite nicely with the above-stated features of caring, and this helps explain the justification of acting in a partial manner. For if caring action is, in general, morally justified, then in seeing the connections between caring and partiality, one goes quite a way in justifying actions done out of partiality.[31] These aspects of partiality are then, first, that an agent is partial to a *particular* person, such as a friend, a spouse, and a child (and even to a group of individuals, such as one's clan or nation, but I am setting these aside). This first aspect of partiality connects with the first feature of caring, namely, that one cares for particular other individuals. Second, partiality typically manifests itself in relationships that are importantly affective, involving emotions and feelings. One is, for example, partial towards a friend or a lover. This aspect connects nicely with the third feature of caring, namely, that caring has an important emotive dimension to it.

Third, an aspect of partiality is that the agent does not typically choose or decide to feel concern for a particular individual. Our partiality for our children, for example, is natural; one does not decide to love one's children. Even friendship and love have this characteristic, since these often exert a pull that makes one feel compelled into them. No doubt, these leave more room for choice than parental partiality (though even the latter has room for choice, such as choosing how best to exhibit partiality and choosing whether to continue to care for a child). This aspect of partiality, moreover, resembles displacement and engrossment, defining aspects of care defined above. Motivational displacement, as we recall, demands adopting and promoting the goals of the cared-for. Engrossment demands a nonjudgmental acceptance of the cared-for and, as a consequence, the possibility of transformation of the one-caring. Because partiality also has this dimension of spontaneity, of some lack of choice, one is led to help the cared-for achieve her goals without judging them. For the very spontaneity and naturalness found in partiality make some conceptual and causal room for accepting another individual and her goals for who and what they are, and the important aspect of concern found in partiality makes conceptual and causal room for helping the cared-for to promote her goals. None of this, of course, denies the need for a critical evaluation of caring relationships, nor does it deny the need to address the question of when partiality ought to be acted upon, a question dealt with in what follows.

The point of the above brief discussion is to highlight some explanatory and justificatory connections between partiality and care, and we should now attend to the issue of conflict between the pull of partiality and that of impartiality. Since we cannot justifiably endorse *all* cases of partial behavior, and since partiality and impartiality sometimes conflict, we need to be able to plausibly situate the former within an overall moral theory. The issue, then, is this: Can virtue ethics supply us with a principled way to justify those cases of partiality that we might reasonably believe to be justified? If virtue ethics can do this, then given its emphasis on the virtue of justice, virtue ethics can offer us one theoretical framework within which our treatment of strangers and intimate others is balanced in a morally justified way. And in so doing, virtue ethics can both incorporate care ethics and improve upon it, in as much as care ethics has emphasized the importance of partiality and has proven to be deficient in treating the claims of strangers on the moral agent in a convincing manner.

First, we should not exaggerate the conflict between partiality and impartiality. For one thing, it is not usual that our attention to our loved ones conflicts with the demands of impartiality, because the moral domains of our dealings with intimates and with strangers are usually separate from each other.[32] It is not typically the case that one is conflicted between the demands of friends and of strangers. Furthermore, even given a duty of general benevolence towards people, this is not usually understood as the claim that we ought to divide our attention to everyone equally. There is a good reason for this, in addition to the fact that it is humanly impossible to do so. In order for individuals to lead happy and rich lives, they need to be able to pursue their own goals, activities, and interests, and this ability would be thwarted were individuals to divide their time and energy equally with others. And virtue ethics certainly recognizes this. In its emphasis on flourishing, virtue ethics gives ample room to the above idea, and insofar as it insists on friendship as an essential factor that goes into flourishing, it also recognizes the importance of having friends and family relationships, and the importance of the attention that such relationships require.

But cases of conflict between the demands of friendship and those of others do arise, and it is important to see whether virtue ethics would adequately deal with such types of cases. The issue here is under what conditions one should heed the pull of partiality. Suppose, for example, I promise a colleague of mine to meet her for lunch at a restaurant, but I get a call that a friend is in the hospital. If the idea behind care ethics' insistence on partiality is that I go and visit my friend in the hospital, even if this results in my breaking my promise to my colleague, then no reasonable philosopher would wish to argue against such a conclusion, and no sophisticated moral theory would, since we recognize that friends have special claims upon us. Virtue ethics is no exception, for surely the virtu-

ous agent would know that her friend requires her attention and so goes
to visit her.

But consider a different case. Suppose I get into a car accident such
that both my spouse and a stranger are severely hurt, require immediate
attention, and I can only attend to one of them. In such a case, care ethics
would surely imply that while impartiality requires that either person is as
worthy of assistance, it is at least ethically permissible that I attend to my
spouse. Again, however, this is somewhat of an uncontroversial case.
While impartiality entails that both are equals as far as their humanity is
concerned, it need not follow that impartiality requires that I attend to
them equally. How can I, given the case? Furthermore, if I attend to my
spouse, my action would be perfectly permissible. Given my love for my
spouse, his importance to my life and to my well-being, I simply cannot
be morally faulted if I help him. This bond between my spouse and I is
the salient feature of the situation that justifies my choosing to help the
spouse. And that virtue ethics accommodates this type of case needs, I
take it, no explanation.

But suppose the case is slightly different. Suppose my spouse is not
hurt, but badly shaken and is starting to show symptoms of entering into
a screaming fit. Should I attend to him, knowing that the other person *is*
in need of immediate assistance?[33] While a virtuous person, in virtue of the
strong ties to his spouse, would surely feel a strong desire to be with his
loved one, he would not act on this desire. Perhaps he might rush to his
spouse and say something to the effect that he will be with him soon. But
surely he would give the necessary help to the stranger, because a virtuous
person is disposed to render help to those who are in immediate need and
to alleviate suffering. And this is the right conclusion to reach, because in
this case the needs of the stranger are more pressing. Such conflict cases
indicate that it is not always morally correct to act on one's desires to help
and care for a loved one. Sometimes strangers (e.g., starving children in
the world) have immediate needs that one is in a position to attend to and
that one should attend to, even if this involves a discomfort to a loved one
or a loss of some material good. Furthermore, a case such as this indicates
that there is no precise *method* of deciding when one ought to help a
stranger and when one ought to help an intimate. There simply seems to
be no "calculus" to decide such things; we need to go by our moral sense
of what is morally right to do in such cases.

Consider one last case, important to highlight that aspect of impartiality concerned with justice. Suppose that because I love my child, I bribe a
school official to ensure her place in the school. Obviously, in doing so I
violate just procedures.[34] Given that I am being partial towards my child,

would it be correct to say that my action is morally permissible? Surely not. For even if my action is done out of care for my child, if Card's (1990) criticism that we need justice to ground our obligations to those we are not in caring relations with has any plausibility to it (and it has), then to argue that my action in this case is permissible, is to reject, in effect, the claims that justice has on us. Furthermore, a virtuous person would surely not act in this way, for she has the virtue of justice, a virtue that covers treating others fairly and according them their dues.[35]

Now it is important to note that once we remember that the virtuous person is just, much of this discussion is put in perspective. For an essential part of the story of what it means to be virtuous is that one has the virtues and that one has practical wisdom that allows the agent to decide on the correct exercise of the virtues given the context. Once this is remembered, it should be realized that not every case of partial action is going to be morally permissible under virtue ethics. Whether it is will depend, partly, on whether it impermissibly violates the dictates of justice. Someone will claim that I am here begging the question against proponents of care ethics. But this cannot be correct. For if they want to claim that partial actions are morally permissible in *all* cases of conflict, then they will be faced—once again—with the objection that this entails the neglect of the important concept of justice. There is, therefore, the need for a way to reconcile the two, and virtue ethics can in principle do this.

Before summarizing the above cases, I wish to make it clear that I am not claiming that in each of these cases the agent *must* invoke some moral principle before acting; to claim this is to go against care ethics' emphasis on acting directly. Indeed, I would even argue that, in the first three cases at least, the agent need not even *deliberate* about what to do (need not have one thought too many, in the famous words of Bernard Williams). A virtuous agent is one who recognizes what place people have in one's life, and when faced with situations such as the above, the agent need only perceive the facts and act. Knowing that my friend is in the hospital I would just go to see her, and would make amends to my colleague later. Seeing that my spouse is in mortal danger I would go and help him. Seeing that he is not in danger but that another is, I would go and help the latter.

To summarize the points about impartiality, I have argued that, typically, conflicts between the claims of strangers and those of cared-fors are rare. In cases in which there are conflicts, one would have to consider the factors involved in each case. Sometimes the claims of strangers are overridden when those near and dear to us require immediate attention. Sometimes the claims of strangers override those who are near and dear to us because the former's are pressing and humanly important, while the latter's can withstand delay of attention. When both are equally pressing and one can attend to only one, then the claims of loved ones take priority. And we morally cannot violate just—and not only legal—procedures simply because this would help the ones that we love. While there are no neat formulas here, the point is that care considerations and partiality cannot simply trump other ones, even if we are in situations in which we are strongly desirous of attending to the cared-for. Even though care comprises an essential dimension of our ethical lives, strangers, acquaintances, colleagues, and others do have claims upon us, and the claims of partiality and those of impartiality need to be balanced against each other.[36]

But—one might object—surely there are cases that contain irresolvable moral dilemmas. The cases I have mentioned so far contain dilemmas, but they all seem to be resolvable. What about the case—and many more can be generated by following its basic recipe—where the agent is the captain of a ship, the ship is sinking, and the only way to save the ship is for the captain to throw out either his spouse or the two other passengers (because the spouse weighs as much as the other two, and a certain amount of weight needs to be jettisoned)? The agent, say, cannot commit suicide in this case because he is the only one who knows how to steer the ship to safety. In this case, the agent should, as captain, save the two other passengers, but, as husband, should save his spouse.[37] Either action is wrong from some point of view. Can virtue ethics offer a principled way of dealing with such cases? And how would it proceed? And wouldn't care ethics have a clear answer to them and thus the upper hand?

Before tackling this objection, we should remind ourselves of the central question of this section, namely, whether virtue ethics can accommodate the insights about the importance of partiality, and whether virtue ethics can avoid strict moral accounts that claim that all persons should be treated equally. Back to the objection: to put it bluntly, it does not succeed. First, while it *might* be true to claim that care ethics has a clear answer to this, it does not follow that its answer is correct. And so it does not follow that we have a case in which virtue ethics cannot accommodate the claims of care ethics. For consider what care ethics is seen to be telling us. On the assumption that care ethics would indeed recommend that the agent save his spouse (and it is an *assumption*, because I doubt that the claim it embodies would command general assent from care ethics advocates), care ethics would nevertheless be giving a controversial answer. Part of the case is that the agent is the *captain* of the ship, and captains have particular duties. The answer that the agent save his spouse cannot be, then, *obviously* the correct answer. *At best*, it is a plausible yet controversial one, and if it is, then it cannot be the case that care ethics has the upper hand here.

Part of the difficulty has to do with the very idea of irresolvable dilemmas, since a few philosophers have denied they exist. What is often involved in denying the existence of irresolvable dilemmas is giving an answer to any offered case and then claiming that the dilemma is not, therefore, irresolvable. But that an answer can be given does not entail that it is the right answer, but rather simply that, depending on one's theoretical commitments or intuitions, one can offer *an* answer. The points in this paragraph and in the one above are, of course, connected. An advocate of care ethics might offer an answer to the above case as being the correct one, but he will do so precisely because he is an advocate of care ethics, and this should indicate that the answer will be controversial.

But what would virtue ethics tell us that the agent should do? Well, the case—and putting its suspicious fictitiousness aside—is an irresolvable dilemma, and I do not think that virtue ethics would—and should—claim that there is one correct answer.[38] We cannot say, for example, that the captain should save his spouse because the other two are strangers. The reason is that the agent is the *captain* of the ship, and being a captain is, in addition to involving duties of particular types, a vocation, and it is one of those vocations whose possessors deeply identify with. To fail as a captain, or—and more in line with the case—to *feel* that one has failed as a captain in such drastic ways is to leave a deep scar on the agent's life. Either option is permissible, but on either one, the agent is going to emerge deeply shaken to the core; whatever he does, his life is marred. So I do not think that virtue ethics has one answer to offer as *the* correct one.

But we should keep in mind to what extent this discussion is relevant to the issue at hand. The issue is virtue ethics' ability to accommodate partiality in morally justified ways, and surely the existence of irresolvable dilemmas does nothing to impugn the conclusion that virtue ethics does accommodate partiality but without neglecting justice, to put it somewhat mildly. The existence of such tragic cases *would* threaten the conclusion only on the assumptions that, first, care ethics gives a clear and uncontroversial answer to the case, and that, second, virtue ethics' answer must depart from that of care ethics. But neither assumption is warranted: care ethics does not give an uncontroversial answer to the case (if it gives one at all), and virtue ethics does not give one answer as *the* correct one, and so does not necessarily depart from the answer given by care ethics. Some of the cases I mentioned earlier involve making decisions that leave the agent with unease, but the answer to the cases were clear, and so they did not constitute irresolvable dilemmas (with the exception perhaps of the case of the car accident in which both one's spouse and the stranger are hurt; I say "perhaps" because, unlike the captain case, the nonspouse person is a stranger to the agent and such that the agent has no specific duties to him, such as those that a captain has to those under his care). In *these* cases, we can see how virtue ethics can balance partiality exhibited in caring and other requirements. But that virtue ethics refuses to say that there is one right answer to cases of irresolvable dilemmas is not a strike against it (indeed, it might be a point in its favor), nor is it a point against its ability to accommodate the concerns of care ethics.

There is one aspect of the partiality debate that I have not yet considered. Sometimes this aspect is stated in terms of universalizability, that is, that some moral actions are done towards particular others in particular situations, and so they need not be universalizable (Meyers 1987; Jaggar 1995). In short, this aspect of the partiality debate is concerned with the rejection of universalizability as a way of justifying actions. Noddings, for example, argues that since universalizability is parasitic on the notion of sameness of situations, and since sameness requires abstracting from the concrete situation, then universalizability is not a desirable justificatory criterion, given the importance that the particularity of the situation has for caring (1984, 84–85).

The issue as far as virtue ethics and care ethics are concerned is this: the former seems to be very much accommodating of universalizability. Or, to put the claim in a weaker way, virtue ethics *can* accommodate universalizability. Care ethics, however, seems to be not so accommodating. If so, then we have on our hands one crucial aspect of partiality on which virtue ethics and care ethics part company. But if this is correct, then it would seem that virtue ethics cannot incorporate care ethics successfully.

First, consider Noddings's argument against universalizability. This argument relies on an exaggerated sense of "sameness." If it means "identical in every respect," then Noddings is right, for no situation would be identical to another (they would at least differ in their temporal properties). But this is not the sense of "sameness" that is usually employed in such situations. The relevant sense is that of "moral similarity." What is crucial for universalizability is that the situations be sufficiently similar in the moral elements involved. In this sense, it is entirely possible that two situations be the same.[39] As George Sher (1987) has argued, surely in thinking contextually one cannot take *every* factor into account but must be selective. And this requires some amount of abstraction. Moreover, it is surely possible that those factors salient in some situation might also be the ones salient in another, and that if the agent's action in the first situation is permissible, then the same action by another in a similar situation would also be permissible.

Next, consider how virtue ethics accommodates universalizability, for it is important to see that it *can* retain universalizability despite its own emphasis on the particular, and it can do so via Aristotle's second condition for virtuous action (that the action be done *because* it is virtuous). The argument is simple in essence. When an agent performs an action *because* it is just, or temperate, or benevolent, the agent would be performing it for *moral* reasons. The virtuous agent, on most construals of virtue ethics, has practical wisdom. Practical wisdom is the faculty that enables the agent to discern what is right to do, given the circumstances. If all is going well, then the virtuous agent's action would be justified. Part of what this means is that any person, in sufficiently and relevantly similar circumstances ("sufficiently" is intended to be broad enough to cover simple and complex cases), would be justified in acting in the same way. And this, it seems to me, gives us the core and essential idea found in universalizability. For example, if in rescuing a child the virtuous agent acts for the reason that a child's life is at stake, then if another agent is faced with a similar situation, her action of saving the child would be justified (even if, by the way, the *latter* agent did it for nonmoral reasons). In short, universalizability is not generality, and hence its compatibility with particularity.

Moreover, even when the reasons for a virtuous action are agent-relative ("Because he is *my* friend"), the "my" is universalizable even though it makes essential reference to the agent: anyone who is in sufficiently similar circumstances can morally act for the same reason, namely, because so-and-so is one's friend. What cannot be universalized is the idea that a reason makes essential reference to a *specific* and particular agent. I mention this point—unoriginal though it may be—so as to highlight the idea that even if virtue ethics countenances agent-relative reasons, there is room for universalizability. This is important for care ethics' concerns, because much of the insistence on partiality connects in essential ways with agent-relative reasons: "Because she is my friend," "Because he is my brother," and "Because she is my child" are all examples of reasons offered for justifying certain actions. If everything else is equal, such reasons are universalizable. They are universalizable because—to borrow and slightly rephrase an argument given by Diane Jeske (2001)—when Matt acts out of concern for his friend Dana, Matt needs to take into account Dana's (subjective) reasons, traits, and/or goals. That Matt *needs* to do so, however, is not a subjective reason grounded in his desires. Rather, it is an objective reason grounded in the very intimacy and friendship that exists between him and Dana. In this sense, "Because Dana is my friend" presents or embodies an objective reason for Matt's actions towards her. But because such reasons are objective, they are in this sense universalizable, even if they embody terms such as "my friend." This, of course, does not entail that Matt should satisfy whatever Dana desires or wants, or that he should support whatever goal she has. For the issue here is not what particular actions Matt ought to undertake, but the general one of the universalizability of reasons stemming from caring relationships.

There are two more points that are important to mention. First, concerns with universalizability need not be explicit as far as the agent's reasons for action are concerned. In other words, the agent need not say to herself, "This action of mine is universalizable." Second, the universalizability test does not entail that in any particular set of circumstances there is *one and only one* right way to act. That there is only one right way to act is sometimes the case, as when one is in a position to rescue a child, or when one has made a promise to another, and there are no conflicts. But sometimes there could be more than one way to act correctly, and each of these ways is universalizable. For example, if a woman is strapped for cash, she may pass by a needy stranger asking for money and not give him any. Her action is certainly not vicious; indeed, it is right. Yet she may decide to give him some money, and in doing so she is acting virtuously, and hence also rightly. And it seems to me that either action is universalizable, because the reasons for either action are reasons that are morally relevant and connect in the right ways to whether someone may give money to the needy.[40]

Now it is true that I have not considered all the arguments that care ethics advocates might invoke against universalizability. But this does not seriously damage the claim that virtue ethics' incorporation of care ethics is successful. For given the importance of universalizability for consistency in action, and given that it is perfectly compatible with the particularity of the context of the action, there seems to be no good reason why care ethics advocates should be set against it. If so, then one worry about virtue ethics' success in incorporating care ethics is removed.

I have so far argued that (i) by construing care as an ethical virtue and incorporating it within the theoretical structure of virtue ethics we are able to preserve the desiderata of care ethics, while (ii) explaining how caring need not clash with the requirements of impartiality and universalizability. I have argued that virtue ethics preserves and emphasizes the social embeddedness of human beings, that it allocates a central role to friendships and family relationships, and that it gives the emotional component of caring actions the importance it deserves. I have also argued that virtue ethics is able to emphasize the importance of partiality in our moral lives so long as partial actions do not conflict with other moral demands, such as those of justice, and that this answer is what ought to be expected from a theory that calls itself "moral." What now needs to be explicitly addressed is whether virtue ethics can accommodate care ethics' claim that care is central to our moral lives.

4. Care as an Important Virtue

What does care, as a virtue, "look like," that is, in what ways does care fit our understanding of what a virtue is? And can virtue ethics offer care the status of an *important* virtue? Unless virtue ethics can do this, then it cannot plausibly accommodate the central concerns of care ethics, given that care ethics advocates have insisted on the importance of care to the ethical life. I will first start with the first issue, of what care as a virtue is, and then move on to the second, since discussing the former sets much of the stage for the discussion of the latter. Regarding the first issue, then, there are four central questions: What emotions motivate caring actions, and which ones does care exhibit? Is care a trait one needs to flourish, to live well, to be *eudaimon*? Does care make one a better human being *qua* human being? Does care fit at least some of the definitions of "virtue"? The first and fourth questions are connected to the nature of the virtues. The second and third questions are connected to ethical naturalism. In addressing them, I will be brief and programmatic, given the complexity of these issues. Specifically, in addressing the second and third questions, I rely on some general considerations about human beings, namely, that they are social and rational creatures, and these are considerations whose elaboration would require another book.

Virtues are dispositions not only to act rightly, but also to feel emotions correctly. Part of what this means is that a virtuous person would feel emotions and/or feelings "at the right times, about the right things, towards the right people, for the right end and in the right way" (Aristotle 1985, 1106b20–23 [see also 1109a28 and 1115b17]). Generosity, for example, is not simply desiring to spend money (and time) on whomever comes in one's way. It involves the desire to give money when the occasion calls for it (e.g., a loved one's birthday), because the occasion deserves it (e.g., birthdays are important events), because the person one is spending money on is worthy of it (e.g., it is one's child), because one's reasons for being generous are right (e.g., one wants to make the other happy, rather than wanting to be in the latter's good graces), and without being lavish (e.g., because one has limited means, because one does not want to spoil the child, or for both of these reasons).

Moreover, if generosity is the disposition to exhibit, correctly, the emotion of affection and/or of liking someone, if patience is the disposition to exhibit, correctly, the emotion of anger, if sexual temperance is the disposition to feel correctly sexual pleasure, and if (to give a fourth example) courage is the disposition to exhibit, correctly, the emotions of fear and confidence, what emotion does care, as a virtue, exhibit correctly? We should not, in answering this question, assume that every virtue *must* have an emotion around which it revolves and/or exhibits correctly. If Aristotle is our source, there is nothing in his views to indicate that he held such a strong position, and, indeed, it is obvious that some virtues, such as justice, respect, and pride need have no emotions attendant to them. What these virtues revolve around is correct *judgment*: in the case of justice, a judgment in regard to what is another's due; in the case of respect, a judgment in regard to the worth of another (or one's self, in the case of self-respect); and in the case of pride, a judgment in regard to one's achievements (or abilities, heritage, and so forth). And, to give one more example, "[T]he virtue of . . . magnificence, which is contrasted with vulgarity and pettiness, is a virtue which consists in correct *judgement*. The magnificent man judges correctly that the expense is worthy of the result and the result of the expense; the vulgar and the petty constantly get this judgement wrong" (Hursthouse 1999a, 106; emphasis in original).

But even with respect to virtues that revolve around an emotion, some virtues, such as courage and generosity, could have more than one emotion attendant to them. Moreover, since caring has often been associated with emotion, there is a strong presumption in favor of thinking that it is one of those virtues that *does* usually revolve around one or more emotions. Now, the difficulty in addressing this issue stems from the fact that "care" as a term is commonly used to refer to actions, attitudes, *and* emotions. Can one then simply state that the virtue of care exhibits correctly the emotions of caring? Not quite, because the claim is not very informative. We need to unpack it, and in order to do so, let us return to the two important components of care: motivational displacement and engrossment.

Engrossment is the tendency to be open to the cared-for, to accept him or her uncritically, and to be willing to be transformed by him or her. Motivational displacement is the willingness to adopt the cared-for's goals and to help promote them. What emotion or emotions of these aspects of care is exhibited and felt in virtuous action? It seems obvious, to me at least, that there is no single emotion that caring manifests (this, again, is not unique to caring; other virtues can exhibit a number of emotions: generosity can exhibit love, tenderness, and joy; and courage revolves around fear and confidence). Rather, the virtue of caring manifests a cluster of emotions, desires, and feelings, such as love, liking, sympathy, compassion, empathy, goodwill, kindness, openness, open-handedness, the desire to help another, and the desire to be with another. This claim, it seems to me, is inescapable given the variety of ways that caring can manifest itself in relationships and actions, and my only reason for it derives from such a variety.

It should also be obvious how each of these emotions can be manifested in inappropriate and appropriate ways. Care, of course, as explicated in this chapter, is a disposition to feel these emotions towards *particular others who are near and dear to us.* Furthermore, which emotion is exhibited and to what degree varies from one type of relationship to another. The desire, for example, to be with the cared-for might better fit caring exhibited in relationships between lovers and friends, rather than that between siblings (and this is a very rough generalization). Now, for care to be a virtue, care must partake in practical wisdom. Part of what this means is that, in conjunction with correct moral upbringing, the agent who is virtuous would be disposed to feel the above emotions at the right times, about the right things, towards the right people, for the right end, and in the right way. But in the case of care, the clause about the "right people" takes an interesting turn. For unlike courage, benevolence, justice, and other virtues, which can be directed at perfect strangers, caring is directed at those who are near and dear to us, usually those people we are in long-term relationships with. And part of what this entails is that exhibiting care towards them will be an essential part of the intimate relationships we have with them. More important, however, is the idea that "right person" does not just refer to someone we are intimate with, but to someone we are intimate with *and* who deserves to be the recipient of care, given our earlier discussion about the role of reason. If my friend turns irrevocably evil, then my friend is no longer the "right person." More controversially, if one's son turns or turns *out* to be evil, then the son is no longer the "right person," no matter how gut wrenching withholding care from him might be.

Of course, actual cases are not so extreme; most likely, most of us are neither fully virtuous nor are we in relationships with people who are fully virtuous. And this is, I believe, what makes caring for others so morally pregnant and interesting. We should also, in the light of the discussion of the regulative role of reason, understand "at the right time," "in the right way," "for the right end," and so forth as not requiring deliberation on every occasion of acting. These conditions would be satisfied once the relationship one is in has been given clearance, so to speak, by the virtuous agent's wisdom and moral commitments. And so, to give a few examples, one might care for wrong person *y* even though *y* is morally corrupt. One might care for *y* at the wrong time when one should, at that time, tend to other things, such as a stranger who is in need of immediate attention (the assumption is that *y* at that time does not require attention). One might care for *y* by promoting the wrong things, such as supporting a project of *y*'s that should not be supported. One might care for *y* for the wrong reasons by giving *y* gifts so that *y* can come to love one. And, finally, one might care for *y* in the wrong way by lying to *y* so that *y*'s fears can be calmed (the assumption is that honesty in this case is crucial). A virtuous person, armed with the virtue of care, would not, under normal circumstances, err in these ways.

Furthermore, even in the extreme case of a parent withholding care from her child because the latter is bad, she is likely to continue to feel the emotions associated with care for her child. This is neither a surprising fact nor a criticism of virtue ethics' approach to care. It might be thought a criticism because in the case of withholding care, the virtuous person— even the ideal one, the one possessing all the virtues to the highest degrees—should not feel the emotions associated with care. But we know that in many cases parents, lovers, friends, and siblings continue to feel kindness, love, and sympathy towards their children, ex-lovers, ex-friends, and siblings after they have withheld care from them. Surely it is implausible to claim that the former are not virtuous. How, then, can virtue ethics be a plausible approach to care?

This objection is unfair. If we are raised correctly, we will be sympathetic, compassionate, kind, and possess all of the emotions associated with caring. When we become parents, we will feel these emotions towards our children not only because we have been taught to have and feel these emotions, but *also* because we are parents, and parents feel these emotions towards their children. Furthermore, we raise our children in a caring manner, not only because to do so comes naturally, but also because we have no beliefs that tell us we shouldn't. We do not, for example, look at our babies and think that they are rotten and do not deserve care. If anything, we look at them and think that they are good, that they are innocent, and thus deserving of the best care. When, then, some of our children turn out to be bad, to be evil, after all the effort to make sure that they turned out good, and when we decide to withhold care from them because we have done all that we can and we can no longer support their ways, it is only expected that parents continue to feel the emotions associated with love and care for them (indeed, it might even be wrong to try to expunge these emotions, but I will leave this issue open). A virtuous mother would surely continue to feel such emotions, and this does not tell against her virtue, nor does this fact tell against virtue ethics. Virtuous people do not possess superhuman strengths, nor are they immune from the luck and tragedies of this world. They are human beings, with all the general frailties and strengths that come with this status.

I have focused on the parent-child example because it presents us with what is thought to be the strongest tie two human beings can have with one another. But much of what I have said applies to other intimate relationships as well. However, to what extent, for example, a lover or friend's continuing to feel positive emotions towards his ex-lover or ex-friend is a sign against his virtuousness will surely depend on the nature and length of his relationship with his ex-lover or ex-friend. It is perfectly compatible with being virtuous for the agent to continue to feel the emotions associated with care after she has withheld care from the one previously cared-for.

Let us now turn to the second and third questions.[41] If care is a virtue, then it should be a trait that one needs to flourish. This means that care would be both a trait that enables its possessor to live well and to be a good human being *qua* human being. The two are connected, of course. For part of what it means for a human being to live well is to be a good human being *qua* being human (if one were—objectively—living well, then this indicates that one is also satisfying the conditions for being a good human being *qua* being human). Conversely, part of what it is to be a good, nondefective human being is to flourish, be happy, and live well (if one were a nondefective human being, then this counts for one's living well). The first question, then, is: Does care enable its possessor to flourish, to live well, to be happy?

The answer is surely affirmative. Caring is essential to intimate relationships. First, we all enter this world as dependent creatures. We need our parents to support us, tend to us, and raise us properly, and these activities require a substantial amount of care. Without care, the likelihood that one will grow up to be morally and psychically damaged is high indeed. Can one plausibly be said to flourish if one, say, lacks affective responses due to lack of care? Can one plausibly be said to be living well if one is morally and psychically damaged? As *recipients* of care, then, care is crucial to the individual's flourishing.

Moreover, as *givers* of care, care is crucial to its possessors. If one is incapable or unwilling to care for others, be they friends, siblings, lovers, parents, and/or children, one is in effect incapable or unwilling to enter into intimate relationships, and it is hard to see how one can flourish without these. We need our friends, lovers, and family for support, to share our joys with, to trust, to engage in enjoyable activities with, and to, simply put, lead a rich life. Care also gives our lives meaning, and this allows an

individual to flourish in no uncertain terms. As David Hume once rhetor-
ically asked, "Destroy love and friendship; what remains in the world
worth accepting?"

There are two more points worth addressing. First, none of the above
remarks deny the possibility of flourishing without care. A hermit, for
example, could very well lead a flourishing life in a remote forest and without caring one jot for the animals and the trees around him. But this does
not impugn the discussion, because the discussion is about care as a *general* trait that people need to flourish. The examples of hermits do not
negate the claim that care is crucial for human beings to flourish any more
than examples of fat, lazy smokers who live up to a ripe old age and who
die of natural causes negate the claim that being healthy is crucial for living to a ripe old age (Hursthouse 1999b, 172–73).

Second, the discussion now is importantly different from the one in
section 2 above. In that section, the issue is whether care is a candidate for
being a virtue. The issue in the present section accepts the claim that care
is a candidate for being a virtue, but is concerned to see whether it can satisfy the two important conditions for a trait being a virtue (benefiting its
possessor and enabling her to be a good human being *qua* being human).
Part of what this means is that we are discussing care as shot through and
through with practical wisdom, not as a trait that can manifest itself
wrongly: towards the wrong people, at the wrong times, and so on. This
point can be clearly seen in terms of how we can handle a worry that Card
has about care as an ethical trait.[42] The worry she has is whether
Noddings's account of caring has anything ethical about it *if* it is understood in isolation from justice. That is, Card accepts the idea that caring
might have something good in it, but she wonders whether this goodness
is ethical if caring is divorced from justice.

The fact that Card agrees that caring has something good in it corresponds—if I understand her correctly—with the point discussed in section
2 that caring is plausibly thought of as a candidate for a virtue. What Card
wants to emphasize is that for caring to be ethical, it must be thought of
in connection with justice. She is right if her claim is simply that caring can
become disastrous (or simply bad) without some other mechanism or ethical concept to regulate it (such as justice), and this is the issue that is dealt
with in section 3.2 in this chapter. Now to construe care as a virtue is to
situate it among a host of other virtues one of which is justice and all of
which are tempered by practical wisdom. In this respect, Card's worry is
alleviated even further. For not only do we secure a sense of justice towards
those with whom we are not in intimate relations, but we also secure good
and successful caring by making sure (theoretically, of course) that care, as

a virtue, is a disposition to care for others *properly*. In this respect, to ask whether care is a virtue is to ask, not whether the tendency to look after intimates is a virtue, but whether the tendency to look after intimates, properly exhibited, is a virtue.

Finally, does care enable its possessor to be a good human being *qua* being human? Do human beings, in other words, need caring in order to live well as human beings? Consider the following thought. Human beings are not only social and political animals, they are social and political animals in a highly distinctive way: through and by being rational. Bees are, in a way, social animals, but bees are so nonrationally. (Indeed, the "in a way" is there precisely because using "social" to describe the life of bees is to extend the application of the word from the lives of rational creatures to those of nonrational ones.) We are rational social animals, and care is crucial for both of these aspects. First, without care we are not likely to grow to be social animals. This is not simply because we will not be involved in intimate relationships. These relationships, after all, do not capture all that goes into what is meant by "social." Rather, without care we are likely to grow to be affectless, morally and psychically damaged beings. And these defects prevent us from entering into *any* kind of social relationship, intimate or not.

As importantly, if not more so, is the issue of how lack of care affects our rationality. If MacIntyre is right, lack of adequate care to human infants exposes them to all sorts of dangers that can affect the healthy growth of their linguistic and mental capacities. The danger here is that human beings can grow to be defective human beings in that they will not have the capacity to be reasoners (1999, 71–79). If we do not have that capacity, we lose an essential trait that we have as human beings. Furthermore, rationality and sociality are necessarily connected: we do not, and even cannot, know what it means to be a human social animal that is somehow devoid of rationality. Any claim that asserts that *we*, human beings, can be social yet nonrational animals is simply nonsense. Care, then, is indeed a crucial trait needed for us to flourish *qua* human beings.

These remarks have focused mainly on human beings as recipients of care; as recipients of care, we need it to flourish *qua* being human. But as *givers* of care, care is just as important to our flourishing. Someone who is either incapable of giving care or not desirous of doing so is someone who is incapable or not desirous of forging, maintaining, and being in intimate relationships. Such a person, according to most psychological theories, is a paradigm example of someone who is a defective human being, defective not necessarily in a biological or physiological sense, but in a mental and rational sense (though of course the former and the latter might be connected causally).

Given that care satisfies the two necessary criteria for a trait being a virtue, then we have excellent reasons for thinking of care, understood as suffused with practical wisdom, as indeed a virtue. Further support for this claim is given in addressing the fourth question: Does care fit some of the definitions of "virtue"? I will stick with the two definitions offered in the introduction. Briefly, consider as a start Aristotle's definition, namely, that virtue is a state involving choice and lying in a mean, with the mean relative to the individual (1985, 1107a1–4). There is no difficulty in thinking of care as an actual state that would dispose the agent to act given the right circumstances. It also involves choice: barring unusual circumstances, the agent is not coerced to care for others; it is ultimately up to the agent to decide whether to withhold or offer care on a particular occasion. Most importantly, caring can admit of a mean, and we have seen what it means to care for the wrong person, at the wrong times, or for the wrong reasons.

Consider now Zagzebski's contemporary definition of "virtue": "a deep and enduring acquired excellence of a person, involving a characteristic motivation to produce a certain desired end and reliable success in bringing about that end" (1996, 137). Details aside, it is no violation of our understanding of caring to think of it as a deep trait of a person, or that it is enduring (a caring person is one who is liable to remain a caring one, everything else being equal). It is also easy enough to think of care as acquired: while we might have the capacity for caring, caring *properly* (virtuously) is a trait acquired by training and good upbringing. Caring can also be easily thought of as an excellence simply because it is a good trait to have. Furthermore, a caring person would be characteristically motivated to care for others, as we have seen, and would, typically, desire to produce a certain end. In general, the end of caring is, as we have seen, the well-being of the cared-for understood via the notions of engrossment and motivational displacement, and this general end can be attended to in myriad ways depending on the specific context: help *y* out, feed *y*, take *y* out for a walk, make *y* feel better, enjoy *y*'s company, and so forth. Lastly, the caring, virtuous person is not a stumbler: with the world hopefully cooperating, he would in general be successful in attaining the ends of his caring actions.

Thus, we have excellent reasons for the claim that care can be a virtue. The issue now is whether virtue ethics can offer care an important status. Otherwise, it would not be able to preserve one central insight of care ethics. For it to do so, it must be able to offer some plausible reasons that care is a crucial virtue for human beings, and it must be able to make plausible the idea that the virtues can be ranked in some sort of hierarchy of importance.

The considerations offered above in regard to the importance of care for human flourishing are sufficient, I believe, to render convincing the claim that care is indeed an important virtue. Furthermore, a glance at the list of Aristotle's virtues should tell us in no uncertain terms that not all the virtues on this list deserve equal ranking. The virtue of wittiness, for example, cannot be plausibly placed on equal footing with that of truthfulness as far as the importance of these virtues for social life and for the agent's flourishing are concerned. Wittiness might benefit its possessor by making her more likeable, for example, and it might very well make her a better human being insofar as its possession reflects a healthy and correct outlook on life. But it cannot seriously compete with caring, truthfulness, and justice. Friendliness, to consider another virtue, might be more important than wittiness, though it might not be more so than courage, and certainly not more so than justice. The point is that these virtues do allow us to offer some sort of rough ranking with respect to their importance. This ranking need not be precise and exact, and it need not be rigid and set in stone; we might be able to imagine cases in which, say, exercising wittiness is more important than being just, the difficulty of imagining such cases notwithstanding.

Virtue ethics is thus perfectly hospitable to the idea of ranking the virtues in terms of their importance. And this entails that, on the hypothesis that care is a virtue, we are at liberty to give it a tentative ranking among the virtues, provided we offer reasons to justify its assigned ranking. And the reasons for giving care a high status among the virtues are the ones already offered in this section, namely, that it is a trait one cannot generally do without if one is to flourish. Thus, not only is it plausible to think of care as a virtue, but it is plausible to think of it as an important one. Alongside justice, honesty, and proper pride, care would take its place as a virtue needed for living well.

5. Noddings and Slote on Care as a Virtue

Nel Noddings denies that care is a virtue (1984, 96). Michael Slote (1998a, *passim*; 2001, chs. 3, 4, and 5) avers that care is a virtue. Noddings claims that care is *the* basic ethical *concept*. Slote claims that care is not just one virtue among many others, but that it is *the* basic virtue. Noddings's claim was published before the criticisms (such as Card's) regarding the importance of justice were offered. Slote, however, is aware of these criticisms and attempts to make a case for his position that is sensitive to them. A critical look at these two accounts will help to support and clarify my own view. Beginning with Noddings, I will address what I take to be the arguments that support her position and will argue that they do not succeed. I will then turn to Slote's account and argue that his also is not convincing.

Noddings's remarks about the connections between care and virtue ethics are brief and somewhat enigmatic. She agrees that she is in part advocating an ethics of virtue (1984, 80), but claims that it is one's commitment to the ethical ideal as one-caring that gives rise to the virtues: "It is not, for example, patience itself that is a virtue but patience with respect to some infirmity of a particular cared-for or patience in instructing a concrete cared-for that is virtuous" (96). The idea here seems to be similar to Aristotle's early denial in the *Ethics* that a good life can be a life of inactive virtue. Aristotle claims that since one can have virtue and yet "be asleep or inactive throughout his life," virtue would be an incomplete account of what the end of the ethical life is (1985, 1096a). Similarly, Noddings seems to be saying that simply possessing virtue is not enough, and that one has to exercise virtue in concrete situations.

Upon closer inspection, however, we see that this is not exactly what Noddings has in mind. For she goes on to claim that we "must not reify virtues and turn our caring toward them. If we do this, our ethic turns inward and is even less useful than an ethic of principles, which at least remains indirectly in contact with the acts we are assessing. The fulfillment of virtue is both in me and in the other" (96–97). The idea *here* seems to be that if we claim that patience or any other trait traditionally dubbed as "virtue" is a virtue, then we somehow get saddled with paying too much attention to our own characters. We start to care for our own traits (hence the "inward" turning) rather than displaying these traits in concrete relationships with others. This is, by now, a usual worry often found in a typical objection to virtue ethics (e.g., in D. Solomon 1997), to the effect that virtue ethics encourages the virtuous agent to pay more attention to her character than to the moral demands of others.

Noddings's argument, then, seems to be the following: because the ethical ideal requires us to be ones-caring—because this is the highest ethical ideal—then any ethical view of the virtues must consider them as instrumental to this ideal. By "instrumental" I simply mean that the role played by the virtues in ethics is secondary; what plays the primary role is the concept of caring (and the concept of the ethical ideal). Patience is a virtue when it is exhibited with respect to some particular cared-for and as part of the agent's ideal of being one-caring. The same holds for the other virtues (although the virtue of justice here would be problematic). Furthermore, the thought seems to be that any view of the virtues that does not regard them as instrumental to the ethical ideal of caring is bound to be problematic since it yields a picture of an agent who is more attentive to his own character and traits than to particular others. What is crucial, then, is the claim that the virtues are secondary to caring, and that, when acted upon, they should be exhibited in caring relationships. This claim brings us back to the most basic issue in Noddings's ethics of care, namely, the claim that care is a primary ethical concept.

There are two reasons Noddings thinks that care is a primary ethical concept, and both work in conjunction with each other. The first is that she considers human beings to be ontologically constituted by relations with others. In this, she is close to Aristotle in his insistence on the social and political nature of human beings. To Noddings, we are not primarily autonomous beings who then choose to enter into relationships. Rather, we are born into relationships and our lives are shot through and through with them. We are, in short, relational beings. Furthermore, and still within the first reason, Noddings thinks of caring relations as ethically basic (1984, 3). They are more important than and prior to other kinds of ethical relationships. And this brings us to the second reason why caring is primary, namely, its innateness: "Ethical caring will be described as arising out of natural caring—that relation in which we respond as one-caring out of love or natural inclination. The relation of natural caring will be identified as the human condition that we, consciously or unconsciously, perceive as 'good.' It is that condition toward which we long and strive, and it is our longing for caring—to be in that special relation—that provides the motivation for us to be moral" (5). Later in her book, Noddings claims "that the impulse to act in behalf of the present other is itself innate. It lies latent in each of us, awaiting gradual development in a succession of caring relations. I am suggesting that our inclination toward and interest in morality derives from caring" (83).

Because we are constituted by relations, and because caring is innate to us, Noddings infers that caring provides the motivation and justification for ethical behavior, thought, and inquiry. Now there is much to be said for some of Noddings's claims. No doubt, caring is important for us in terms of survival and growing up to be healthy individuals. Caring is also innate to us, at least in the sense that we have the capacity for it, and, more importantly, its very innateness might provide a reason in its favor. Furthermore, Noddings might also be correct in claiming that we are ontologically relational beings. All of these claims might be true, and whatever is plausible in them goes a long way to account for the importance of care in our lives.

But they do not, individually or jointly, license the inference that our ethical ideal should be constituted solely by caring. For the fact that caring is a generally good thing to have, because—perhaps—of its innateness, does not entail that *every* caring relationship is a good one. As we have seen, depending on whom we care for, caring can be corrupted and can take morally undesirable forms. If so, then caring cannot be the sole ethical constituent of our ideal. Indeed, and as I have been stressing, one crucial advantage of thinking of care as a virtue, understood along the lines of neo-Aristotelian virtue ethics, is that it would have to partake in wisdom, much like any other virtue. In this way, we can preserve the intuitive and realistic distinction between virtuous caring and corrupt forms of caring, while also being perfectly comfortable admitting the general importance of care to us human beings.

We are then led to conclude that Noddings is wrong in thinking that *ethical* caring constitutes our ethical ideal. It is best to think of it as one virtue among many others that go into the making of a virtuous and ethical agent. However, Noddings explicitly rejects the claim that caring is a virtue (96). Her reasons for doing so, however, are not clear. My conjecture is that *because* she thinks of the virtues as being instrumental to the ethical ideal of caring, then caring itself is not a virtue. And *because* she thinks of caring as a basic, natural, and innate sentiment, whereas the other virtues are not, she withholds the label of "virtue." However, this is partially a matter of terminology and partially a matter of the issue of how primary care is as a concept. When one reads Noddings's discussion of actual care-taking, one cannot but be struck by the similarity to how we think virtues usually operate. The attention to detail in virtuous action, the narrative component found in ethical thinking, the importance of contextual factors in moral deliberation, and the primary role given to the presence of emotions are the hallmarks of Noddings's examples of caring action and thinking. It is for this main reason that I attribute to Noddings the claim that care is a virtue, despite the fact that she denies it.

Let us now turn to Slote's account. Slote (1998a) attempts to make the concept of care the sole foundation of a comprehensive, virtue-based moral view. If Slote's account is correct, then my own view that care is one virtue, albeit an important one, among others would be false. Hence, arguing that Slote is mistaken would further support my own position. Furthermore, Slote's mistakes are instructive: they warn us against the dangers lurking in handling the concept of care and in how we are to unpack it.

One of Slote's motivations for embarking on his attempt is his belief that care ethics can answer the charges that it is, on its own, deficient as far as comprising a comprehensive moral theory. This, we have seen (especially in light of Card's objection), is especially pertinent when it comes to issues of justice (Slote 1998a, 171; 2001, 93). For care ethics to answer these charges, it is best, according to Slote, to articulate it in a "virtue-ethical manner," specifically, as a form of virtue ethics that Slote calls "agent-basing." To Slote, care ethics evaluates actions in terms of how they exhibit caring motives, and so care ethics does not emphasize the consequences of actions. Insisting on the primacy of motives, Slote states that care ethics is a form of agent-based virtue ethics, which "treats motivation or motives as the ultimate basis for evaluating actions and, as we shall see, institutions, laws, and whole societies as well" (1998a, 173). This idea should not be surprising given agent-based virtue ethics: a virtue ethics is agent based if "its ethical characterizations of human actions are derivative from independent and fundamental aretaic characterizations of (the motivations, dispositions, character, or other inner traits of) agents" (1998a, 173). So the moral goodness or rightness of actions depends on whether these issue from good motives. Regarding care, the rightness of actions would depend on whether these express a "sufficiently" caring attitude on the part of the agent. In addition, and since the practical attitude of caring need not be grounded in other facts, such as the consequences of caring actions, Slote thinks that an ethic of caring can be a distinctive moral view that can stand on its own. As such, "it can regard caring as an overarching and ideal moral virtue whose status as such is intuitively plausible in its own right" (1998a, 173).

The crucial issue now is how Slote's conception of care ethics deals with justice. Slote states that the relationship between the laws, customs, and institutions (henceforth abbreviated as "laws") of a society and its members can be thought of as analogous to the relationship between an agent and his actions: "The laws, customs, and institutions of a given society are, as it were, the actions of that society—they exhibit or express the motives (though also the knowledge) of the social group in *something like* the way actions express an agent's motives (and knowledge), though in a more enduring manner that seems appropriate to the way societies typically outlast the individual agents in them" (1998a, 186; 2001, 99; emphasis in originals). And so on this view, the laws of a society are morally good and "positively and admirably just" if they express caring motives on the part of the lawmakers. They will be bad and "unjust" if they express "morally bad or deficient" motives (1998a, 186; 2001, 100). The reason for making such a claim is based on the idea that just as we are supposed to care for those individuals who are near and dear to us, we are supposed to "love and care" about our own country more than other countries. The idea is that as far as entities larger than individual people are concerned, "there can be moral requirements both of depth and breadth, and I propose to use this parallelism or similarity to move toward an account of the social virtue of justice that naturally complements the morality of caring" (1998a, 182).

So just as an individual, according to agent-based virtue ethics, is good if she has good motives, a society is morally good (just) if the motives of its people are good: "Thus . . . the justice of a society will depend on whether (enough of) its members have (motivation that is close enough to) the kind of motivation recommended by the caring ethic expanded or reconfigured so as to include concern for one's own and other countries along the lines indicated above" (1998a, 187; 2001, 101). In short, whether a society is socially just depends on the motives of those who enact its laws.

There are at least five basic problems with Slote's views. First, the form of virtue ethics as agent-based is implausible. Second, other than care, there is no use of virtue- and vice-related terms. Third, the concept of care employed is too broad. Fourth, and related to the third point, the concept of care used by Slote is packed with too many other concepts, to the point where one wonders whether it really is just the concept of care that is doing all the theoretical work. Fifth, the claim that a society is just if its members are caring is, simply, implausible. Since arguing that agent-based virtue ethics is implausible will consume too much space and is unnecessary for our purposes, and since the second point requires only a brief treatment, I will focus on the last three problems. But before turning to these, let me say this about the second point: it seems that any account that goes by the name of "virtue ethics" ought to make some essential room for the use of virtue- and vice-related terms. I am unsure how Slote will do this since on his account care is the most important concept we need in our moral theorizing. In this respect, I think that Slote needs to answer some questions about the role of other virtues in his account. And if other virtues play no essential role, then one wonders why even claim that his view is a "virtue-ethical" one. But rather than speculate about these questions and their possible answers, I will move on.

The third point is that Slote's concept of care is too broad. Slote does not confine himself to the use of the concept that is applicable to the relationships between intimates ("care *for* X"). He rather bases his account on the concept of caring *about*, and he frequently uses "concern" as a synonym. This shift from "caring for" to "caring about" should be treated cautiously since caring for intimates is very different from caring about abstract issues such as political causes, laws, and customs. Slote is aware of this shift and attempts to defend it: "This idea goes beyond Noddings's own *theory* or *conception* of caring, but the ordinary *concepts* of care and concern in fact allow us to speak of caring or concern about what happens to strangers and distant others. . . . In regard to anyone's relations with other people, we can distinguish between *depth* of concern or caring and *breadth* of concern and caring" (1998a, 180; emphasis in original).[43] Noddings focuses on the former, but Slote thinks that we can, and should, focus on the latter when it comes to larger social issues.

But this will not do. First, "caring about" does not involve those very aspects that some have found desirable about care ethics, namely, the contextuality, the particularity, and the psychological and emotional intimacy of caring relationships. While it might be coherent to use the notion of "caring about" as a basis for morality, one should not claim to be extending care ethics to social issues while *in effect* removing from the concept of care what has been thought essential to it, especially when doing so ushers in moral discrepancies. For example, partiality is crucial to Noddings's notion of care, but any attempt to extend partiality to "caring about" and then apply this latter concept to social issues such as justice would be disastrous. Second, even if the "ordinary" concept of care allows us to discern elements of depth and breadth within it, this does not mean that moving from "caring for" to "caring about" is not problematic, because ordinary concepts often disguise a number of different ones within them, and common usage of a word is simply not a reliable guide to how the concept ought to be used in philosophical settings.[44]

Related to the above problem of Slote's use of the concept of care is the fourth point mentioned above. The problem here is that using the concept of "caring about" might end up being simply a matter of nomenclature if the concept is going to be packed with too many others that do particular types of philosophical work. This can be easily seen in Slote's use of the concept. For instance, Slote discusses the possibility of legislators who work under self-deception: while their real motives in enacting laws are to pander to their political constituencies, they think they are working for the good of the country. Slote claims that they are deceiving themselves and ought to know better. If so, then they are not "really, or at the deepest level," concerned with the good of the public (1998a, 190). So now, apparently, "caring about" should be understood to include a dimension of self-knowledge required to avoid self-deception.

Continuing with the above case, Slote discusses the possibility that legislators are misinformed about what it takes to attend to the good of the public. To remedy this, Slote requires that genuine caring should include knowledge of relevant facts: "Thus, if legislators are *fully* concerned with

the public good . . . they will try to inform themselves before passing leg-
islation intended to benefit (the people of) the country" (1998a, 191;
2001, 105; my emphasis). So now genuine concern requires knowledge of
facts. But we have now opened the floodgates to what such a concept will
require if it is to do the work Slote wants it to. What if the legislators are
concerned with the public good, but because they are afraid of individuals
with political clout they pass laws appeasing the latter? Perhaps genuine
caring will now require the *courage* to act on one's concern. What if they
are genuinely concerned with issues about health, medicine, and education, but are too philosophically ignorant of the important distinctions and
other issues surrounding these fields? Will theoretical knowledge, or a certain amount of philosophical thinking, be required as part of the concept
of care? (This point, furthermore, does not embody a philosophically fancy
example. Just consider the current debates conducted by non-philoso-
phers—especially politicians—about such issues as cloning, euthanasia,
abortion, gay marriage, gays in the military, and just consider how their
views are sorely lacking in important distinctions that are the stuff of philosophical discussions.) What if the legislators are not disposed to be truth
tellers? Will honesty be a requirement of genuine caring? The point is not
that these requirements are outrageous to impose on a governing body
(they may be perfectly reasonable), but that without packing in other
virtues—ethical and intellectual—"caring about" is too impoverished to
do the work that Slote thinks it can. But if we enrich it in the ways just
described, then the concept loses its force and becomes—perhaps—simply
a shorthand term for what would be a more robust virtue ethics approach
to social issues about justice.

　　I am not denying that care, as a *virtue*, is inextricably linked with other
virtues (and this, of course, raises the issue of the unity of virtues). Caring,
for it to be successful and good, requires the assistance of a host of other
moral and intellectual virtues, such as honesty, courage, patience, generosity, trust, hope, and knowledge of the cared-for (to this effect,
Mayeroff's discussion of these connections is superb [1971, ch. 2]).
Furthermore, this reliance on and codependency with other virtues
exhibits, in a slightly different way, the role of practical wisdom in bringing a number of different virtues to bear upon a single course of action or
in mediating and coordinating these virtues. But this does not weaken the
force of the criticism against Slote, because it shows him to be clearly
guilty of running together concepts and features of caring and other
virtues that ought to be kept separate.

　　The last point regarding Slote's general proposal is that it is implausible to claim that a society is just if its members (or lawmakers) are caring.

Consider, for instance, how Slote handles the case in which the legislators are misinformed about facts and that, despite their best efforts, end up with unjust laws. Slote states that "our agent-based theory will (have to) say that the laws they pass as a result of being misinformed are, morally speaking, just, even if they turn out to have unfortunate results that are the very opposite of what the legislators intended" (1998a, 191; 2001, 106). Indeed, "if the society is just, if the legislators are duly elected, if they make their best efforts, and if the laws they pass reflect all those facts, then there is nothing morally to criticize about those laws, on an agent-based view, and I think this conclusion is fairly intuitive" (1998a, 191; 2001, 106). One can say here that Slote is not only biting the bullet, but a whole salvo of shells. Putting aside the problem of how Slote can call such a society "just" when it has laws that yield "unfortunate results," the claim that there is nothing morally to criticize is simply false. The fact that the laws have these results is enough to morally criticize them because they will, presumably, end up mistreating in one way or another a segment of society. It is simply not true to claim that the laws are just, even if *on agent-based virtue ethics* it might be intuitive that the laws are morally in the clear. Good motives are simply not sufficient for securing social justice. There is nothing, for example, to prevent legislators with good motives from instituting highly paternalistic laws that consistently violate the autonomy of individual citizens (didn't Plato propose this in the *Republic?*). They could have all the knowledge they need of facts and yet could subscribe to a theoretical view of what is good for human beings such that, out of good motives, they enact laws based on this theoretical view. Slote's program will simply not work on a number of fronts. Indeed, the problems that beset Slote's position are very similar to those that beset Noddings's for the simple reason that both Noddings and Slote want the concept of care to do too much. While care is an important disposition and virtue, it should not be burdened with work better left to other virtues and other moral concepts.

6. The Inadequacy of Alternative Approaches

Before concluding this chapter, I want to discuss briefly how my approach to the debate surrounding the status of care ethics in moral theory is better than other approaches offered in the literature. Specifically, virtue ethics avoids the shortcomings of other accounts that have been given regarding the relationship between care and justice reasoning.

So, for example, one account has it that these types of reasoning cannot be seen simultaneously in a given situation; they are like the duck-

rabbit gestalt switch: one sees the situation in terms of either care or justice (Gilligan 1987). But this is surely false. Not only is it conceptually possible to see one and the same situation in both terms, it is also
psychologically possible.[45] I can see attending to my spouse as a matter of
care while also seeing that I can infringe upon the injured stranger's
demand upon me to attend to him instead, given that both are injured and
I can attend to only one. Also, while I can see that care for my child to
attend school makes me entertain ideas of possible bribery, I can see that
doing so would violate just procedures. A virtuous person would not see
each of these situations as being simply one of justice or care, but would
see both elements and their moral weights.

Another approach to the connections between care and justice reasoning is that each has its own separate domain of application (Blum 1980,
1993). While this approach is tempting, especially in light of the remarks
that partiality and impartiality typically do not conflict, it should be
resisted because it is false that friendship and family relations are domains
in which the notions of fairness, justice, and duties do not arise.[46] As some
have argued (Annis 1987; Stocker 1987; Okin 1989; Friedman 1993, ch.
5), friends have duties to each other, and justice within the family is a
moral necessity. And although I have not discussed this issue in this chapter, virtue ethics can do justice to it. A virtuous person would be fair to her
children, for example, and would not treat them with favoritism (not
unless the case is special, for instance, if one of the children is evil, à la
Damien in *The Omen*). Also, while I might not be in the mood to help my
friend move his furniture to a new house (is anyone ever in the mood for
this?), I would still do so because he is my friend and has special claims
upon me. I am, of course, not claiming that considerations of justice are
all that enter into intimate relationships. After all, if the relationship
between two spouses is reduced to nothing but talk of justice, then this
would be a sign of real trouble between them. My claim is simply that such
considerations are necessary to intimate relationships but not exhaustive of
them.[47]

Indeed, although Aristotle claimed that "if people are friends, they
have no need of justice" (1985, 1155a27), this remark should not be
understood to mean that justice has no role to play within friendships.
(And, understanding *philia* broadly, we should not understand the remark
to mean that justice has no role to play in love affairs, loving marriages,
and sibling relationships.)[48] It should be understood, rather, to mean that
friends have no need to have recourse to principles of justice to settle issues
between them and to regulate their friendships. There are two reasons for
my claim. First, Aristotle had in mind here friends who are virtuous, and

this means that they would already possess the virtue of justice. This implies that they would not treat each other unjustly; that their just treatment of each other is taken for granted. Second, in the *Eudemian Ethics*, Aristotle explicitly states that those who treat each other unjustly cannot be friends and that "if one wishes to make men not wrong one another, one should make them friends, for genuine friends do not act unjustly," and he even concludes by stating that justice and friendship are "either the same or not far different" (1984, 1234b24–30). And all of this confirms my contention that Aristotle considered virtuous friends to be just to one another.

Finally, another approach is to simply claim that care ethics does not in any important way necessitate a re-visioning of traditional moral theory (Sher 1987). Thus, one can argue that no justice tradition has ever asked us to not take into account the moral complexity of the situation, that no such tradition has ever asked us to neglect the domain of the family and of friends, and that no such tradition has ever required us to act as calculating robots, with no emotive dimension to our actions. While I agree with this general reasoning, my worry is that some traditions have not given theoretical emphasis to care ethics' concerns, and I have tried to argue that virtue ethics does this in a unified moral framework. For example, while consequentialists might argue that caring relationships are conducive to overall better states of affairs, the theoretical priority is still given to the latter. Thus, caring actions would have to be considered instrumentally good. Virtue ethics, however, gives theoretical priority, via its emphasis on flourishing, to intimate and caring relationships.[49]

The fact that subsuming care ethics under virtue ethics is an approach to salvaging care that is superior to other approaches should not be surprising. Virtue ethics is a powerful theory that contains a rich array of virtue and vice terms. By subsuming care ethics under virtue ethics, we do not just supply the one-caring with wisdom as a regulative method with which she can scrutinize her relationships, nor do we just allow caring actions, in all their emotiveness, to be in harmony with virtuous reasons for actions, nor do we just fasten upon a theory—virtue ethics—that gives due importance to the role that caring plays in a flourishing life. We also imbed care, as a virtue, among a host of other virtues (and they need not be confined to those on Aristotle's list). With a suitable account of the unity of virtues, caring becomes part of a virtuous character that is courageous, kind, honest, sensitive, fair, temperate, friendly, proud, modest, self-respecting, dignified, and wise. With such richness, one wonders why so much ink has been spilled over the status of care in moral theory.

By way of conclusion, I would like to respond to one possible objection (an objection, I should add, that may be raised against the main conclusions of the next two chapters and so is worthy of attending to). It might be thought that the account I offer of care ethics' relationship to virtue ethics is not only too sketchy, but also—on some points at least—solves problems by waving them away. So, for example, one might object that I do not go into the nitty gritty of virtuous action, how it can be caring, and how it can preserve both acting for virtuous reasons and being emotive. Also, it might be thought that in dealing with the issue of warding off evil relationships, claiming that reason has a regulative role to play is simply waving away the problem (and calling reason "wisdom" won't do much to alleviate this worry). And, in dealing with the issue of partiality, the objection continues, I again wave away the problem by simply declaring that virtue ethics has an in-principled way of adjudicating between partiality and impartiality, and that the virtuous person's wisdom allows her to do this.

In one way, the objection is quite correct. I indeed do not enter into the nitty gritty of virtuous, caring action and how it is harmonious with emotion; I do not document a large number of cases of such actions, nor do I imagine them and offer them to the reader in rich detail. But the reason is simple: doing this is not part of my project, which is to locate a theoretical framework within which care ethics can be adequately housed. As is known, according to virtue ethics what counts as a virtuous action cannot be simply read off from a moral principle or codex; the virtuous response to a moral issue depends on the wisdom of the virtuous agent and the situation she faces. Thus, any discussion of how virtuous action operates in specific cases requires a discussion very different from mine. Moreover, I do not need to enter into such detailed discussion of cases, because my point is about what it would take to salvage care ethics.

However, the objection is, in another way, not correct. Calling a mechanism by which one regulates one's caring, intimate relationships "wisdom" is *not* waving the problem away. The word "wisdom" does not mean what "cleverness" or "deviousness" or "cunning" or "intelligence" means. Within virtue ethics, it has a more or less specific meaning, namely, the ability to plan and deliberate about one's life and actions within the constraints of what is moral, good, and right. Thus, to speak of having moral wisdom is not simply to hide behind a label. An agent who is virtuous has a much better method by which she can regulate her intimate relationships than an agent who lacks wisdom, and who is, say, happy-go-lucky, or morally indifferent, or stupid, or vicious. What I do not do is enter into detailed cases, and this might give the impression that my claims are superficial. But discussing detailed cases is not my aim. It is true that having wisdom and reason is no guarantee that one will not encounter misfortunes, that what one thought was a good relationship is actually nasty to the core. In this sense, wisdom can only do so much. But then again, nothing human can give us such guarantees.

2

Love

Romantic love has a very strong hold on our lives and thoughts. Much of popular culture concerns romantic love, from music to television shows to movies. Moreover, many people would agree that romantic love is an ideal that they aspire to. It is a commonplace that romantic love is very important to our lives, and that people who do not have it in their lives are somehow objects of pity. But despite this hold, the connections between romantic love and morality are often not clear. Some believe that somehow the claims of romantic love override the claims of morality. But others maintain that romantic love is itself somehow a moral notion. It is the task of this chapter to make sense and to organize these claims, especially in regards to two issues: the connection between romantic love and virtue, and the importance of romantic love to a well lived, flourishing life.

It is often customary in philosophical discussions of love to begin by doing two things: first, to note how thorny the topic of love is; second, and partly because of this thorniness, to delimit the topic of discussion in some way, usually by focusing on one type of love. I will not depart from this custom. A moment's reflection should reveal that love raises a plethora of conceptual and normative questions, such that the connections between them are difficult to trace and answers difficult to come by. Second, my focus in this chapter is on erotic love, often also called "romantic love," "passionate love," and even "personal love" (but see my note on terminology in the paragraph after the next), to be distinguished from other types of love such as parental love, friendship and sibling love, and universal love for humanity. *How* these are distinguished from each other is a matter of dispute. For example, some argue that what sets erotic love apart from the rest—Freudians notwithstanding—is the usual presence of sexual desire (see Newton-Smith 1989 and Martin 1996, 12). But other candidates are also offered, such as exclusivity, constancy, and desire

85

for reciprocation (on this, see, for example, Caraway, chs. 36 and 39, and Soble, ch. 38, all in Soble 1997b).[1]

Given the tremendous difficulties in defining "love," I will take the cowardly yet sagacious way out and not offer a definition. Suffice to say that the type of love I am speaking about is "the love that one person has for another person (usually not a blood relation); that may exist between two people when it is reciprocal (which is often, but not always, the case); that today often leads to marriage or cohabitation (but obviously need not); that often has a component of sexual desire (in varying degrees); and that, occasionally, for heterosexuals, eventuates in procreation" (Soble 1990, 2). It is characterized by the following—hopefully noncontroversial—features on the part of the lover (and vice versa): concern and care for the beloved, affection for the beloved, desire for the flourishing of the beloved for the beloved's own sake, and the desire for some type of commitment with the beloved (Newton-Smith 1989; Stafford 1977).[2]

Before continuing, a note on terminology is in order. What I quoted in the above paragraph from Soble is, strictly speaking, Soble's characterization of *personal*, not *romantic*, love. There is good reason for this distinction. For while the notion of romantic love might have strong connections to and affinities with personal love, it might also be characterized differently. For example, one can claim that unlike personal love, romantic love has its origins in the courtly tradition. This is a historical point. But one can also offer the conceptual point that romantic love is characterized by the fact that the lovers aim at union with each other, that it arises (and disappears) mysteriously, that it is ultimately selfish, and/or that the lover can fall in love with the beloved without having reasons for doing so. Insofar as these need not characterize personal love, then romantic love might very well diverge from the type of love under my inquiry. However, I will continue to the use the label "romantic love" to refer to the love I discuss here for one main reason. The label is commonly used among people to refer to the type of love under discussion. This is no accident, of course, because romantic love is indeed closely affiliated with other types of erotic love. Unless one is a professional philosopher, using other adjectives, such as "erotic," "personal," and "passionate" might be misleading. Furthermore, the features thought to set romantic love from other types of personal love are controversial, and I'll briefly discuss some of them in this chapter. Given that they are controversial, if it turns out that such features are indefensible, then romantic love becomes more and more similar to personal love. Because I do believe that these features are indeed indefensible, I do not hesitate to use "romantic love" to refer to what many would consider to be personal love.

My *primary* aim in this chapter is not to offer a conceptual analysis of the concept of love. A conceptual analysis of love, broadly construed, embodies a large number of issues, such as what types and varieties of love there are and how to distinguish them; whether love is essentially an emotion or something else (such as a desire, an attitude, or a virtue); how and in what ways love is different from other emotions—if it *is* an emotion, and if indeed it is different from other emotions; what essential features love has (Is it exclusive? constant? reciprocated?); how the beloved can be loved for himself despite the fact that the qualities on which the lover's love is based are found in others; and the connections between love, on the one hand, and sex, marriage, monogamy, and other related topics, on the other.

My primary aim, rather, is to address two normative questions. The first can be put as follows: What are the connections, if any, between romantic love and the virtues? We can be more specific and break the question into a number of more focused ones: Is romantic love a virtue, and how do we go about arguing whether it is or isn't? If romantic love is not a virtue, what is its relation to virtue? Is romantic love *structured* by the virtues? Or is it *enabled* by them? Or are romantic love and the virtues antagonistic, with the presence of one sitting in tension with the presence of the other? Notice that the very first question—whether romantic love is a virtue—is a conceptual one because it inquires into the nature of romantic love. This does not go against what I have claimed is my primary aim, however, since it is a necessary question that clears the ground for the other ones. My answers to these questions, roughly, are that romantic love is not a virtue, and that romantic love is not structured by the virtues but enabled by them. In this respect, romantic love is certainly not antagonistic to a life of virtue. These are the questions I will be addressing in the first three sections of this chapter.

In the first section, I examine the possible connections between romantic love and morality, concluding with the claim that romantic love is an essentially moral concept due to its reliance on the concept of concern or care for the well-being of the beloved. In the second section, I address the issue of the connections between romantic love and virtue. I argue against positions that claim that romantic love (i) is not an emotion, (ii) is (to be identified with) a desire, (iii) is structured by virtue, and (iv) is a virtue, concluding with the thesis that romantic love is enabled by the virtues. It is important, moreover, to note *why* I engage in these arguments. Because I believe that the popular opinion about romantic love being an emotion is basically correct, it is crucial that I argue against positions that conclude otherwise. Since the usual view about romantic love

is that it is an emotion, it is plausible that the onus of proof falls on anyone who wishes to argue otherwise. By arguing against such latter positions, and by stressing, while doing so, the similarity of romantic love to
other emotions, one is able to preserve the idea that the former is an emotion. Once this idea is preserved, one can go on to ask about the connections between romantic love and virtue. It is important for me to evaluate
in detail such positions in order to come to an accurate conclusion about
what romantic love is before we can look into its connection to virtue. In
this respect, I also want to defend the popular claim that morally good
romantic love is the love that issues from a morally good person (i.e., the
thesis that the virtues enable romantic love). Thus, romantic love is not
morally good simply in virtue of its being romantic love. In the third section, I develop the thesis that romantic love is morally good when it is
enabled by the virtues and defend it against two objections.

I address the second question of this chapter in the final section: How
necessary is romantic love to a flourishing life? This question does not ask
whether romantic love is a *basic* good or value without which one's life
would be deeply hampered. The answer to *this* question is clear: romantic
love is not a basic good or value, and so differs from basic goods such as
minimally decent health, liberty, and minimally decent economic means.
While these are necessary for a decent life, romantic love is not. Nor does
the question ask whether romantic love is intrinsically good or only instrumentally good. Perhaps romantic love *is* intrinsically good, yet it would not
follow from this that it would be indispensable to a flourishing life. There
are plenty of things in life that are intrinsically good, yet not all are necessary for a well-lived life (e.g., eating ice cream, watching a performance of
Swan Lake by the Bolshoi Ballet, etc.).[3] Rather, the question asks about the
dispensability of romantic love to a *well-lived* life. My conclusion is inspired
by Aristotle's views, namely, that what is essential for a flourishing life are
relationships characterized by intimacy, trust, closeness, and affection.
Romantic love will be necessary for a flourishing life insofar as it contains
these elements. However, it should be clear that romantic love construed
in this way is a species of friendship, differing from friendship in the
degrees to which it instantiates intimacy and the other factors in a relationship, and *these degrees* are contingent. So romantic love, as such, is not
necessary for a flourishing life, and when one claims that it is, one does so
because of socially contingent features that happen to emphasize romantic
love rather than friendship.

Before we begin, the reader should be aware that in this chapter I make
use of two important claims from the previous one. First, I rely on the concept of care, specifically, on the idea that romantic love is a concept that

essentially contains that of care. Second, I rely on the defense of the claim that friendships are necessary for a flourishing life.

1. Romantic Love and Morality

In this section, I discuss some of the connections that contemporary philosophers have discerned between romantic love and morality, and then mention a few things lacking in these accounts. I then argue that romantic love is not a virtue, first by arguing against some accounts offered in the literature on this issue, and then on more general grounds. Next, I will turn to the connections between romantic love and virtue.

1.1. Some Connections between Romantic Love and Morality

A number of contemporary philosophers have claimed that romantic love is importantly connected to morality. Others have claimed that, in one way or another, romantic love and morality are in tension. In some cases, the author does not espouse the claim, though the very logic of the position commits him to it. I will begin with such a position. Looking at a sample of these positions allows us to derive some important lessons about romantic love and morality.

Laurence Thomas (1991) argues that the event of falling in love does not admit of justification, but only of explanation, because the lover's reasons (explicit or implicit) for falling in love are not subject to rational assessment. John can love Eva for Eva's moral character, and Ellen can love Tim for Tim's beautiful eyes, and both John and Ellen are equally "rationally correct." Strictly speaking, Thomas does not deny that romantic love can be subject to moral evaluation, for he claims that sometimes the *object* of love can be morally inappropriate, as when a man falls in a love with a child (470). Moreover, sometimes the lover's explanations for falling in love can also be morally evaluated (472–73). To Thomas, then, "being justified" means the same thing—at least in the context of that particular essay—as being rationally correct (468); it does not mean "morally justified." On the face of it, then, Thomas's position does not seem to belong in this discussion.

But Thomas, I believe, is pushed to accept the claim that romantic love is indeed immune from moral evaluation. One reason is found in his comparison of romantic love with anger. He argues that whereas the former does not admit of rational correctness, the latter does. If John feels anger at Eva, then John "needs to tell a story which rationally justifies his anger—if at least he is to be seen as a reasonable individual" (468). Immediately, Thomas goes on to claim that this is different from morally evaluating the anger. The idea is that once a story is offered, we can *then* go on to morally evaluate the anger as being excessive, deficient, or appropriate (468–69). In other words, while telling a story is sufficient for meeting the requirement of rationality, it is not sufficient for meeting the requirement of moral assessment. This, however, is a very puzzling position for Thomas to hold, especially as far as romantic love is concerned. For if "rationality" here means simply "telling a story which justifies" the agent's emotion, then the same requirement can be as forcefully applied to romantic love. Typically, when one falls in love with another, if one persists in claiming that one does not know why one fell in love, we think something is amiss. We think either that one is simply not able to access one's reasons, or that—at worst—one is being—yes!—irrational. People who fall in love *do* give stories for why they fell in love. If this is what rationality amounts to, then romantic love is as rational as anger.

Thomas faces a serious dilemma. Either anger is rational simply in the sense that angry people are required to tell a story, or it is rational in the stronger sense that the anger needs to be morally justified. If the former, then romantic love is as rational as anger and people in love can be and are beholden to the very same rationality requirement. If the latter, then Thomas will have to take back his point that romantic love is subject to moral evaluation (and he shouldn't, because it *is* subject to moral evaluation). But the idea underlying my discussion of Thomas's position is that "telling a story" is too weak a requirement when we speak of justified anger (as Thomas does). Indeed, when we speak of justified emotions, we mean emotions that are appropriately felt, given the occasion, and this is what Thomas *should* mean by it. But if so, then romantic love is just as susceptible to such justification. Hence, Thomas's claim that romantic love is not rationally justified comes awfully close to the claim that it is not subject to moral evaluation.

But there is a major reason why Thomas, given his reasoning, is pushed to divorce romantic love from moral evaluation. The reason is found in Thomas's claim that what differentiates anger from romantic love is that the former is "conceptually tied" to beliefs, whereas the latter is "tied" (the word "conceptual" does not appear here) to a "desirous feeling to interact with a person in a certain way" (470). Thomas understands romantic love as being essentially based in desires rather than beliefs: the desires to engage in "mutual caring, sharing, and physical expression with the individual in question" (470). The problem here is that desires, at least the desires found in romantic love, are typically tied to beliefs. I say "typically" and not "conceptually" because I want to leave room for the possibility of cases in which John feels merely (and magically?) pulled to be with Eva, to kiss her, to hold her hand, and so forth. But these cases are rare enough. Typically, one's desires to "care, share, and physically express" with one's beloved are strongly tied to beliefs to the effect, say, that the beloved is gorgeous, that she is a brilliant conversationalist, that she is a "man" of letters, and so on. And once we see this, then we see not only that romantic love is subject to rational evaluation, but also that it is subject to moral evaluation. If we go Thomas's way, then, given the strong connections between desires and beliefs, not only must we chuck the rationality of romantic love, we must also do away with its moral justifiability or unjustifiability. In short, Thomas's position that romantic love is not rationally justified, in conjunction with his understanding of romantic love, if correct, strongly supports the conclusion that romantic love is also immune from moral assessment. As will shortly be obvious, this is a starkly wrong conclusion.[4]

Unlike Thomas's position that happily though somewhat incoherently allows for connections between romantic love and morality, Robert Ehman's view sets romantic love in opposition to morality.[5] According to Ehman, this opposition, moreover, is not accidental or due to contingent factors; it is rather due to the very natures of romantic love and of morality. For on the one hand, the former is exclusive: "The fundamental requirement of love is to raise the beloved above others and to give her a privileged status in our life so long as she retains the personal style of life which serves as the ground of our love for her" (1989, 260). Morality, on the other hand, requires us to treat everyone equally. Hence, there is a necessary conflict between the two. Indeed, the conflict is also severe. Ehman claims that from the point of view of romantic love, the demands of others count for nothing (260), and this is because romantic love cares nothing for fairness and principles: "it singles out an individual for special concern simply on the basis of her personality and of the delight we take in being close to her" (260).[6]

But the conflict between romantic love and morality is not just seen in terms of what these two *require*, but also in terms of what they *aim* at. According to Ehman, the aim of romantic love "is achieved when the lovers retreat by themselves to a personal world apart from the world of everyday social and moral life" (265). Morality, however, is "in principle" opposed to such a retreat to a personal, private world given its aim to constitute a "common social world in which each person is recognized as being of intrinsically equal worth and treated in a manner valid for anyone in the same circumstances" (265). Hence, we get another necessary tension between romantic love and morality.

Ehman, I fear, has gotten the picture of the relationship between morality and romantic love wrong. To put it in a more cautious way, Ehman offers a simplistic and so highly controversial picture of this relationship. It might be correct to claim that in romantic love "the beloved has a value for the lover above that of others and that the lover regards his relation to his beloved as more important than his other relationships" (256).[7] But this entails neither that the lover also does not recognize the requirements of morality nor that he should not. The claim that Eva is the most valuable thing in John's life is fully compatible with the claim that John recognizes that he might have to act in ways contrary to his love for Eva if morality so requires, and with the claim that John should do so, given the circumstances. This is not, of course, to deny that there easily could be cases of tension between the claims of romantic love and those of morality. Newton-Smith puts the point nicely. He does not accept the claim that "in 'true' love, commitment to the beloved must take preference over all other commitments," but that "in the case of love there are these tensions, and this displays the extent to which love involves a commitment" (1989, 205–6).

From the other side, one can argue that morality does leave room for partiality and for a retreat to a personal world. This claim is not to be understood along the lines that our lives are divided between heeding the demands of morality, on the one hand, and frolicking and loving freely in a nonmoral space, on the other. Rather, the claim is that morality allows us a space within which we can love, care, and tend to particular others. The arguments here are the same ones from the last chapter regarding the partiality of caring. Given the importance of intimate others in life, morality allows for a good measure of partiality. The point is not that there is *no* conflict between romantic love and morality. Rather, it is that the conflict is contingent, not necessary. It surfaces in particular cases such as when our duties to others and to our loved ones directly clash, when we find ourselves in dilemmas, whether resolvable or not, and when we are tempted to violate justice (or the greatest good) in order to preferentially treat our loved ones.

The conflict, as I stated, is not necessary. The demands of romantic love conceptually leave room for morality, and vice versa. For even if we accept Ehman's claim that the fundamental conceptual requirement of romantic love is to raise one person above the rest, this requirement does not entail that we do so at any cost. In other words, the demand of the requirement can be fulfilled without necessarily violating the dictates of morality. As for his reason that romantic love cares nothing for principle and fairness, it is false. Strictly speaking, romantic love is not the kind of thing that cares or does not care. It is lovers who fit this type of description. And whether a lover cares about fairness or not has nothing to do with the fact that she is a lover, and everything to do with whether she is virtuous or not. In general, a virtuous person would not, and need not, jettison the requirements of morality, while a vicious person would (but much would depend here on the particular vicious person). If morality allows for a measure of personal freedom and partiality, then we can see that the conflict is not necessary but simply contingent.

It is difficult to find in contemporary moral philosophy ethical theories that so starkly deny the claims of romantic love, as Ehman seems to think (his essay, however, was originally written before such current accommodations of partiality by moral theories). Kantian ethics leaves much room for the personal and the partial, as long as it is subject to general requirements of duty. Virtue ethics, of course, leaves room for friendship and love in the agent's life. Common-sense morality certainly leaves room for partiality (indeed, with a vengeance, if Michael Slote [1992] is right). Not even consequentialism—the theory which has been most criticized as far as the issue of partiality and favoring loved ones is concerned—need require its agents to act with an eye to treating everyone equally. Indeed, it might allow for the idea that agents treat loved ones with the usual favoritism on the grounds that this is the best way to maximize good states of affairs in the long run.[8] So the requirement that Ehman attributes to morality must be taken very cautiously, keeping in mind which theory we are talking about and at which level we are doing so, that is, whether we discuss that theory at the level of its foundations, at the level of its assessment of actions, or at the level of what it tells us is required of agents in their actual thinking, motives, and behavior.

1.2. Romantic Love as a Moral Concept

In this section, I will argue that because the concept of romantic love includes the notions of care for the welfare, the well-being, and the happiness of the beloved, the concept of romantic love is essentially a moral concept. Moreover, the concern and care that I have in mind are robust; that is, they are not ultimately selfish. This is not to say that all the instances of romantic love are morally good (after all, romantic love can be bad), but that the concept of romantic love is not a morally neutral concept.

The preceding discussion brings up the issue of the grounds on which morality can justify romantic love. In section 2 in the previous chapter, I appealed to Aristotle in justifying friendship: without friends, it is difficult for one's life to flourish and prosper. Can we plausibly apply this to romantic love also? It seems not. For romantic love does not seem to be *merely* a species of friendship, though it has strong affinities to it. Lovers often put their beloveds before their friends; lovers spend a lot more time with each other than with friends; they often live together, sleep together, eat together, and engage in a lot more activities together. An Aristotelian might consider romantic love to be a form of friendship with sexual activity added to it, given Aristotle's requirement that friends live together. I will return to this issue below. For now, it is important to note that *we* think of romantic love and friendship as being different from each other not only in degrees, but also conceptually and morally. We might think, for example, that romantic love conceptually requires passion and exclusivity, whereas friendship does not. We might think that, morally speaking, beloveds come before friends and that our emotional reactions to the death, betrayals, sicknesses, and so forth of beloveds are, and should be, stronger than those of friends. Furthermore, while romantic love might not be a basic value, it is hard to claim that friendship also is not one. Whether these claims are true is not the issue. The issue is that they do reflect our prevalent beliefs, and thus indicate that romantic love might not be simply a form of friendship. If so, romantic love cannot be morally justified in the same ways that friendship is.

But this argument is not valid. For from the fact that romantic love and friendship are importantly, and even essentially, different it does not follow that their moral justifications must be different. If, for instance, romantic love and friendship play the same basic roles in human life, then, and despite the differences in their concepts and in some of their moral dimensions, the same type of justification might do as well for each. Suppose, then, we make the following plausible claims. First, romantic love is a more or less universal human phenomenon, meaning that any one can experience it. Second, romantic love is not inherently antimoral or immoral. It is true that lovers often commit immoral acts in the name of and/or because of romantic love, but this is not inherent to the nature of love (below, I will address an argument, however, that concludes that romantic love poses a serious threat to morality). Third, lovers, precisely because romantic love is different from friendship in important ways, provide the kind of support and opportunities for sharing that friendship does not; friends who are not also lovers rarely cuddle, sleep next to each other, or accompany each other through life's daily trips and journeys; lovers do. *If* this is so, then the intimacy found in romantic love is much stronger and more prevalent than that found in friendship. And this indicates that romantic love contributes to the prosperity of life in basically the same ways that friendship does, but in stronger, deeper, and more pervasive ways.

The first two claims shift the burden of proof to those who want to deny that romantic love is morally justified. It becomes their problem, so to speak, to show why it should not be morally justified, or, at the very least, why there are serious obstacles to justify romantic love morally. The third claim, however, assimilates romantic love to friendship in terms of the *roles* both play in a human life, and adds that romantic love performs this role in deeper ways than does friendship. So if the justification offered for friendship in the first chapter is plausible, it should even be more plausible when offered on behalf of romantic love. We need not, then, worry too much about how morality allows for romantic love.[9]

However, the connections between romantic love and morality can be, and are, much stronger than simply that morality leaves room for romantic love. We can begin to see this by noting the importance of care (or concern) to romantic love. In section 2 of the previous chapter, I claimed that a romantic love without care (or minimal care) is not really a love at all. If the lover has no concern for the well-being and flourishing of the beloved, it is hard to see how he can justifiably claim to *love* his beloved. Alan Soble, using the example of Humbert Humbert from *Lolita*, claims that we can agree that Humbert is enchanted with Lolita or that he desires her sexually, but that it is much harder to agree that he loves her. The reason is simple: he is insensitive to her flourishing (1990, 257). In Raymond Carver's "What We Talk About When We Talk About Love," a short story structurally and thematically similar to Plato's *Symposium* (though not without some elements of parody), Terri tells us of her ex-boyfriend, Ed, who loved her so much that he tried to kill her: "He beat me up one night. He dragged me around the living room by my ankles. He kept saying, 'I love you, I love you, you bitch.' He went on dragging me around the living room. My head kept knocking on things." (1989, 138). Mel, Terri's current boyfriend, denies that this is love. He thinks that in the love *he* is talking about one does not go about trying to kill one's beloved. But Terri insists that Ed loved her. Whether it is Terri or Mel who is right is a matter that cannot be settled without more information. Terri might be right if Ed's beating her were an isolated incident. This is not to justify his behavior, of course, but to make the point that love can tolerate a few incidents that are incompatible with the flourishing of the beloved (excuse the banality, but human beings are complex entities; they sometimes intentionally do destructive things, both to the ones they love and to themselves). However, if Ed's behavior is recurrent, then Mel would be right. Subjecting Terri to conditions under which she might be killed or maimed is sufficient, though not necessary, to render Ed uncaring about Terri's flourishing. And if Ed does not care about *that*, then he does not love her.

We have seen what caring must essentially include in the previous chapter. What needs to be emphasized is that this caring is not selfish; the lover does not care for the beloved simply to get something in return. Furthermore, the caring must leave room for the lover to sometimes sacrifice his good for the sake of the good of the beloved. And, in tandem with the discussion in section 1 of the previous chapter, the care is not just for the good of the beloved as the beloved sees her good, but must be for the good of the beloved objectively. If the lover tended to the good of the beloved only as the latter sees it, this opens the possibility that the beloved is mistaken. If she is mistaken, then what she sees as good might be actually bad for her. So if the lover were to promote that apparent good, even though he realizes it is not actually a good for the beloved, this would not be consistent with claiming that the lover is concerned for the *flourishing* of the beloved. No doubt, there must be a balance struck, for heeding the beloved's wishes is also respecting her autonomy, and her autonomy is crucial to her flourishing. I will not go into the intricacies of defending and elaborating these claims.[10] The point that I wish to make, rather, is that if we agree that concern or care for the flourishing, well-being, and good (and I am using these interchangeably) of the beloved is intrinsic to the very idea of romantic love, then the concept of romantic love will turn out to be an inherently normative and moral concept. Not only do the demands of romantic love and morality not necessarily conflict, but the concept of romantic love necessarily relies on some basic moral concepts.

Because this conclusion underlies much of what I have to say below, and because it is essential for the ensuing arguments and discussion, it needs to be strengthened further. This can be done by way of a reply to a possible and important objection. My treatment of it will be somewhat brief, since it has been adequately addressed in the literature (Soble 1990, ch. 12). Nevertheless, because the objection is a famous and an important one, it needs to be attended to. The objection can be dubbed the "realist objection," and it goes as follows. Romantic love is not really a type of love at all, because, at best, it does not involve an interesting or nontrivial type of concern towards the beloved, or because, at worst, it does not involve any such concern. The underlying idea is that romantic lovers are simply motivated by egoistic concerns, and hence the so-called concern for each other is not morally interesting in any morally important sense.[11]

The objection derives strength from two observations. First, in romantic love, the lover falls in love with the beloved based on certain preferential concerns. In other words, because the beloved's properties, such as wit, dry humor, sarcasm, and pessimism, meet the needs of the lover, or, at the very least, delight the lover, the lover "chooses" the beloved, from a large number of other people. But since the lover fastens upon *this* beloved because *this* beloved suits the needs and the temperament of the former, romantic love is egoistically motivated. John loves Eva because Eva meets John's general "needs." While one does not need to be an advocate of *agapic* love to raise this observation, the observation can nevertheless be highlighted by comparing romantic love to *agapic* love. In the latter type of love, one loves another not because of any specific properties that the beloved has, but simply because the beloved is, say, a human being. And this is in stark contrast with romantic love.

Second, the objection can be further strengthened by pointing out that, typically, when a (romantic) lover desires that the beloved flourish, and when he or she desires that the beloved be well off, the lover is not simply concerned that the beloved's well-being be attended to by just anyone. Rather, the lover desires that *he* (or she), be the one to attend to the beloved's well-being. Consider a simple example that also reflects a very prevalent type of case. Sarah (romantically) loves, and is in a relationship with, Mona. Mona likes sex a lot, and Sarah wants Mona to be happy and sexually satisfied. Yet Sarah bristles at the thought of someone other than herself giving Mona sexual pleasure. *She* wants to be the one giving Mona sexual pleasure and so make her happy. It is observations such as this one that give strength to the objection. Such observations seem to indicate that romantic lovers are indeed egoistically motivated, and if this is so, then the type of concern in romantic love is not morally important. Lovers are concerned for the welfare of their beloveds because, ultimately, it satisfies their owns needs and egos.

If this objection is plausible enough, then my view that the concept of romantic love is essentially a moral concept would be implausible, to say the least. Thus, the objection needs to be addressed. I will do so in two ways, the second of which is more decisive. The first way of responding to the objection goes as follows: the objection does not square with an important fact about how many lovers behave, which is that they are often willing to make huge sacrifices for each other. Of course, there are lovers who are egoistical in the sense intended by the objection (Humbert Humbert is one example). But not all lovers are like this. Oftentimes, a lover is willing to sacrifice her life to preserve the life of her beloved. A lover is willing to relocate to another geographical place and to another job for the sake of her beloved. This indicates in a straightforward manner that lovers are willing to make, and do make, important sacrifices for the sake of their beloveds, and this does not seem to be egoism.[12] Of course, an advocate of the objection can reply that ultimately such sacrifices bring the lover pleasure or contentment. Indeed, even in the case in which a lover sacrifices her life, the reply would be that were the lover not to do so, she would not be able to "live with herself." So ultimately such sacrifices are egoistical.

This response is not convincing, however, because it assumes that being satisfied with one's actions is a form of morally bad egoism. But does one really want to claim that when a parent makes sacrifices for the sake of his children, he is egoistically motivated, at least in a morally pernicious way? At the very least, one cannot simply assert this claim, which seems to go against what we observe. But then why make an exception in the case of romantic lovers? This brings me to the second response to the objection. Briefly, the objection seems to ride roughshod over an important distinction, namely, that between selfishness and self-interest. At best, what the objection shows is that romantic lovers are motivated by self-interest. What it does not show, however, is that they are motivated by selfishness. While selfishness, almost by definition, is morally bad, self-interestedness is not, or, at the very least, need not be. Selfish people ignore the goods and interests of others in pursuit of their own goods and interests. At best, selfish people take the goods and interests of others into account only as a way to promote their own goods and interests. But one can pursue one's own goods and interests without ignoring those of others. And one can pursue the interests and goods of others, as an end, because this is what one is committed to do. Not doing so would make one unhappy, and perhaps feeling shame. This is a form of self-interest. Yet it is a far cry from selfishness. That romantic love can, and does, make people happy is perhaps a given. That we are interested in being happy is also a given. But that our interest in and pursuit of happiness is morally problematic is not a given. And it is this last point that the objection needs to convince us of. John loves Eva because, as the commonplace goes, "Eva makes him happy." But that John's desire to be happy is, as such, incompatible with robust concern for Eva, and so morally problematic, remains to be argued for. Hence, the objection is not convincing. If so, then the claim that the concept of romantic love is essentially tied to that of concern for the flourishing of the beloved is not shown to be in danger of being morally trivial. If so, then the claim that the concept of romantic love is essentially moral in an interesting and robust sense is certainly highly plausible.

However, it is important to show how self-interest can be, not only morally permissible, but also morally good. Since I will be here relying on—and somewhat simplifying—an argument given by Neera Badhwar (1993), I will be brief. Typically, when we think of egoistic acts, we think of them as acts that are calculated to bring about not very wholesome moral ends, such as money, pleasure, and fame. However, first, people are often interested in maintaining other important goods, such as their integrity, their commitments, and their ideals. Second, people need not act in a calculating manner to maintain such goods (indeed, maintaining these is at odds with calculating the effects of one's actions). Rather, oftentimes people's actions are an expression of such goods. If these two claims are correct, then we achieve something important, namely, dislodging the picture of the self-interested act as being necessarily morally suspect. But now consider someone who is morally good or virtuous. Such a person has moral commitments and ends, such that, acting on these commitments is an expression of who she is as a person and of her integrity, her desire to see to it that she maintains her virtue and her sense of self. When faced, for example, with a situation in which others need help, especially at some risk to her, she would help them. Not doing so would not only go against what her goodness impels her to do, but would also result in feelings of shame and guilt. She would help the people because she is interested in maintaining her moral self. What motivates her to act is the plight of the people, and her desire to help is an expression of her commitment to and her desire to maintain her moral self. If this is correct, then we can see how a self-interested act can be not only morally permissible, but morally good. If so, then we would have given one strong consideration to show that self-interest and robust concern for the welfare of others not only need not be incompatible, but often work in tandem.

One might object, however, that the example I have chosen in the above paragraph is ill suited for romantic love. After all, it might be true that self-interest and morality need not conflict in some case (for example, helping strangers), but this does not show that this is also true of the concern found in romantic love. The idea is that because in romantic love the lover falls in love because of particular traits that the beloved has and that the former finds desirable, this ushers in the possibility that the concern in romantic love does not fit the morally good type of self-interested action. The reason is that what would motivate the concern for the beloved would be ultimately a form of selfishness: x is concerned for y because y's properties make x happy or satisfied, and this concern seems to be instrumental, and not robust.

Perhaps some romantic lovers are like that. But the above argument cannot be true of all lovers. For if one were a good and virtuous person in general, then it is implausible to claim that when it comes to the area of romantic love, suddenly this virtuous person's commitments to the beloved take on the selfish guise. That in romantic love (and in friendship) we associate with certain people rather than with others is a given. But that this shows that a person's concern is ultimately selfish is certainly not a given. For instance, a good person would be moved by the sufferings of others. But he would also be moved by the suffering of his beloved. Why the latter must be a form of selfishness requires further argument, if it is conceded that the former is not selfish. In other words, the claim that one can show genuine compassion to strangers and yet selfish compassion to his beloved is very implausible and thus requires defense. And any such defense must take into account the fact that accusations of selfishness do not typically fit the descriptions of romantic lovers who care for their beloveds. Moreover, we associate with specific people because these people make us happy, comfortable, satisfied, and joyful to be alive. But this is not, as such, selfishness. If everyone who desired to be happy were selfish, then we certainly would have an entirely new meaning of "selfishness" on our hands. Thus, preference for others is not, as such, a form of selfishness.

While the above is sufficient to dispose of the first observation in support of the realist objection, it does not seem to be sufficient to dispose of the second observation, namely, that it is the *lovers* who want to be the ones to secure the happiness of their beloveds. Contrast this with the example of helping others. If I were to see a stranger drowning, I would not—unless I had a warped sense of myself or an ulterior motive (for example, a desire for a reward)—feel jealous or angry were I to step aside and allow a more efficient swimmer to save the drowning person. This is the case because when helping strangers, we have their good primarily in mind, and not so much who safeguards or promotes that good. Granted, Eva's romantically loving John because he makes her happy need not be a form of egoism. Yet the issue remains that Eva wants to be the one to promote John's welfare and happiness and does not want others to do so.

There are two points to make here. First, the second observation needs to be handled carefully. For it is not true to claim that lovers desire to be the source of every avenue that leads to the happiness and welfare of their beloveds. If John works, then Eva would be extremely psychologically troubled were she to feel upset that *she* is not the one who pays John his monthly salary. Lovers are rarely upset or jealous if they find their beloveds laughing at jokes told by someone else, or if they find that their beloveds like to play sports or, indeed, engage in many sorts of activities with people other than themselves. This indicates that lovers tend to be upset about not being the source of their beloved's welfare and happiness in some, and not all, areas, such as sexual pleasure, the amount of time spent with the beloved, and being the primary, or one primary, object of affection of the beloved. This, I think, shows that when one is confronted with the second observation as a way to argue for the egoism of romantic love, one must be careful to attend to those specific areas in which lovers especially feel upset or jealous when they are not the source of the happiness of their beloveds.

I will not address such areas specifically. I will, however, offer the following suggestion (this is my second point): the areas in which lovers feel especially desirous of being the source of their beloveds' happiness seem to be directly related to the very love between them. Sexual activity and sexual pleasure, intimacy, the amount of time spent together, and other such areas are the core of a successful romantic love relationship. If so, then when lovers feel upset that they are not the sources of their beloveds' happiness that comes from such activities, they may be morally justified. For this might threaten *their* (the lovers') happiness and welfare, in as much as such happiness and welfare are invested in their love relationships. And their happiness is not, as we have seen, as such a matter of selfishness or egoism, but a matter of self-interest. Moreover, this form of self-interest is morally good. As Jean Hampton rightly observes (1993), part of what goes into the notion of self-respect is that the agent has a good and healthy sense of what he needs to flourish, both as a human being as such and as the particular person that the agent is. Included in the latter are the agent's plans, goals, and commitments. And one primary example of these is the agent's decision and/or desire to not only prefer one person to be in love with, but to also decide to maintain his relationship with that person. Thus, because Eva decides and chooses to maintain her relationship with John, because this choice is an expression of Eva's autonomy, and because some areas in her relationship with John require that *she* be the one to tend to John's needs, Eva's desire and decision to tend to these needs are an expression of Eva's autonomy and sense of what she needs to flourish as the particular person that she is. Thus, the desire by the lover to tend to the needs and desires of the beloved need not be a form of egoism. It might be a form of morally good self-interest. Needless to say, this desire must be subject to moral constraints. Moreover, some forms of jealousy or protectiveness are either simply inappropriate or excessive, and such instances can be morally evaluated case by case. But this does not show that lovers' concern for the sources of their beloveds' happiness and well-being are always morally unjustified because they are egoistical. So we can safely put the realist objection to the side.

There are two important points to keep in mind at this juncture. First, that the concept of romantic love necessarily contains that of care or concern does not mean that the care we are speaking of is the *virtue* of care, because, as we have seen from the last chapter, care as a virtue requires the participation of practical wisdom and the cooperation with other virtues. But one could love another, and so care for him, in all sorts of unvirtuous and corrupt ways. This brings me to the second point. To say that romantic love is necessarily a moral concept does not entail that love can never be bad. I am not, in other words, understanding "romantic love" in such a way that bad love is ruled out by fiat. The reason is that the care for the beloved can manifest all sorts of defects: it can be, to give a few examples of its failings, twisted, psychotic, irrational, ignorant, irresponsible, and/or suffocating. To say that romantic love essentially embodies a moral dimension is simply to say that when we claim that Ellen loves Tim, we are essentially—though not exhaustively, of course—claiming that Ellen is concerned for Tim's welfare and good. And this says *nothing*, on its own, about whether Ellen's concern is manifested in good ways or in defective ones.

The preceding two points and the claim that romantic love is essentially a moral concept can be further illustrated by taking a brief look at Irving Singer's position. Doing so also allows us to see that the issues here can be very tricky. Singer guardedly agrees that care is essential to romantic love, but goes on to claim that in romantic love the lover nevertheless need not act the way morality requires:

> It is almost impossible to imagine someone bestowing value without caring about the other person's welfare. To that extent, love implies benevolence. And yet the lover does not act benevolently for the sake of doing the right thing. . . . If we offer help, we do so because *he* wants to be better than he is, not because *we* think he ought to be. Love and morality need not diverge, but they often do. For love is not *inherently* moral. There is no guarantee that it will bestow value properly, at the right time, in the right way. (1984, vol.1, 11; italics in original)

First, Singer claims that insofar as love is the bestowal of value—the thesis at the heart of Singer's characterization of romantic love—it relies necessarily on the notion of care, and this implies that the concept of love necessarily has a moral dimension. Second, Singer claims that it is possible and even frequent (love and morality "often" diverge) that when the lover tends to the welfare of his beloved, he need not be acting morally. This is because the lover would be acting in order to fulfill the *desires* of his beloved, not because he *ought* to. This illustrates the point of how love can go morally bad, because the assumption seems to be that acting morally requires acting in the way one does because this is what morality demands on that occasion. In other words, one's reasons for action must be moral reasons. But here we have to be careful. What Singer is after, I believe, is the worry that if the lover were to act towards the beloved because he *ought* to, then he would be acting out of duty or some other moral reason, rather than out of affection and love. This, it seems, is the explanation that Singer gives to account for how lovers need not act morally. But this might not be true if it turns out that morality need not require that one's reasons for action must be moral ones in every case of morally good actions. In other words, if one can act morally and yet do so out of love-related reasons, then Singer's explanation would not be exhaustive. In the next section, I will examine an argument that concludes that romantic love is not a virtue based on an account similar to the one Singer gives. For now, suffice it to say that this explanation is misguided.

I have examined some contemporary philosophical positions on the connections between romantic love and morality primarily in order to derive a few lessons that help pave the way for the discussion of romantic love and virtue.[13] One important lesson is this: how we understand romantic love is crucial in shaping our position on the connections to morality. This can be tricky. In the case of Thomas, Thomas thinks he is able to preserve the connections, but, as I have tried to show, the logic of his position impels him to sever these connections. In the case of Ehman, Ehman's distorted understanding of romantic love and morality leads him to falsely put the two in necessary opposition to each other. With Soble and common sense, we have reached the conclusion that romantic love is essentially a moral concept in its reliance on the notion of care for the flourishing of the beloved. And herein lies the second, more important lesson: the concept of romantic love, because of its embodiment of that of care or concern, will turn out to be dependent on a large number of other moral concepts. When we speak of romantic love and its successes and failures, a crucial and essential dimension will be a moral one. In the next section, I will begin investigating this claim by turning to the connections between romantic love and virtue.

2. Romantic Love Is Not a Virtue

My main aim in this section is to defend the view that romantic love is an emotion and not a virtue. Moreover, I will argue for the latter claim—that

romantic love is not a virtue—indirectly by defending the usual view that
romantic love is an emotion. Since emotions are not virtues, it follows that
romantic love is not a virtue. I will also argue for it directly, by arguing
that, first, romantic love does not fit the definition of "virtue" and that,
second, it does not satisfy the criteria for a trait's being a virtue. It is important to note that the argument that romantic love is an emotion does not
only serve to establish the claim that romantic love is not a virtue. It also
helps strengthen and clarify the claim, discussed further below, that the
virtues enable romantic love.

Most contemporary philosophers writing on romantic love deny that it
is a virtue, either explicitly or by implication. Alan Soble (1990) accepts the
claim that romantic love is an emotion, and so by implication—though
Soble himself does not state this—denies that it is a virtue, perhaps because
of the plausible and prevalent claim that virtues and emotions are not identical. Mike Martin (1996) claims that romantic love is an attitude, and so
claims, explicitly, that it is not a virtue (given the plausible claims that
virtues are not attitudes). O. H. Green (1997) argues that romantic love is
a desire, and this implies that it is not a virtue.[14] Philip Pettit (1997) explicitly denies that romantic love is a virtue. I will first attend to Pettit's argument (the one that I alluded to above in connection with Singer's
explanation as to how acting in love because one *ought* diverges from the
requirements of romantic love). I will argue that, while its conclusion is
true, the argument is itself defective but that its defects are nevertheless
instructive. I will then go on to argue that romantic love is not a virtue. I
do so first, indirectly, by defending the position that it is an emotion and
by arguing against the positions that it is a desire and an attitude, and second, directly, by arguing that it neither fits the definition of "virtue" nor
satisfies the criteria of what a virtue is. My position, basically, is that romantic love is not a virtue because it is an emotion, not because it is a desire or
an attitude. This position relies on the view that virtues are not identical
with dispositions, emotions, desires, or attitudes.

2.1. Romantic Love Is Not a Virtue: Pettit's Argument

Pettit's argument has a simple form. It offers a picture of what the structure of virtue is, claims that romantic love does not exhibit that structure,
and so concludes that romantic love is not a virtue. Consider fairness and
kindness, two examples of virtues which Pettit offers. We may readily
explain an agent's action by saying that she did it because it is fair: "the fact
that someone believes that the option is fair will serve to explain the choice,

to the extent that we think the person is fair and we expect fair people to
be moved by that sort of belief" (154). Kindness is a bit more complicated,
according to Pettit, in that the agent's belief that an action is kind will not
explain the agent's choice to act in that way were we to think her kind:
"For we expect kind people to be moved, at least in most cases, not by the
belief that this or that option is kind—that is too reflexive for comfort—
but rather by the belief it has those features that happen—and the agent
need not be aware of this—to ensure that it is kind" (154). Notice how
justification and explanation come apart: the justification of the action lies
in the fact that the action is kind. Its explanation, however, lies in the fact
that the agent is kind and in our belief that kind agents are moved by the
belief that the option has such and such features, features that in the right
context make the choice a kind one (154).

Acting out of romantic love, however, does not exhibit this structure
of explanation, according to Pettit. That Beth loves Julie may justify Beth's
action towards Julie. We might be tempted to explain an agent's action as
being done out of romantic love because, like kindness, it involves sensitivity to features that make the act a loving one. But, according to Pettit,
we should resist this temptation: "Someone may be sensitive to features
that make acts loving in relation to someone, not because of being truly in
love, but rather because of being committed to behaving in a loving way:
not because of a lover's commitment, as we might put it, but rather
because of a commitment to love" (155). A kind person is committed to
kindness; she will notice kindness-related features of a situation because of
this commitment. If we were to transfer this reasoning to romantic love,
we would have to say that the lover notices love-related features because
of her commitment to love. But this turns the lover into someone who is
committed to an ideal, or a value, or a concept, rather than to the beloved
(155).

How, then, *do* we explain a lover's loving actions towards the beloved?
It is, simply, the fact of loving her: "Thus my loving someone will be naturally invoked to explain my keeping note of her birthday, my giving readily of my time to help her, and perhaps my sharing all that I have with her.
The idea is that loving the person makes those responses easy and even
compelling. . . . To act out of love, as we might put it, is to be moved by
love and not by the recognition of being in love" (155–56). What has the
same structure as that of virtues such as fairness and kindness is the commitment to love, not the lover's commitment to her beloved.

Despite its ingenuity, the argument is not convincing. It is not convincing for one simple reason: if accepted, it turns many actual lovers into
shams; in other words, it does not fit with lovers' actual experiences. First,

it is not *that* implausible to think of lovers as being committed to love. This need not entail that their behavior is done out of some duty to the notion of love or out of some love principle. Rather, it might simply entail that, when in love, they want to monitor their behavior to make sure that they are not acting selfishly, insensitively, unkindly, and so forth towards their beloved. There is nothing bizarre or rare about such a phenomenon, either. The agent need not have a bad character to think along these lines and to attend to his actions in this reflective manner. Indeed, any love that is not attended to is liable to become defective. The point is that it is false to place a person's commitment to romantic love in opposition to his acting out of love in the way that Pettit thinks real lovers usually do. The former entails only a *general* attention to one's loving actions and attitudes and not a motive to act out of a duty to love or an adherence to some principle that tells Beth that she ought to love Julie.

Second, it is not strange to claim that lovers can be sensitive to features of the situation. Consider a kind agent K who performs a kind action A. According to Pettit, we explain K's action by saying that K is moved by the belief that her choice to do A is due to the features of the situation, which, in that context, make A a kind action (without K necessarily thinking that A is a kind action). But suppose we ask K why she did A. Suppose she answers by giving us one or more of the following answers (the list, of course, is just a sample): "It will ease its pain" ("its" refers to, say, a lion which has a thorn in its paw), "Doing this will help her move on with her life," "Because this will allow him to finish his work without having to worry about those other things," "It will give her much pleasure." Now I admit that these answers might serve as justifications for K's action. But they also serve as explanations as to why K did what she did, and they all appeal, implicitly or explicitly, directly or indirectly, to features of the situation.

Suppose now we ask a lover, Beth, why she did B, where B is an action performed for her beloved and done out of love. Suppose Beth were to give us one or more of the following list of answers: "Because it's her birthday," "Because she likes lemon pie," "It will make her happy," "Because she is feeling down," "She will get such a kick out of it!" "Because she is busy and this will allow her to focus on her work." Will anyone believe that such answers detract from the lover's commitment to her beloved? Most lovers offer such explanations for their actions towards their beloveds, and people have no difficulty in accepting them. Yet they all embody references, explicitly or implicitly, directly or indirectly, to features of the situation, which, in the context, make the action one of romantic love. Indeed, one wonders how an act can be truly loving if the lover were somehow to act without heeding the features of a situation.

In this respect, a lover is liable to notice and to be moved by features of the situation that, in the context, make the action one of romantic love. It seems simply false to claim that if a lover were to be moved by considerations such as these then he is committed to love rather than to his beloved. A kind person would undertake steps to comfort person *y* were he to perceive that *y* is in pain. He need not, as Pettit rightly observes, say to himself, "This calls for kindness," or "I should be kind," but he would notice the feature—pain in *y*, for example—that would motivate his kind action. Let *y* now be the agent's beloved, and keep the pain and the desire to comfort as part of the case. Is there anything amiss in the lover's noticing the pain of *y* and being motivated to ease it? Surely not. In this regard, Pettit's claim that "someone may be sensitive to features that make acts loving in relation to someone . . . because of being committed to behaving in a loving way" is true only if the sensitivity ranges over not just the features, but also the consciousness that one's act is loving. But this cannot be what Pettit means, because if it is, then the case would not be parallel to that of kindness, and Pettit's denial of that parallelism would not go through.

Otherwise, his statement is, on an obvious reading, false. A lover may be sensitive to features of the situation without having to be committed to an image of himself as a lover. And even if the lover—as I said above—is committed to love, this commitment need not be operative in every case of action. It might simply be a background evaluational standard to which he appeals every now and then in reviewing his life with *y* and his love for her.

There is then no good reason to believe that romantic love is not a virtue on the grounds adduced by Pettit. Acting out of romantic love may exhibit the same type of structure as acting out of kindness, and, because of this, we have a reason to think that romantic love is, after all, a virtue. The general lesson we can nevertheless derive from the discussion of Pettit's argument is this: any attempt to argue that romantic love is not a virtue grounded in the difference we want to impose on (or find in) *actions* done out of romantic love and between ones we want to impose on actions done out of virtue are bound to face severe difficulties. The reason is simple: actions done out of romantic love can be accommodated within a general Aristotelian account of virtue, as we have seen in the discussion of care and Aristotle's conditions of acting virtuously. What the conditions of virtuous action require is the subjection of one's life and actions to a *general* scrutiny of reason, and this does not entail that every action must be deliberated, or that every action must be done under a description employing sophisticated moral concepts. In this respect, it would be difficult to show that loving actions cannot conform to such a picture. One can do so only if one offered an implausible account of loving actions, such as an account that would require that no action (or that very few actions) done out of love is deliberated, or done under the knowledge that it is a loving action; or an account which required that all or most loving actions be spontaneous, or impulsive, or washed over with emotion, and so on. But the reasons why such accounts are implausible are, I take it, obvious.[15]

In summary, while it might be true that romantic love is not a virtue, Pettit's reasons for this claim are the wrong ones. Let us turn next to an argument that concludes that romantic love is a desire. By rejecting this argument, we help to get closer to the claim that romantic love is an emotion.

2.2. Romantic Love Is a Desire: Green's Arguments

How can we go about finding out whether romantic love is or is not a virtue? Here is a seemingly simple way: given the commonsense view that romantic love is an emotion, and given that virtues are not emotions (virtues are dispositions to exhibit emotions and actions correctly), we can easily infer that romantic love is not a virtue. This way is, as I said, seemingly simple. If there are good reasons to think that romantic love is *not* an emotion, then we cannot assert so straightforwardly that it is not a virtue. I will examine two arguments, both given by O. H. Green, to the effect that romantic love is not an emotion. I will argue that the arguments are not successful and so, because his arguments are part of a general way of thinking about romantic love, we have no good reasons to claim that romantic love is not an emotion.[16] While this conclusion takes us one step further in the direction of asserting that it is not a virtue, it also helps in making the case that romantic love is an emotion by warding off arguments (Green's) that it is not an emotion, which, in turn, helps to clarify and strengthen the claim that the virtues enable romantic love. I mention this so as to respond to the possible worry that a discussion of Green's arguments is unnecessary. The worry is that since Green concludes that romantic love is a set of desires, and since virtues are not to be identified with desires, then Green's conclusion does not threaten the claim that romantic love is not a virtue. But, like I said, a discussion of Green's arguments helps support the claim that romantic love is an emotion.

Both of Green's arguments are simple in structure. The first is that for something to be an emotion, it is necessary that it be based in beliefs. Since romantic love is not always based in beliefs, then it is *not always* an emotion. His second argument is that even in those cases when we are tempted to think that romantic love is an emotion, we are mistaken because, unlike emotions, beliefs and desires are never sufficient for romantic love. Let us consider these arguments in some detail.

The first argument relies on two crucial premises, namely, that beliefs are necessary for emotions, and that romantic love can be belief-less, that is, that beliefs are not necessary for romantic love. The evidence, however, which Green offers in support of the claim that romantic love need not be based in beliefs is flimsy at best. He states that "Common enough is the case of the girl . . . [who] sings, 'I love him because he's . . . I don't know . . . because he's just my Bill.'" (1997, 211). That is, what is common, according to Green, are cases in which lovers have no beliefs that provide reasons for loving the beloved. But what is weak about this support is not only that Green uses *one* case and confidently tells us that other cases like it are common; but that the support is not really support at all. Supposedly, Green's premise asserts that romantic love need not be based in beliefs. Thus, we need plausible cases of romantic love in which it is not based in beliefs. But what we are offered instead is a case in which the *lover* is either *unable* to find reasons for loving her Bill or has not looked into herself deeply enough to find those reasons. But that lovers are sometimes (and commonly enough, to satisfy Green's intuition) unable to give reasons for their love or have not introspected deeply enough for these reasons does not entail that romantic love is not based in beliefs. This epistemic veil does not entail an ontological love not based in beliefs.

But perhaps we should not make too much of this. Perhaps we should grant Green the premise that some romantic loves are not based in beliefs. After all, it is just as difficult to argue for the opposite claim. That is, it is as difficult to argue that, conceptually or logically, romantic love is belief-based; that there are no, nor could there be, cases in which Leo loves Dan, yet Leo's love is not based on beliefs having to do with Dan's properties or attractions, as Green puts it (211). So we can admit of the possibility of non-belief-based romantic love. Still, what remains troubling is Green's insistence on the first premise, namely, that emotions are necessarily belief-based. He defends this claim by arguing that without it, it is difficult to see how we can make sense of the idea that emotions can be assessed for their rationality and irrationality, that is, that without beliefs it is hard to see how an emotion can be rational or irrational.[17] For example, if one were to claim that my fear of all snakes is irrational, then one would have to attribute to me some belief or other to the effect that I believe that all snakes are fatally dangerous. Without such a belief, it is hard to see how one can evaluate my fear as being irrational. Green, moreover, defends the claim that all emotions are belief-based on other grounds, namely, by appealing to our intuitions regarding the difficulty of explaining how one can feel an emotion without the requisite beliefs.

It seems, however, that Green's first premise is not true. Consider, for example, a case of someone who is thoroughly familiar with snakes, their types, their species, and so forth, and yet nevertheless feels fear when a snake is near him or slithers around his feet, even if he knows that that particular snake is harmless because he knows what type it is and so what it can and cannot do to him by way of harm. Or consider someone who is gripped by fear and cannot sleep every time he watches *The Exorcist*. He need not believe in God or Catholicism, let alone demon possessions. Surely these are plausible cases of emotions that occur without their possessor having the requisite beliefs (that snakes are dangerous or that this snake is going to bite me; that demon possessions occur frequently enough or that there is a good chance I will be possessed by a demon fairly soon, and so on).

Green can always respond by arguing that the person experiencing the emotion has the requisite beliefs, but that these beliefs are hidden, or are unconscious, or are implicit. Or Green can respond that the above two cases mischaracterize the psychological states of their agents. What these agents are feeling are not emotions, but something else, like moods. But neither of these two responses is convincing. Consider the second: the agents in both examples phenomenologically feel what it usually feels like to be in fear. They exhibit the usual range of reactions that are typical of fear. And if asked what they are feeling, they would respond with, "Fear." Furthermore, and unlike moods, which are usually characterized as having no objects, the two agents' psychological states in the two examples do have objects, namely, snakes and demon-possessed girls.

The first possible response by Green is also not convincing. Other than trying to save the view that *all* emotions are belief-based, what reason can one offer to the effect that we know that these beliefs are there somewhere in the person's mind? Perhaps what is correct about the idea behind Green's view is that emotions are necessarily *cognitive*. But to claim this is not to claim that they necessarily involve *beliefs*.[18] All that they need involve are *thoughts* or images about their object, without necessarily having such thoughts be beliefs. In this respect, one can experience an emotion, tell us plausibly that it is fear, and yet have no beliefs to the effect that the object of the emotion is dangerous. If the object is associated in the person's mind, for example, with fearful experiences, then the person might very well experience fear. Consider a more specific example involving the emotion of revulsion. Suppose that Steve had dinner at a restaurant one night, and that, because something was wrong with the food or with him (or a combination of both), Steve stayed up all night throwing up. The night was, by all measures, miserable for Steve. As a result, Steve simply cannot bring himself to eat at that restaurant again. Even though he has been told that the place is clean, that the chef has been replaced, and so on, and even though Steve believes these claims to be true, he nevertheless feels revulsion at the mere idea of going to that restaurant. His emotion is not based on any beliefs or propositions, but simply on cognitive images of the place, images the content of which is taken up by the agent. The upshot is that not all cases of emotions need involve beliefs; perhaps they all need to involve cognition and/or images of some sort (they are not raw feelings). And if we keep this in mind, then romantic love will not be anomalous in this respect. Surely romantic love is cognitive in the weak sense that the lover's emotion involves thoughts about her beloved.

However, one can ask, "What exactly is the difference between beliefs and thoughts?" The answer, in the words of Noel Carroll, is that "to have a belief is to entertain a proposition assertively; to have a thought is to entertain it nonassertively. Both beliefs and thoughts have propositional content. But with thoughts the content is merely entertained without commitment to its being the case; to have a belief is to be committed to the truth of the proposition" (1990, 80). In the snake example, I entertain the proposition that snakes are dangerous, but I am not committed to believing that snakes are dangerous. Thus, emotions need not contain beliefs. All they might contain are thoughts. That Green has beliefs in mind, and not *also* thoughts, is evident from his argument that without beliefs we cannot assess the rationality of emotions, because were he to include thoughts within the class of objects to which "belief" refers, he would not have insisted on the requirement of rationality. For once we bring thoughts into the picture, the question of the rationality of emotions cannot be raised in every case of having an emotion. Consider the snake example again. I believe that snakes are not dangerous, yet I fear snakes due to my thoughts about them. Is this fear rational or irrational? On the one hand, and because of my belief that snakes are not dangerous, my fear seems to be not irrational, for it does not rely on a false belief. Yet its rationality does not exactly shine, either, precisely because of my belief that they are not dangerous. The point here is that once we allow for thoughts to be constitutive of emotions, the rationality of emotions is not as clear cut an issue. Because Green does not raise this question, this indicates that he did not include thoughts within his view of beliefs. And if this is so, then his claim about the necessity of beliefs for emotions is false.

But we are not out of the thicket yet, because Green has another argument whose conclusion is that romantic love is not an emotion. Recall that the conclusion of his first argument is that romantic love *need not* be belief-based, and this leaves room for the possibility that some cases of romantic love are, and could be, belief-based. What Green's second argument is designed to do is to, if not eliminate it, put this possibility into serious doubt. Green argues that in general both beliefs *and desires* are "required" for emotion. For example, "If *A* . . . is glad that *p*, [then] *A* believes that *p* and *A* desires that *p*; and if *A* is sorry that *p*, [then] *A* believes that *p* and *A* desires that not-*p*" (214). Notice Green's wording: these claims, in addition to his use of "required," are stated in such a way as to indicate that being glad and being sorry are sufficient for the beliefs and the desires, and that beliefs and desires are necessary for the emotion. But notice how he continues with romantic love: "Suppose that *A* believes that *B* is beautiful and *A* wants to be with *B*. There is so far no emotion which *A* has in virtue of his belief and desire" (214). But this way of putting it is in terms of the *sufficiency* of beliefs and desires for emotion, not their necessity. What Green should have said is this: "If *A* loves *B*, then *A* believes that *B* is so-and-so and *A* desires to such-and-such with *B*." But had he put it this way, there would be nothing implausible about it. After all, he is discussing a case of romantic love based in beliefs, and so we would expect *A* to have beliefs about his beloved. As to desiring *B*, surely a lover would have some such kind of desires. And even if he were not discussing a case of romantic love involving beliefs, there is nothing implausible about the claim that *A*'s love for *B* entails beliefs about and desires for *B* on behalf of *A*.

Perhaps then Green's claim is in terms of the sufficiency of beliefs and desires: if *A* believes that *p* and desires that *p*, then *A* is glad that *p*.[19] When it comes to romantic love, Green's claim would be much more plausible than the one about necessity of beliefs and desires. For if *A* believes that *p* (about *B*) and desires *B*, then it does not follow that *A* loves *B*; *A* could be only sexually desiring *B*. Indeed, *A* could even *hate* *B*, given the appropriate background story. This argument, however, is convincing only when pitched at the general level at which Green pitches it. To see this, consider someone, Adam, who is, say, at a party and who forms the belief that he was insulted by Janet (whether Janet insulted him or not is irrelevant; what is relevant are Adam's beliefs and desires). Suppose that Adam, being morally healthy, desires not to be insulted. Given the belief that he has been insulted and his desire not to, what emotion should Adam feel? Anger? Sorrow? Sadness? Despair? Frustration? Embarrassment? Surely we need to know more about Adam to answer this question.

I am not arguing that beliefs and desires are not sufficient for emotion; I am arguing that, *assuming* that beliefs and desires are sufficient, we need to know quite a number of Adam's beliefs and desires before we can decide what emotion Adam would have. If Adam believes that Janet is his friend, for example, Adam might feel sadness, rather than anger. If he believes that Janet is his friend and that she has been insulting him at parties for quite over a period of twenty years now, he might feel despair. The point is obvious. It does not threaten the belief-desire sufficiency account of emotions, but it reveals the weakness in Green's application of this account to romantic love. For it is easy to claim, at a general level, that Leo can desire Dan and believe that Dan is so-and-so, and yet not feel love towards Dan. But it is important to see that once we start adding more of Leo's desires and beliefs about Dan, then, depending on these desires and beliefs, it might turn out to be a deep puzzle why Leo, indeed, does *not* love Dan. Suppose, for example, that Leo believes that Dan is attractive, is smart, is his soul mate (this does not beg any questions), is morally good, and has good taste. Suppose Leo desires Dan sexually, desires to spend time with Dan, desires that Dan share his time with *him*, desires that Dan reciprocate whatever Leo desires about Dan (this is too crude, of course, but it should serve the point), and desires that Dan fare well in life and flourish for his (Dan's) own sake. Suppose after all of this, Leo tells us that he nevertheless does *not* (romantically) love Dan. I take it that we would be puzzled at this; we would find that Leo's claims are somehow amiss. Given his beliefs and desires, we expect love to follow.

In short, Green's position faces a dilemma. Either the argument is pitched at a general level at which we speak only of "belief that *p*" and "desire that *p*" or it is pitched at a level which allows for a listing of the individual beliefs and desires. If the former, then it is hard to see how beliefs and desires can be sufficient for a type of emotion, and so even though they would not be sufficient for romantic love, they would also not be sufficient for a plethora of others, such as anger, sorrow, despair, frustration, pride, hope, and elation. If the latter, then beliefs and desires would be sufficient for emotions, but it would also be obvious that depending on which desires and beliefs are listed, we may or may not expect to find love, and so the account would apply equally plausibly to romantic love.

Green's own preferred position is to identify romantic love with a set of desires (*sans* beliefs, of course): "Love is identical with a set of desires: desires are constitutive of love, not just caused by love; and desires are essential to, not just typical of, love" (216). He goes on to identify romantic love with three kinds of desires: the desire to "share an association with" the beloved that typically has a sexual aspect, the desire that the beloved "fare well" for her own sake, and the desire that the beloved reciprocate the desires for association and welfare (216). Green offers this account as one of identity, which implies that the desires are individually necessary and jointly sufficient for romantic love. No doubt, such desires play an important and perhaps essential role in romantic love.[20] But we need not claim that romantic love is not an emotion in order to preserve this role for desires. For emotions—and Green, of course, agrees with this claim—are composed of cognitive and desiritive (and affective) components. So if romantic love were an emotion, then desires would still play an important role. The point is that we need not deny that romantic love is an emotion in order to preserve an important role for desires.

I have argued that Green's attempts to show that romantic love is not an emotion fail. Moreover, since it is difficult to see how else—other than by denying that it is anchored in beliefs—one can deny that romantic love is an emotion, the conclusion that Green's arguments fail is not a minor victory. It renders the claim that romantic love is an emotion extremely plausible, and it does so by arguing that the one hopeful way of denying romantic love's status as an emotion is not promising. If emotions are constituted by beliefs, desires, and affective states, then romantic love seems to be as much of an emotion as any other usual candidate. Moreover, if romantic love is an emotion, we are then in a strong position to see that it is not a virtue.

2.3. Romantic Love Is an Attitude: Martin's Argument

Mike Martin (1996) denies that romantic love is an emotion, and instead claims that it is a type of attitude. Martin's book is devoted to showing that, and exploring how, romantic love is structured and enabled by the virtues. The aim, then, is not to define "romantic love" or to give an account of romantic love's nature (Martin uses the term "love" in its sense of "genuine" or "true love," a sense in which romantic love is moral and virtuous). Still, Martin's remarks to the effect that romantic love is an attitude are sketchy and somewhat enigmatic. But let us see what we can make of them.

Martin claims, in a number of places, that romantic love is "primarily a set of virtue-structured ways to value persons" (6).[21] He "suggests" that, instead of thinking of romantic love as a feeling or an emotion, romantic love is "primarily an attitude and a relationship. A commitment to love is a commitment to sustain an attitude of valuing the beloved as singularly important in one's life" (57). Elsewhere he adds that "genuine love is guided, structured, and partly defined by virtues" (135), and that "love, after all, is not an uninterrupted feeling of affection. As an attitude, love embodies the full gamut of human emotions, including moments of depression, annoyance, anger, and even hate" (135–36).

A few things are clear from these quotations. First, Martin does not think that romantic love is a virtue.[22] Whatever it is—and we should keep in mind that "structured" is a rather nebulous term—romantic love is structured or constituted by some virtues (and enabled by others). Second, Martin does not think that romantic love is an emotion. Early in the book, he claims that there is a sense of "true love" that is simply classificatory, a sense that simply describes a person's feelings or attractions towards another (12–13). Perhaps in that sense, "romantic love" refers to an emotion. Nevertheless, Martin wants to claim that according to the sense he is using, a sense that refers to the virtues that underlie and constitute romantic love, we should think of it as primarily an attitude rather than an emotion. Third, romantic love is an attitude in which another person is valued as "singularly" important, and which is supported and constituted by the virtues (or some of them).

Why does Martin think of romantic love in this way? Sometimes it appears that he prefers to think of romantic love as an attitude so as to avoid objections against romantic love that can be successful only if it is an emotion (56). But I think that there are three more important reasons why Martin thinks of romantic love as an attitude. The first can be gleaned from the last quotation given above: "love, after all, is not an uninterrupted feeling of affection" (135). Perhaps Martin is worried that if romantic love were construed as an emotion, then we would land ourselves in a serious puzzle: How can Melissa claim to love Dan if Melissa's *emotion* is not always present to and in her? The idea is that when Melissa claims to love Dan, she is referring to a longstanding, long-term commitment of sorts to her beloved. But we know that emotions are not always present in us. If Melissa loves Dan, then, except perhaps for the initial stages of the affair, Melissa would not be constantly thinking of, dreaming about, and fantasizing about Dan (hopefully, she would have a job which requires a bit of her attention). But we want to say that Melissa's romantic love for Dan does not disappear during those times when (on the job, for instance) she is not thinking about and desiring Dan. However, if we think of romantic love as being an emotion, then we would be forced to make such claims. It is important to mention that nowhere in his book does Martin explicitly entertain this worry. It is one which I attribute to him given some of his remarks (such as his implicit equating an emotion with a "momentary feeling," [57]) and given his desire to think of romantic love as structured by virtue.

But this is not a real worry. If it were, then many of those mental phenomena that we consider to be emotions would turn out not be emotions. People take pride in all sorts of things; yet they do not spend every hour of the day thinking about them. People are often angry with other people. Yet the former—except perhaps for the early stages of the anger (or unless they are deeply troubled)—do not spend their time mulling over their anger. People often hope to achieve certain things, to be certain types of people, to have a certain job or status. But unless they are all pre–princess stage Cinderellas, they would not continuously dwell on such hopes. The same point applies to a range of other emotions, such as hate, gratitude, concern, envy, pity, compassion, sympathy, resentment, and fear. If the worry I attributed to Martin were sufficient to convert an emotion into an attitude, there would be precious few emotions.[23] There is, however, the possibility that Martin understands an attitude to be a longstanding, dispositional emotion. This is a crucial possibility and one that I will address shortly. For now, suffice it so say that Martin does not explicitly offer this understanding of "attitude."

The second reason why I think that Martin prefers to think of romantic love as an attitude rather than an emotion is linked to the one above but is also essentially different. It is his implicit belief that unless we think of romantic love as an attitude, we would not be able to capture its constancy, its pervasiveness in the lives of the lovers, its ability to change people's lives, and a host of other features and abilities commonly attributed to romantic love. A commitment to romantic love, according to Martin, implies a commitment to being responsible for a relationship, and this is not something to be taken lightly. Perhaps if romantic love were an emotion, it would not be able to conceptually support such heavy duties and concerns.

But the problem with this account is that it is difficult to understand romantic love as an attitude unless it is understood, fundamentally, as an emotion. Martin suggests that we think of romantic love as "primarily" an attitude. It is not clear whether this word is meant to merely shift the emphasis from thinking of romantic love as an emotion to thinking of it as an attitude (without denying its emotiveness) or, more strongly, to displace romantic love as an emotion by romantic love as an attitude. But even if we go by the former and weaker suggestion, without emphasizing that romantic love is an emotion we cannot get very far. For one thing, "attitude" sometimes refers to purely intellectual mental postures, as in, for example, the expression, "One can have at least three different attitudes towards the idea that mental states are brain states." Such an understanding of the notion of attitude is ill suited for its application to romantic love. For another thing, to say that romantic love is "an attitude of valuing the beloved as singularly important" would not take us very far; this is how the Count de Monte Cristo regarded his enemies, one by one, until he was able to satisfy his lust for revenge.[24] As the narrator in George Eliot's *The Mill on the Floss* states, "Anger and jealousy can no more bear to lose sight of their objects than love" (1998, 100). The point is that the person whom one values singularly could be the object of one's hate, envy, jealousy, sympathy, benevolence, and so on. We need to find a better specification of valuing and regard by speaking specifically to the desires, beliefs, and affections that structure them so as to be able to place a tight grip on both the valuer and the valued. But understanding the beliefs, desires, and affections of *x* regarding *y* comes awfully close to understanding *x*'s *emotion* towards *y*. In short, where emotions are present, the notion of attitude is parasitic on that of emotion. What attitude *x* has towards *y* depends essentially on what emotion or emotions towards *y* that *x* has. Thus, Martin cannot simply decide to shift the emphasis from emotions to attitudes.

Another way to make the above point is this: it could make perfect sense to speak of romantic love as an attitude were we also to claim that attitudes, in general, are longstanding emotions and so need not exhibit themselves at every moment of the agent's life. In other words, romantic love is an emotion that need not exhibit itself in action and feeling constantly, but at a number of moments or intervals in the lover's life. If we accept this claim, then romantic love would indeed be an attitude, but only in the sense that it is first and foremost an emotion, and that it is that kind of emotion which can exist in an agent for long periods of time yet not constantly exhibit itself in action and feeling. This would be a plausible picture to give of romantic love, at least in the sense that it squares with many lovers' lives. But it would also be a picture that is inconsistent with Martin's claim that romantic love is not an emotion. At best, it would not be an emotion like that of anger. For anger is not the kind of emotion—putting unusual cases aside—that is longstanding. It might endure for a while, but it usually goes away after a brief period of time, either simply on its own, or after reparations have been made to the one who is angry, or after the latter's beliefs change requisitely. Though it differs from anger and some other emotions in this respect, romantic love would still be essentially an emotion. Moreover, further support for the claim that romantic love would still be an emotion even though it differs from anger in this respect—support in addition to the fact that it coheres with lovers' actual lives—is the fact that there are many other emotions which are longstanding, such as hate, envy, jealousy, and admiration. These are obviously considered to be emotions, they can be part and parcel of an agent's life for long periods of times, and they need not exhibit themselves in actions and feelings constantly. Thus, a longstanding emotion is dispositional. If, for example, hate is such an emotion, then if Jim hates Bob, (i) Jim has the emotion of hate for Bob for a long period of Jim's life, and (ii) Jim would not constantly feel and/or mentally dwell on Bob; he would feel the emotion under certain conditions, such as seeing Bob, being reminded of him, and hearing Bob's name. It should be noted, however, that though some emotions, such as hate, jealousy, and romantic love, can be longstanding emotions, they need not be. They can be also momentary.[25]

The third reason why Martin thinks of romantic love as an attitude rather than an emotion has to do with his specific thesis that romantic love is structured by the virtues. His thought might be that were romantic love to be thought of as an emotion, it is difficult to see how it can be structured by the virtues. In this, Martin would be fully correct. On the Aristotelian definition of "virtue," emotions cannot be structured by the virtues, since it is the former that—to put it loosely—enter into the latter, rather than the other way around. So if we want romantic love to be structured by virtues, we had better not claim that it is an emotion. But then again, I do not think that we want to make this claim, the main reason being that no convincing argument has been offered in the literature to the effect that romantic love is not an emotion. And if so, then perhaps we had better stay on the side of common sense. In connection with Martin's view, rather than argue that romantic love is structured by the virtues, we are better off arguing that it is enabled by them. And to make *this* claim, there is no need to deny that romantic love is an emotion. I will explore the view that romantic love is enabled by the virtues in the next section, where I will also return to Martin's views on this issue. For now, I want to offer two more direct arguments to the effect that romantic love is not a virtue and then explore a position which claims the opposite.

2.4. Romantic Love Fits Neither the Definition of Nor the Criteria for Virtue

In this section, I will attempt a more direct way to argue that romantic love is not a virtue, by arguing that it does not satisfy well the definition of "virtue," and by arguing that it also does not satisfy the criteria for being a virtue.

Let us suppose that romantic love is *not* an emotion. Let us further suppose that it is a candidate for being a virtue (understood along the same lines as care being a candidate for a virtue, from section 2 of the previous chapter) in that it is a disposition of sorts (a longstanding disposition), keeping in mind that something's being a disposition does not entail that it is also a virtue. Let us also keep in mind the crucial point that the type of love under discussion is erotic or romantic love, not sibling, parental, or friendship love. And let us now consider the issue, along the lines of section 5 from the previous chapter, as to whether romantic love can satisfy the two conditions for a trait being a virtue. To recollect, the two conditions are, first, that the trait benefits its possessor and, second, that it enables her to be a good human being *qua* being human. Moreover, it will not do to answer these questions by saying that romantic love can be corrupt, bad, misguided, etc. For we are to assume that romantic love is shot through with practical wisdom and so dons a good garb. The question is, then, whether, and given these assumptions, romantic love can satisfy the two conditions for being a virtue.

It is difficult to answer this question in a fully convincing manner, but there are some good reasons for answering it in the negative. First, consider whether romantic love benefits its possessor. The answer to this question is contingent: it depends on the person's life and situation. While the virtues are crucial for the flourishing of individuals, romantic love need not be. One can barely live decently without the virtue of caring; without honesty, people would not trust one; without courage, one is much likely to lead a highly impoverished life; and without generosity, others are liable to shun one, and unlikely to show one consideration and gratitude. Again, the claim is not that one *cannot* live a decent life without one or more of the virtues. Rather, the claim is merely that the possession of the virtues enables one to lead a good life because they benefit one. (If the claim were put in terms of the impossibility of living decently without the virtues, then we could not speak of "benefit" and would have to speak, instead, in terms of necessity.)

It does not, however, seem to be the case that romantic love is beneficial in such ways. People who do not fall in love, or do not experience the emotion of love, or who forgo romantic love, are not, because of these facts, unreliable, morally off, defective, and so on. It is true that often enough the inability to, or desire not to, romantically love can be signs of deeper faults; one might, for example, not want to love because one is arrogant: one thinks no one is quite good enough for one. But this is not an invariable law, nor does it imply a conceptual connection. It is caring which is really the crucial disposition here: insofar as one is able and willing to care, then one shows others one's nondefectiveness, so to speak. The point can be put in this way: as far as the issue of benefiting the agent is concerned, the virtues are basic to the agent's life in that it is difficult for her to get on without them. The virtues benefit her because without them she is very likely to find life difficult to live, given the way human beings are and how they relate to each other. Whether one should be virtuous does not depend on the agent's own valuational scheme; it is, simply, rational to be virtuous given our humanity. This is not so with romantic love. Whether it is rational to be in love, and so whether romantic love benefits the agent, depends on the specific circumstances of the agent and her life plan. In this respect, romantic love's benefits, unlike those of the virtues, do not *ground* the agent's values and plans.[26]

Turn next to the issue of whether romantic love is necessary for the agent's goodness as a human being or *qua* being human. The answer is "no." Human beings do not need romantic love in order to grow up to be healthy social and rational animals. Indeed, it is *usually* the case that by the time human beings reach the age at which they can fall in love and experience its passions and upheavals, they would already be at an age when their characters and intellects are more or less formed. Of course, romantic love can later in her life make the agent a better human being. But the frequency of this is an issue difficult to determine. Even if we are discussing romantic love as being directed by practical wisdom, its effects on the agent's rationality and sociality are ambivalent. They could lead human beings to desire isolation from society so as to create a world for themselves and their beloveds. More generally, romantic love, as such, does not seem to be necessary for human life to go on in smooth ways. It is often said that being in love makes one a better human being, and one contemporary philosopher states that "love makes us better. Because loving involves actively helping the other, it fosters our virtue" (Kupfer 1993, 116). I am never sure what such claims mean, but if they mean that one becomes more caring, more sensitive, more giving, and so on, then I have my doubts. At least, if one were not already to some extent good and virtuous, then the effects of romantic love may not be so laudable. If this is correct, then we can roughly state that whether romantic love makes one a better human being depends to a large extent on one's prior goodness. I do not wish to deny the *possibility* of cases involving bad human beings turned good by romantic love. Rather, I am doubtful regarding their frequency. After all, if the virtues and vices are deep character traits, and hence difficult to change, then the case of a bad person turned good through romantic love would be rare indeed. In this respect, unlike the virtues, romantic love does not make one a better human being; it makes one a better human being if one is good to begin with (it "*fosters* virtue," as Kupfer himself puts it). The point is that whereas the virtues, given the right environment and the requisite external needs, *unconditionally* make a human being a good one *qua* being human, romantic love does not do so in this way. It usually requires the agent to be good for it to make her (the agent) a better human being (this claim will be fleshed out further below).

The conclusion we can reach is that at worst, romantic love does not satisfy the conditions of a trait's being a virtue. At best, we can say that it is difficult to make a case for the claim that romantic love satisfies these two conditions. This is not to say, of course, that romantic love is not necessary for flourishing, because it might still be an external good, such as friendship and a moderate amount of wealth, which are necessary for an agent to lead a flourishing life. (I will address this issue in the final section of this chapter.)

But there is also another argument to the effect that romantic love is not a virtue: it does not fit well the definitions of "virtue." I will focus on the two definitions offered in the introduction. Let us start with Aristotle's: virtue is a state involving choice and lying in a mean, with the mean relative to the individual (1985, 1107a1–4). To begin with, while romantic love might be a dispositional state in that it disposes its agent in all sorts of ways towards the agent's beloved, it nevertheless seems not to be a virtue on this definition. The reason is that because romantic love does not seem to issue in actions that can be plausibly classified as "love actions." True enough, there are actions done out of love—done out of the emotion of love—but these do not belong to one type of action; they are "love actions" because they stem from the emotion of love. To see this point, consider the goods that other virtues revolve around. Courage, for example, revolves around the protection of important goods in the face of adversity. Caring revolves around the support and promotion of the ends of the cared-for. Justice, to give one last example, revolves around what others are owed. But love does not seem to have a unique good around which it revolves. To say that it revolves around the well-being of the beloved is not narrow enough, for a number of other virtues (caring, courage, justice, and generosity, to give a few examples), can have the well-being of another as their goal. Well-being, in short, is too broad to do the job. Because of this fact about the virtues, it makes sense to speak of corresponding "caring actions," "courageous actions," and so on. However, to speak of "loving actions" means—at best, as far as the issue of virtues is concerned—to speak of loving actions that are caring, or that are wise, or that are fair, and so forth, but that are directed at the beloved.

Now on the face of it, there is nothing in the Aristotelian definition that rules out romantic love. It is a state, and a dispositional one at that, that also might involve choice. But the part of Aristotle's definition where romantic love ultimately falters is the notion of the mean. Because acting correctly, as the mean clause stipulates, requires situational and contextual ways in attending to moral values and goods, and because acting out of romantic love does not target a moral value or good unique to romantic love, acting out of romantic love does not fit this part of Aristotle's definition well. In acting out of romantic love, I may act courageously, fairly, wisely, charitably, or temperately. In doing so, I will be acting virtuously and so as the mean requires. Yet none of these actions involve any moral goods unique to romantic love. What rather makes them romantic love actions is that they stem from the emotion of romantic love and are directed at the beloved.

Furthermore, it is also clear that some predominant conceptions of romantic love do not sit well with that part of Aristotle's definition about "involving choice." For part of these conceptions is that romantic love "washes over us," that we have no control over falling in love. Now it may not be true that romantic love is *never* a matter of choice. Nevertheless, the fact that many instances of romantic love do not involve choice implies that romantic love does not fit this clause of the definition well at all. However, if this clause of the definition is better construed as referring to actions, namely, in this case, actions done out of love, then there is no good reason to claim that romantic love would not fit it. For obviously, many actions done out of love are the result of choice. And if so, then romantic love would also fit the clause about the mean (just as caring actions can be done at the right time, for the right reasons, and so on, so can ones done out of love). What is crucial, however, is that for these clauses about choice and the mean to lend support to the idea that romantic love is a virtue, what must first be shown is that romantic love issues in virtuous actions that are specific to itself, because these clauses are reliant on the idea that the virtues target unique moral values and goods. And *this*, I contend, is difficult to show.

Next, recall the contemporary definition of "virtue" given by Zagzebski: a virtue is a deep and acquired excellence of a person, involving a characteristic motivation to produce a desired end of a worthwhile type, reliable success in bringing about that end, and a characteristic disposition to react emotionally to one's situation. As far as romantic love is concerned, all is not smooth with respect to this definition. The stumbling block is the notion of an end. First, if we understand "end" to refer to the *types* of ends that each virtue in general has, then we get a discussion very much similar to the one above. Consider, as comparative examples, the virtues of honesty, courage, kindness, justice, and caring. Each of these revolves around a certain end: honesty revolves around the end of truth telling; courage around defending important goods; kindness around helping others; justice around upholding rights; and caring around promoting the goals of intimate others. But what is the end around which romantic love revolves? There does not seem to be any specific one or ones.

For example, promoting the well-being of the beloved as an end of romantic love is too general to be of any help, given that nearly all of the virtues have it. Union with the beloved is certainly a famous and traditional candidate offered for being the end of romantic love. However, the notion of union in this context is a mysterious one. If it means something innocuous, something along the lines of shared activity, then it is not specific to love. Friendships—even Aristotle's friendships of pleasure and of utility— and other associations have it. If it means anything more substantial, such as shared identity (Solomon 1990 and Nozick 1991), then it would run into some logical difficulties. If the identity in question means that both lovers, *x* and *y*, have numerically identical properties, then union would be an impossible goal, because it would entail that two different people have the goal of merging into one. This is not only physically impossible, but also goes against the very phenomenon of love, since romantic love as an emotion is directed towards another person and is often realized between *two*, not one, people. If the identity in question means that the lovers would have nonnumerically identical desires, thoughts, feelings, and other psychological traits, then union would not be impossible. Obviously, some people can, in principle, achieve it. But then this end would not be unique to romantic love, for it can then characterize the goals of (at least some) friendships. Furthermore, understanding "union" in this way would have the result that most lovers have never achieved, do not achieve, and probably will never achieve this goal. For it is obvious that many couples whom we call "lovers" do not fully have such identical psychological states. They share *some* identical states, but not all of them. This means that either we should reject describing these couples as lovers or reject union as a goal on the grounds that it is *practically* almost impossible to achieve. I would go with the latter option, since it is obvious, to me at least, that many people are romantically in love even though not all of their psychological states are identical. We should also keep in mind the different point that any substantial notion of union would be subject to the severe objection that it precludes robust concern for the beloved. I will not go into this last point, however, since it has been adequately dealt with (Soble 1997c).

Second, if by "end" we were to refer to particular goals issuing from particular actions, then, again, romantic love would not fit this part of the definition. For actions done out of romantic love do not carve for themselves a specific domain to the exclusion of other ends in other types of actions. Suppose, for example, Brad buys Yoni an ice cream cake out of love. Suppose the reason Brad does this is because it will make Yoni happy, or because Yoni loves ice cream cakes. Whatever reason we can cite, it can be subsumed under another type of virtuous action, such as a caring one. This indicates that romantic love does not fit this clause of the definition well.

At this point, we should also remind ourselves that the above discussion was conducted under the crucial assumption that romantic love is shot through and through with wisdom and so comes in a good form. I have made this assumption in order to show that even under this strong assumption, romantic love is not a virtue. But we can now relax this assumption. Once we do so, we will see that romantic love would easily not fit the above two definitions of virtue. For then it would not be necessary that it lie in a mean (Aristotle's definition) or that it is an excellence (Zagzebski's definition). It would be an emotion, and, like most other emotions, it can be good or bad, depending, to a large extent, on whether its possessor is good or bad.[27]

Let us tentatively conclude, then, that romantic love is not a virtue.[28] The word "tentatively" is meant to capture the ideas that the above arguments are certainly not conclusive or exhaustive. There might be other arguments that show that romantic love is not an emotion, and the arguments I have offered to show that it is not a virtue certainly leave much room for dissent. Before we can be content, after all this detailed assessment of some arguments, that romantic love is an emotion, we need to address one position that argues that it is, indeed, a virtue. To this I now turn.

2.5. Romantic Love Is a Virtue: Solomon's Argument(s)

An interesting approach to the issues at hand is to accept the idea that romantic love is an emotion, but to nevertheless argue that emotions can be virtues. If this approach is viable, then one can argue that romantic love is an emotion but that it is also a virtue. My task is to argue that this approach is difficult to undertake.

Robert Solomon's aims in his essay are to broaden our view of ethics and to "understand" erotic (or romantic) love as a virtue (1991, 492). After distinguishing erotic love from other types of love (sexual desire is central to the former), and after arguing against the view that erotic love is selfish, Solomon discusses three possible reasons why philosophers do not consider romantic love a virtue. The first is that it might be reduced to mere sexuality and "philosophers . . . tend to see sexuality as vulgar and not even a candidate for virtue" (496). The second is that romantic love may be thought of as an emotion and philosophers consider emotions irrational and unruly in all sorts of ways. And the third reason why romantic love fails to be a virtue is that some see it as involving the selfish indulging of the lover's desires. This is in contrast to virtue, which is often thought of as useful to others.

Solomon claims that the above reasons are misguided. Specifically, he argues that ethical evaluation requires the emotions; that they are, to some extent, within our control; and that they are neither irrational, nor disruptive, nor intrusive, nor stupid, nor stubborn, nor pointless, nor distortive of our experiences. It is obvious that Solomon considers romantic love to be an emotion. But how can one do so and yet claim that it is a virtue? Easily (or so it seems): Solomon asserts that not only dispositions are virtues; emotions can also be virtues: "Even Aristotle . . . insisted that only states of character, not passions, can count as virtues" (496), thus implying that Aristotle was wrong. Later he states that "against much of recent 'virtue ethics,' love seems to show that virtues should not be understood as traits" (516–17). In order for Solomon's claim—that the virtues need not be confined to being character traits—to be non-question begging, Solomon's reason for it, namely, that love is a virtue, must be true or at least plausible.[29] My contention is that it is not.

How is romantic love a virtue? To Solomon, emotions are complex: they involve judgments, desires, and values. Romantic love is no exception. In terms of desires, the one that best characterizes the concept of romantic love is the desire for shared identity, for "ontological dependency" (511). He states that "shared identity is the intention of love, and the virtues of love are essentially the virtues of this intended identity" (511). Solomon proposes to look at the virtues of romantic love itself (as opposed to its good consequences), but he then launches into a discussion about the nature of shared identity in love (512), presumably as a way of answering the question of how romantic love is a virtue. He claims that romantic love is "just this determining of selfhood":

> A person's character is best determined by those who "really know him," and it is not odd to us that a person generally known as a bastard might be thought to be a good person just on the testimony of a wife, a husband, or a close friend. . . . When we talk about "the real self" or "being true to ourselves," what we often mean is being true to the image of ourselves that we share with those we most love. We say, and are expected to say, that the self we display in public performance, the self we present on the job, the self we show to acquaintances, is not real. (512)

As far as romantic love is concerned, it is a process of "mutual self-identi-fication"; in it, selves "merge" into each other, and romantic love is a way of smoothing out the incompatibilities between these selves: "The development of love is consequently defined by a *dialectic*, often tender but sometimes ontologically vicious, in which each lover struggles for control over shared and reciprocal self-images, resists them, revises them, rejects them" (513, italics in the original).

I have quoted Solomon at some length so as to capture, in his own words, the essence of his position. It is more or less obvious—and Solomon never comes out and says this directly and explicitly—that romantic love is a virtue, according to him, because it is a determinant of selfhood. Indeed, it is not just *a* determinant of selfhood; it is one of the "best" determinants. If we are, then, to assess Solomon's claim that romantic love is a virtue, we need to assess the claim that it is a determinant of selfhood. But it should be obvious that his account is beset by some severe difficulties. I will discuss two.

First, it is not clear whether Solomon is discussing an ideal conception of romantic love or romantic love as we generally find it in our daily lives. It seems that he is discussing the latter, given his emphasis on certain claims such as the fact that our society distinguishes between the public and the private (512), and that we can no longer understand the virtues communally as, according to Solomon, Aristotle did (512). These remarks indicate that he is concerned with the way romantic love is actually found in our society: "In a fragmented world so built on intimate privacies, love even more than family and friendship determines selfhood" (512). But this is flagrantly false as an account of the actual ways people love or live. Go back (in the previous paragraph) to his remarks about how romantic love is a dialectic: it is obvious, I think, that many couples who fall in love do not satisfy this Sartrean process of taking control of self-images until some sort of shared identity is formed. At the very least, they do not do so consciously. If they do so unconsciously, then Solomon needs to give an argument for this stronger claim. This is not to deny, of course, that some lovers (consciously) try to dominate each other along such lines. But it is to deny that this characterizes romantic love and the way people love each other.

The mistake is found at the very basis of Solomon's view, namely, the conviction that somehow our intimate selves are more authentic, more real, than our public selves. Indeed, on Solomon's account, it turns out that people are quite split in their personalities. For Solomon seems to want to maintain a drastic difference between the way people show themselves to intimate others and the way they present themselves to strangers, colleagues, and acquaintances (as is evidently shown in the above quotation). But the price for this is simply too high: we emerge as schizophrenic people, shuttling between the most public and most private selves, and all the gradations between them. Moreover, we do not need to pay such a philosophical price, for Solomon's view is exaggerated and false.

It is not typical that we reveal secrets and intimate information about ourselves to strangers. And we *often* do not reveal these to colleagues and to acquaintances. Furthermore, we do things in front of our lovers, family members, and intimate friends that we would feel ashamed to do in front of strangers and colleagues and acquaintances, such as picking our noses, going to the bathroom with the door open, and releasing flatulence. In this respect, most of us are not, fortunately, Homer Simpsons. But we should not infer from such observations that people have different personas. Would a colleague of mine, upon knowing that I am, say, sexually into men who are clad in thongs or jockstraps come to the conclusion, "Heavens to Betsy! Raja has a whole new persona to him!"? Surely not; at least, not unless I have carried myself in such a way as to give her the idea that I am asexual. People know that people keep things private and secret, yet from this they do not infer that they have different personas. The distinction between the private and the public does not map onto the distinction between different personas.

But the second error in Solomon's account is this: even assuming that romantic love is the best determinant of selfhood, it does not follow that romantic love is a virtue. Having a determinate self is no doubt a (qualifiedly) good thing—one does not want one's self perforated and indefinitely plastic for the duration of one's lifetime! But it is quite another to claim that romantic love is a virtue because it is the best vehicle for this job of determination. For one thing, consider again the dialectical process by which romantic love determines selfhood: in his own words, Solomon describes the process as "ontologically *vicious*," characterized by struggles over control, revision, and rejection of self-images. How such a vicious process can be also a virtue is difficult to fathom. If the end result—determination of selves—is sufficient to make the process a virtue, then I wonder what happened to Solomon's claim that he is about to consider romantic love in itself, apart from its results (512).

Even if the end result is sufficient to make a vicious process a virtue, we may question why this should be so. The thought is this: it is, as I said, a good thing that selves get to be determined. But the worry is that romantic love may not be one of the *best* ways to do this. Unless the selves that go into the dialectical process are good and minimally decent, there is the worry that the other self who is going to help determine my self is a corrupt self, a bad self, or an evil self. We are, in a way, back to the problem which Victoria Davion had posed for Nel Noddings's position on care: allowing oneself to be transformed by another cannot be an absolute value. Solomon does not claim that romantic love is an absolute value, and he explicitly states that it is not a trump virtue (516). Still, it is difficult to see how he could maintain his claim that romantic love is one of the best ways of determining selfhood, when the two selves—or at least one of them— can be bad to the bone. Solomon does not claim that the selves that go into the process of romantic love are formless and indeterminate; indeed, he states that most people fall in love at an age when their selves are "full-formed" (513). Nevertheless, the danger is still there: unless those full-formed selves are good, the process of forming a shared identity can be morally dangerous.[30]

Yet Solomon does not shy away from danger: "Of course to deny that love can go wrong . . . would be absurd. It can destroy as well as conjoin relationships, and it can ruin as well as enhance a life. Yes, love can be dangerous, but why have we so long accepted the idea that the virtuous life is simple and uncomplicated rather than, as Nietzsche used to say, a work of romantic art? For love is a virtue as much of the imagination as of morals" (517). I am not sure what to make of the claim that romantic love is a virtue of the imagination in light of what Solomon has been claiming. The thing to notice is that Solomon accepts the idea that romantic love can be dangerous. But he goes on to equivocate on "love as a virtue is dangerous" and "the virtuous life is dangerous." These two claims do not mean the same thing. The latter is about the *life* of the person who is virtuous, not his *virtues*, and Nietzsche was not the only one to tell us that the virtuous life is not simple. Aristotle spent quite a bit of space in his *Ethics* discussing the role of external goods and misfortunes in a virtuous life.[31]

There is, however, a sense in which I have not yet touched upon the core of Solomon's position. The core can be captured by the claims that romantic love is an emotion, that traits need not be the only types of things that can be virtues, and that it is possible for emotions to be virtues also. If we set aside romantic love in its neutral form (which can render this business of determining selves quite morally dangerous) and consider it in its form as moderated by practical wisdom or, to put this in a slightly different way, as found in a virtuous character, the claim that romantic love is a virtue becomes plausible. In order to investigate its truth, it becomes necessary to investigate why it is not plausible to identify the emotions with virtues. (If we investigate instead the claim that traits need not be the only types of virtue, then even if we conclude that this claim is true, we will not be able to conclude that romantic love is a virtue. For we would still need to look into the claim that the emotions can be virtues. So we might as well cut to the chase.)

Why, indeed, did Aristotle (and he is not alone in this) not consider emotions to be virtues? There are three important reasons that we can ascribe to Aristotle even though he never mentioned them himself (and, in any case, my point is conceptual, not historical). The reasons are complex enough to take us into some deep issues that I will not discuss at length because they take us beyond the scope of this book. But one crucial assumption underlying all three is this: both Aristotle and many contemporary philosophers know very well that emotions are cognitive; they typically involve beliefs, judgments, or, at the least, thoughts about particular objects. In this respect, many emotions are intentional. To offer two brief and common examples, if Paul is angry at Newt, then Paul believes that he has been unjustly treated by Newt and desires some sort of reparation from him. If Michael is afraid of Ariel, then Michael believes that Ariel is dangerous and desires not to be harmed.

Virtues are dispositions to behave and emotionally react in the right ways. This does not mean that in actual instances of behavior there are no thoughts about particular objects and people (far from it). Rather, we need to ask about what thoughts and beliefs are involved in the *virtues*, not instances of acting from virtue or virtuously. The answer is difficult to come by, but it must involve the idea that insofar as the virtues are pervaded by practical wisdom, and insofar as practical wisdom is not just about discerning what to do in particular situations but also about what is important and worthwhile in life, then the virtues must embody thoughts about these. Thus a virtuous person will have thoughts—though they need not be articulated in any sophisticated and peculiarly philosophical way—about the place and value of things, people, emotions, and action in a decent and good life.

Partly because of the types of thoughts involved in the virtues (and partly because they require a type of education that spans years), the virtues are more entrenched in a person's life. That is why they are often defined as deep and settled traits. They are not easy to change, and one reason is that the beliefs, judgments, and thoughts they involve are about general values and their place in a good life. In this respect, they contrast markedly with the emotions, and the contrast emerges in the idea that emotions are more easily malleable than the virtues. If Joanna believes that Nick has insulted her and is angry, then once Joanna comes to realize that Nick has not insulted her (and that she misperceived the situation), she is liable to simply not have the emotion any more. I do not mean to claim that every single instance of an emotion is tractable in this way; perhaps there are emotions that are not based on beliefs. Nor do I mean to claim that once a belief is changed, then the emotion is immediately dispossessed. In some cases, such as those of romantic love, the emotion takes much time to be shed, although there are plenty of cases in which romantic love turns sour pretty quickly upon the formation of some new belief or other. In other cases, such as those of a parent's caring for his or her offspring, the emotion might even never go away. The general point, however, is that emotions are typically cognitively based and that they are usually shed when the belief is shed. Both of these aspects are common to the virtues, but change is more difficult in the case of the virtues. To change a virtue, what is required is to change the underlying valuational belief system of the agent. This is no easy feat, because these systems are about general, deep, and basic values and thoughts about what is important in life. They do not involve beliefs about *particular* objects.[32] This is not to say that virtuous people do not become vicious or indifferent, but that it will require much, much more than changing a belief or two about a particular object. The first reason, then, as to why emotions are not virtues is that emotions, whether occurrent or longstanding, often involve beliefs about particular objects or persons, such that once these beliefs are shed, so are the emotions. This is in marked contrast with the virtues, which often involve beliefs, values, and aims concerned with general objects, not particular ones.

Solomon is at pains to emphasize the idea that it is *good* that the emotions are intractable: "It is true that the emotions are stubborn and intractable, but this—as opposed to much less dependable action in accordance with principle—is what makes them so essential to ethics. . . . One trusts a person fighting in accordance with his passions far more than one fighting for abstract principles" (501). Whether Solomon is right about the issue of trust can be set aside.[33] The point is that Solomon does not seem to seriously consider that the intractability of the emotions is dependent on the beliefs which partly constitute the emotion, *and* that, given that the beliefs in emotions are typically about particular objects, they are more easily changed than the beliefs and values involved in virtue. In this respect, the virtues are more reliable than the emotions; they do cut to the core of a person's character.

But there is a sense in which Solomon is correct, and this sense gets us to the second reason as to why emotions are not virtues. Certain types of people are liable to feel certain types of emotions rather than others. Perhaps, for example, good people do not feel envy (which is not to be identified with jealousy). Perhaps bad people, or some of them, never feel compassion. In this respect, we are not speaking of emotions, whether occurrent or longstanding, as being exhibited about particular objects, but about emotions that people of certain characters are liable to feel. One might then think that these types of emotions are virtues. However, this will not do, because *this* kind of claim about the emotions, namely, that some people are liable to feel some emotions but not others, conceptually comes after the claim about the virtues. For unless the person is psychologically ill (for example, a psychopath), it is only after a person has formed her values and beliefs about the important things in life that we can confidently make claims about what emotions she is liable to have, and only then will her emotions reveal to us what she *really* thinks and values, and so, in this sense, cut to her core.

We can then see the second reason why we do not equate the emotions with virtues. For them to be reliable indicators of a person's character, they require the previous formation of the person's beliefs, values, and tendencies. Whether we are speaking of occurrent or longstanding emotions, the point is that *what* emotions an agent has and is liable to experience, and *how* they are experienced depend on the agent's beliefs, values, and tendencies. These three are conceptually basic in the agent's emotions. Because emotions are constituted by cognitive states and desires (in addition to affective states), to assess the goodness of emotions requires an assessment of the beliefs, desires, and values that constitute them. In this sense, the virtues are more basic to an agent's character. My point is not that one cannot have good emotions without being virtuous; obviously one can. My point is, rather, that the goodness of emotions is conceptually parasitic on the values that constitute emotions. Virtues are not identical to values, of course. But because virtues embody the agent's basic valuational outlook, they are more basic than emotions. And because, in sum, the virtues are conceptually more basic than emotions in the assessment of character, it follows that it is wrong to equate emotions with virtues.

The third reason that emotions cannot be virtues is because virtues, on a plausible understanding of them, are dispositions to feel and exhibit the right emotions, at the right times, towards the right objects, and so forth. As one author puts it, "[virtue] lies in the way in which an emotion is felt, not in the simple feeling of the emotion as such" (Carr 1999, 417). It would not, according to this understanding of what a virtue is, make much sense to claim that emotions are virtues. For consider what claim we would end up with, namely, that "emotions are dispositions to feel and exhibit the right emotions." This would be patently circular. At the very least, Solomon owes us a plausible conception of what a virtue is such that under that conception, having emotions be virtues would amount to a sensible, or, at the very least, noncircular claim. The underlying thought behind this third reason is that having and exhibiting an emotion, as such, is not necessarily morally good. People have and display emotions all the time, and yet in many cases they are morally at fault for doing this in the ways and on the occasions that they do. Without the interference of practical wisdom, and without having the disposition to have and display the emotions in all the right ways, how could an emotion be a virtue? And if Solomon intends the claim that emotions can be virtues to mean that they are dispositions to feel and exhibit the emotion in question in the right ways, then how would his proposal differ from Aristotle's? After all, and as we have seen, Solomon takes himself to be disagreeing with, and adding to, Aristotle's views.

If my reasoning is correct, then Solomon is wrong to think that emotions can be virtues. Emotions and virtues are conceptually distinct types of entities. We can then safely conclude, given the arguments of this section, that romantic love is indeed an emotion, though it is not a virtue. I turn next to its connections to virtue.

3. The Virtues and Romantic Love

In this section, I explore two ways in which romantic love and the virtues are possibly connected. The first is that the virtues structure romantic love. The vagueness of the term "structured" notwithstanding, I will argue that this claim is false. Instead, I will argue for the second way in which romantic love connects with the virtues, namely, that the virtues enable romantic love.

3.1. The Virtues Structure Romantic Love

Romantic love is an emotion; it is not a virtue, nor is it simply an attitude. Romantic love as an attitude is conceptually and causally parasitic on the emotion of romantic love. What romantic love as an attitude, given Martin's (1996) claims, amounts to is the idea that romantic love is not fleeting: it is a way of life in and by which two people relate to each other. In this sense, romantic love is consuming in that it takes up an important dimension of lovers' lives. The beloved's ends and goals, for example, become part of the goals and ends of the lover's. They *constrain* the latter's life plans and aspirations. They do so, of course, not in the negative sense of coercing the lover to heed the demands of her beloved, but in the sense of the lover wanting and desiring that the beloved's goals and aims be promoted and the lover realizing that her well-being is bound up with the well-being of her beloved. In this respect, caring and concern for the beloved's well-being are concepts that are essential to that of romantic love.

Martin's main thesis in his book is that if we are to speak of true romantic love, of a love that truly promotes and protects the well-being of the beloved, then the language of virtue becomes indispensable: "Love is internally connected with morality, but primarily in terms of virtues and ideals rather than duties" (178). To this end, we can distinguish, according to Martin, between virtues that structure or constitute romantic love, and virtues that enable it. I will first explore this distinction and then argue that it cannot be maintained on the grounds that Martin offers.

Martin claims that some virtues structure romantic love simply in the sense that when we speak of true love, reference to moral terms is ineliminable: "Moral values define love as ways to value persons" (10), and "Moral values enter into the very meaning of genuine love by structuring relationships and shaping experiences" (15). Examples of such constitutive virtues are caring, faithfulness, honesty and fairness (57), and wisdom, given that wisdom enters all the virtues (133). To Martin, caring is *the* essential virtue in true love, given that it is the virtue that targets people in their full individuality and tends to their well-being (42), and faithfulness is not the same as sexual fidelity, which is narrower in scope. Viewing romantic love as structured by these virtues implies that, if x loves y, then x cares for y, x "makes a sustained effort to understand" y, x respects y, x is willing to trust y, x is honest with y, x is grateful for the joy y brings x, and x summons courage in times of crisis (139).

By contrast to the constitutive virtues, there are the enabling virtues, such as sexual fidelity (75), courage (149), prudence, perseverance (57), and gratitude (164) (what complicates matters are Martin's claims, on pages 149 and 164, that courage and gratitude are *also* constitutive virtues). To claim of some virtues that they enable true love is simply to claim that they play an important role in allowing the love to succeed or fail, but that this role is of guidance and providing motivation for good conduct that allows the love to flourish. Sexual fidelity, for example, is an enabling virtue because it is *one optional* way that couples can enhance and protect the commitment to love each other (77). It is an enabling virtue, then, because it is not necessarily part of the primary commitment to love each other; some couples may have recourse to it as a way to protect and enhance this commitment, but other couples may fasten on other ways.[34]

But I wonder whether the distinction between constitutive and enabling virtues can be maintained. Consider how Martin handles an objection to the effect that his use of the example of Ingmar Bergman's *Scenes from a Marriage* does not vindicate his thesis that the virtues of caring, faithfulness, respect, honesty, fairness, courage, and gratitude are constitutive of romantic love, but that they only enable it. In response, Martin states,

> To the extent these virtues are present, their [Marianne and Johan's] love is present, vibrantly alive; as these virtues recede, their love shrivels. The love shrivels not as a causal aftermath of the virtues' absence, but as part of the meaning of the *relationship* defined by those virtues. That is obvious with regard to caring. Without deep caring the relationship might involve pleasant coexistence but not love. But in addition, the caring is embedded in many of the other virtues. . . . Again, try abstracting from the virtues of respect, honesty, and fairness and see if the *marriage* would amount to the same thing. These virtues structure and define what their love is (20–21, my emphasis).

It should not take much philosophical acumen to notice that this response by Martin is not an adequate reply to the objection. Not only does it merely reiterate Martin's position, it actually unwittingly both makes the objection plausible and leads to the collapse of the distinction between constitutive and enabling virtues. First, in stating that the love of Marianne and Johan shrivels as part of the meaning of—as Martin should have said— "love" and not as a causal aftermath, Martin merely reiterates his own position in the face of the objection.

Second, Martin uses the words "relationship" and "marriage" instead of "love." This is a serious error, because it ends up strengthening the objection: the objection requires an explanation as to how the virtues structure, rather than enable, romantic *love*. For we already know that a good *relationship* is one whose parties are honest, fair, respectful, caring, and so on to each other. When Martin uses "relationship" instead of "love," he is in fact giving the objection more ammunition by not telling us how romantic *love* rather than a relationship is structured and constituted by virtues. The fact, moreover, that Martin explicitly uses "love" in his book to refer to attitudes and relationships (57) does not get him out of this difficulty. For there is a sense of "true love" which does not refer to relationships or attitudes: it refers, simply, to the emotion and its attendant desires. How many times have we heard it said that in true love one desires to benefit one's beloved, to protect him, to be honest with him, to respect him, and so on? Yet this sense does not refer to relationships, but to the emotion and its desires: when *x* loves *y*, *x* desires to do so-and-so to *y*. It is this other common usage of "true love" that the objection could be construed as referring to, and Martin's response to the objection does not evince an awareness of this sense, let alone a mention and a discussion of it. It does not, in short, tell us why the virtues are constitutive of this sense of romantic love rather than simply enablers of it.

Moreover, Martin's response leads to the erasure of the distinction between constitutive and enabling virtues: if we speak of relationships and marriages, then it is hard to see *what* virtue could be an enabling and not a constitutive one. Martin gives courage and gratitude as examples of enabling virtues, yet he also claims that they are constitutive ones, and his discussion of them, both in their respective chapters and in the example of Marianne and Johan, focuses on their constitutive role, without clearly telling the reader how either virtue functions or can function as an enabling one. Furthermore, it is difficult to see how Martin *can* discuss them as enabling virtues given his response to the objection. For it is hard to see how taking courage or gratitude away from a relationship would *not* make the relationship shrivel, and this is the criterion that Martin uses to argue that the virtues are constitutive of romantic love.

The only virtue that Martin is able to make a good case for as an enabling one is that of sexual fidelity. It is enabling, as I said, because it is optional: a couple may use it to protect and strengthen their commitment to love each other. This makes sense as far as sexual fidelity's role as an enabler of romantic love relationships and marriages are concerned. Yet Martin's choice of sexual fidelity as a *virtue* faces a different kind of difficulty: it is not clear why it is a *virtue* to begin with, rather than a good policy, or a rule, or a habit for some couples to adopt to protect their love and relationship. Martin never argues for the claim that sexual fidelity is a virtue or that it can be plausibly thought of as one, and it is hard to see how he could do so. Virtues are universal human traits and so their moral value and importance do not vary from one individual to another or from one society to another. Simply put, if a trait is a virtue, then it is morally and rationally desirable to have (Martin's discussion of pluralism, moreover, does not commit him to a relativism of the virtues; indeed, he expressly denies relativism on page 27). But then if sexual fidelity is a virtue, how can some couples dispense with it? This shows that sexual fidelity is better thought of as, for some couples, a good habit to cultivate or a good rule to adopt. Nor is it clear how Martin could think of sexual fidelity as a virtue given his understanding of virtues as "patterns of character." Sexual fidelity is a way of conducting oneself given a decision to keep one's relationship sexually exclusive. In this respect, it is not easy to see how it can be a pattern of character, given the thought that one can be sexually faithful but be so begrudgingly.

It seems, then, that Martin's view faces difficulties for two main reasons. First, his position that romantic love is an attitude or a relationship is, even though it captures one sense of "romantic love," unconvincing because it does not seem to capture the essence of this attitude, which is love as an emotion. Second, because Martin understands "love" in terms of relationships and actual attitudes, he fails to make the distinction between constitutive virtues and enabling ones convincing. However, there is one crucial truth to Martin's claims, which is this: it is indisputable that in order to make a romantic love *relationship* successful and fulfilling, the parties in the relationship must act and behave in ways that the virtuous person would. I have put this claim in terms of acting and behaving because of one slight worry I have with respect to couching the discussion in terms of relationships. The worry is this: if we speak of relationships, then, with the possible exception of caring, all that it takes for a relationship to be successful is that the parties in it are *continent*. Continent agents can be honest, wise, brave, faithful, fair, and so on in their *actions*, and so *act* as a virtuous person would. But, given the usual definition of "continence," they would have to struggle against contrary desires in order to act properly. No doubt, were the parties to be virtuous, they would have a morally better relationship. But the point is that when we shift the discussion to relationships, we need to be very careful, because continent agents can successfully fit Martin's views about what a morally good romantic love relationship is, and this ushers in the danger that Martin ultimately fails to use the notion of the virtues in the best possible way. Once this is conceded, and once it is also conceded that romantic love is an emotion, it becomes difficult to see how the virtues can structure romantic love, given that it is more plausible to claim that emotions partly constitute the virtues, rather than the other way around. (I am not advocating this latter claim, because it is not clear to me what it really means. My statement that it is more plausible to make this claim is simply due to the fact that it seems closer to the claim that the virtues dispose their agents to exhibit emotions appropriately.) So I turn next to the claim that the virtues enable romantic love.

3.2. The Virtues Enable Romantic Love

As we have seen, speaking of moral romantic love in terms of relationships ultimately falls short of giving the virtues the best role to play in a discussion about moral romantic love, because relationships can be morally successful even if the lovers (or one of them) are continent. They can be fair to each other, they can tell each other the truth, they can be courageous in facing adversity, and they can be faithful to each other. They can act in these ways and yet do so, to put the point in simple terms, grudgingly, without desiring to do so, as continent agents act and feel. So we need to bring in the virtues into this discussion in a different way.

There are two other ways to think of the virtues as enabling romantic love. Romantic love is an emotion and so it can be generally thought of as being constituted by beliefs and desires. It is a dispositional emotion, and usually a longstanding one. If one essential desire in romantic love is the desire to promote and protect the well-being of the beloved, then the lover would be disposed to act on this desire. The virtues would enable romantic love in the sense that they would morally guide the lover to feel and act on this desire in morally appropriate ways. And if the beliefs of romantic love are about the properties of the beloved, then the lover would be disposed to accept well-grounded beliefs about his beloved. The virtues would guide the lover to accept those beliefs that he can back and justify. Moreover, romantic love, like care, involves the disposition to be receptive and open to the needs and desires of the beloved. The receptivity of romantic love also disposes the lover to appreciate the beloved. In the virtuous lover, the virtues would morally guide this dispositional receptivity and openness. The idea here is not *only* that the virtues would perform these functions in actual relationships, but also that they offer romantic love a morally appropriate shelter in the body and psyche of the virtuous person.

In sheltering the desires and beliefs of romantic love in a morally appropriate abode, the virtues not only imply that the moral health of the beloved would be sought after in appropriate ways, but also that the moral health of the lover and of those people who are neither the lover nor the beloved (third parties) would also be sought after in such ways. In the remainder of this section, I will elaborate on these two theses, and I will further discuss them in the face of two objections. The first objection argues that given the possibility of a limited unity of the virtues, the second thesis cannot be sustained. The second objection is the Stoic-inspired one that romantic love is inimical to the virtues, and so neither thesis can be sustained. I will reject both of these objections.

Let us call the first thesis the "virtuous love thesis." The virtuous love thesis simply states that as far as the beloved is concerned, for romantic love to be good, it needs to issue from a virtuous character. As Gabriele Taylor puts it, "So there lurks the Aristotelian thought that only the good man can offer a love which is not defective" (1979, 180). The "only" in Taylor's formulation is too strong: the virtuous love thesis should certainly not be construed as sufficient for good love. For it is obvious that x's romantic love, despite x's virtuousness, can meet with misfortunes (for example, x can become clinically depressed), and so there goes the sufficiency claim. Whether the virtuous love thesis should be construed as necessary for good love is harder to decide. One can argue that it is possible that x's romantic love can be good (by luck or by accident) even if x is not virtuous, and so the virtuous love thesis is not a necessary condition for good love. I am not convinced that such a possibility exists. Nonetheless, perhaps we should keep the possibility open, especially when doing so does not lead to a substantive loss in the content of the virtuous love thesis. Let us then construe this thesis as a probability claim: being virtuous makes romantic love's goodness, as far as the beloved is concerned, highly likely; and the fact that x's love for y is good indicates strongly that x is virtuous. But let us now say a bit more about the content of the virtuous love thesis.

Let us look at some of the desires found in romantic love.[35] Suppose that if Roxane loves Issa, then she would desire to protect and enhance his well-being (flourishing), she would desire his company, she would desire Issa to reciprocate her love, and she would desire to make him happy (in terms of *feeling* happiness, as opposed to *flourishing*). This list is not exhaustive, of course, but it does contain four desires that can be plausibly thought of as typical of romantic love. And some of the desires, such as the first and the fourth, are intimately connected: promoting one's well-being is one way to render one happy, and making one happy is one way to promote one's well-being. Nevertheless, the two are not the same as can be obviously seen in cases in which one's well-being does not coincide with one's feeling happy. Now the virtuous love thesis states that all of these desires would be attended to well, in morally good ways, were x—Roxane—to be virtuous.

To be virtuous is to have and exercise the virtues. The virtues include moral wisdom that pervades the rest (a bit more on this below), which orients the virtuous person towards the good, and which allows the agent to act rightly and perceptively. What the virtuous love thesis requires us to accept is its underlying claim that romantic love is not an anomalous or a unique event in the virtuous person's life *in the sense* that it would not lead the virtuous person to behave out of character (the second objection I will discuss, however, targets this very claim). When the virtuous person falls in love or when she is in love, she might of course experience the euphoria and joys of romantic love, its attendant feelings of elation and happiness. In these respects, romantic love would be a unique—or a rare—event in the agent's life. But as far as virtue and acting virtuously are concerned, the virtuous person would not alter her moral behavior and thought in any serious way (again, I will come back to this issue when discussing the second objection).

An important implication of the virtuous love thesis is that the virtuous lover would tend to her romantic love-desires in a virtuous way. So, for example, regarding the desire to protect and enhance Issa's well-being, Roxane would do so in an objective sense, at least in an objective sense as compatible as possible with Issa's own desires, assuming that these desires depart from what she perceives to be Issa's good. This requires that Roxane attend carefully to what Issa's good consists in and to what is needed to protect and promote it. And all of these require the exercise of wisdom, and attention and sensitivity (to Issa's needs), and sometimes honesty (no deception about what Issa needs or lacks), courage (to face what might be difficult truths), perseverance, patience, and a host of other virtues. Similarly, in attending to Issa's desires in order to make Issa happy, Roxane would do so with an eye for his well-being, to make sure that his desires are at least compatible with what is good for him, while at the same time satisfying some of his desires (after all, attending to Issa's desires, even if these are inimical to his objective good, are part of Issa's autonomy).

Consider Roxane's desire to be with Issa or her desire for his company. Again, the virtuous lover would satisfy this desire in virtuous ways. Roxane would not, for example, exert pressure on Issa when she knows that he is busy or needs to attend to other matters. The general idea is that despite Roxane's desire for Issa's company, if Issa's needs require that Roxane spend less time with Issa, then she would temper her desire to be with him in the appropriate ways (and this applies as much to the case when they live together). Lastly, consider Roxane's desire that Issa reciprocate her love: again, given Issa's needs and circumstances, Roxane would not attempt to satisfy this desire at any expense. One can see in this discussion that Issa's well-being is primary in that it regulates how Roxane is to act on her other desires with respect to Issa. This should not be surprising, of course, given our earlier conclusion that concern for the well-being of the beloved is an essential feature of the concept of romantic love. One way in which one can love badly—morally badly, that is—is if one were to be unable to allow the beloved's well-being to temper one's other desires towards the beloved. In this respect, Roxane's virtues play the important role of allowing her to heed Issa's well-being appropriately, and in doing so, to regulate her acting on her other desires regarding Issa.

Turning now to beliefs, we are often told that even when romantic love is belief-based (*x* loves *y* for such-and-such reasons or because of such-and-such properties), there is no logical limit on what these reasons or properties might be. Eric, then, might love Elizabeth because she is smart, but David might love Mark because Mark can wiggle his ears. But as far as moral issues are concerned, "the logical 'anything goes' does not entail a 'moral anything goes'" as Soble puts it (1990, 282). Roxane, our virtuous agent, would love Issa for the morally right properties. It is hard, of course, to make a distinction between those properties that are morally appropriate and those that are not. But a plausible proposal is to restrict them to those nontrivial properties that capture the identity and core of the beloved. This would be the first restriction. A way to restrict them even further is to include in the latter set only those properties that are also *generally* worthwhile. This would be the second restriction. So, for example, Roxane might love Issa for his looks, and, in the case of Issa, his looks do form his core and his identity given that he has been a model and an entertainer for almost all of his adult life. But if we were to go by the further restriction, then this romantic love might not be fit for a virtuous person given that looks might not be worthwhile and important human properties.

My aim here is not to decide the issue, but to indicate in what ways a virtuous agent's romantic love might track certain types of properties rather than others. Furthermore, there are good cases to be made for each of the above restrictions. For instance, regarding the first restriction, since romantic love is thought of as being not only a nonfleeting emotion, but a longstanding one, one might argue that Roxane's loving Issa because of his identity properties makes it more likely that her love for him is durable since her reasons for loving him are anchored in properties without which Issa would not be Issa.[36] Regarding the second restriction, one might argue that what makes a romantic love good is not just the fact that Roxane loves Issa because of his identity-conferring properties, but also because these are important in general. Identity-conferring properties distinguish silly and shallow romantic loves from serious and deep ones, which are usually more lasting.

But what has virtue got to do with all of this? The idea is simple: the virtuous person is oriented towards the good. She knows, given her wisdom, what is worthwhile and what is not, what is shallow and what is not, what is important to keep and to defend and what is not. Her valuational system, we might say, is correct. And romantic love is no exception: a virtuous person's love would simply not be ultimately based on qualities that she deems unimportant. This parallels to a good extent Aristotle's discussion of pleasure: "In fact, however, the pleasures differ quite a lot, in human beings at any rate. For the same things delight some people and cause pain to others. . . . But in all such cases it seems that what is really so is what appears so to the excellent person . . . what appear pleasures to him will also *be* pleasures, and what is pleasant will be what he enjoys" (1985, 1176a10–19). Commenting on Aristotle's views, Julia Annas states, "For Aristotle, one cannot pursue pleasure regardless of the moral worth of the actions that are one's means to getting it. Rather it is the other way around: it is one's conception of the good life which determines what counts for one as being pleasant" (1980, 288).

Aristotle makes two points in the above quoted passage. First, that pleasures cannot be compared on a single scale because they differ in as much as the activities on which they supervene differ. Second, that what is *really* pleasurable is decided by the virtuous person.[37] The virtuous person's decision is not arbitrary, of course, but correct since such a person uses wisdom to arrive at his knowledge. What this claim implies, and what is of concern to us, is that the virtuous person would simply not find certain pleasures to be pleasures. At the very least, if the virtuous person were unable to expunge his desire for such pleasures, he would nevertheless not pursue them. Whether this amounts to a form of objective correctness (Aristotle's second point) is an issue I will set aside. The point I want to apply to romantic love is the much more easily acceptable one that the virtuous person would not find certain qualities in others conducive to loving these others because she would not find them constitutive of good reasons to love.

It is important, however, to clear away certain misconceptions. First, that the virtuous person would not find that such-and-such properties to be good reasons to love does not entail that falling in love or loving *y* is a matter of choice for the virtuous person. The idea is not that *x*, where *x* is a virtuous person, can decide, based on reasons, as to whether she is to love *y*. The idea, rather, is that *y*'s unworthy properties would not serve as the *ultimate* reasons as to why *x* loves *y* because these properties are not ones that *x* finds worthwhile to begin with. Thus, the insight that falling in love is not a matter of choice can be preserved on this view (although one could argue, of course, that this insight is false and need not be preserved).[38]

Second, and connected to the first point, we must keep in mind that we are speaking here of *love*, and true love at that, not of infatuation or crushes or bouts of lust confused with love or even short-lived love affairs.[39] The virtuous person is not immune to these. Even though she has wisdom, this does not mean that she can never be infatuated with someone just because of the way he sits at her local café, or that she can never have a crush on someone just because of her good looks, or that she can never confuse love with sex, or that she can never be misled into thinking that *this* love is going to last for a good amount of time. Indeed, such features might *cause* a virtuous person to fall in love in the first place. But what they cannot do is play the role of the ultimate justificatory reasons on which the virtuous person's romantic love is based. And, we may add, what her wisdom and virtue imply is that she would be serious about checking on the truth of her beliefs and feelings before she allows herself to get serious with another (more on this shortly).

Third, and connected with the second point, it is crucial to keep in mind that the picture of virtuous, romantic love being presented here does not entail that the virtuous person cannot or does not feel passion. Falling in love (as opposed to infatuation, lust, and having crushes) is often (not always) experienced very passionately. Lovers feel euphoria usually unparalleled in other experiences, they desire to be with each other constantly, and they tend to play down the importance of the rest of the world. Fortunately for the rest of the world, however, this feeling of passion does not last, though the love—though not in every case—does. The point to keep in mind now is that nothing I have written about virtuous, romantic love entails the denial of virtuous people experiencing this passion. Furthermore, much as unworthy properties of a beloved can *cause* the virtuous person to be infatuated with him or her, so can they cause the virtuous person to feel the passion of love. In this respect, the virtuous person is not immune from making mistakes. Indeed, the virtuous love thesis does not deny the possibility that a virtuous person x would fall in love with y even if x saw y for what y truly is (unworthy of love). Because the very properties that can cause x to be infatuated with y can also cause x to fall in love with y (assuming that there is a defensible distinction between infatuation and falling in love), x can, while seeing that y is a scoundrel, fall in love with y because of y's good looks. Rather, the virtuous love thesis claims that, probably, such a falling in love would be of the kind that does not last, precisely because the initial causes cannot serve, for the virtuous person, as justificatory reasons for the love. To deny that virtuous people can fall in love despite the beloved's general unworthiness would be, no doubt, to assert an interesting and meaty claim. But the price for doing so would be too high. It would go against many examples that abound in our world, literature, and movies, and it would turn the virtuous person into someone who is immune to the contingencies of life, a false picture of the virtuous to say the least.

Fourth, nothing follows from what I have said about the virtuous person's ability to "have fun." The fact that virtuous people romantically love (and are in love) for certain reasons and not for others does not entail that the activities they engage in with their beloveds (or others or by themselves, for that matter) are restricted to serious sessions of reading Marcel Proust, or to bouts of attending lectures on the fate of the cosmos, or to hopping from one art gallery to another. Of course, such activities are enjoyable, but the idea is that virtuous lovers can also enjoy the usual, non-intellectual type of fun activities. They can run along the beach, they can ride roller coasters with the usual fits of screaming and laughter, they can have their occasional banana splits, and they can nibble on each other's toes.

There is another point to be made about the beliefs in romantic love. If Eric's beliefs about Elizabeth, the beliefs that ground Eric's romantic love, are negligent, are arrived at or formed superficially, then this is a moral fault, and not simply an epistemic one, because as far as Elizabeth is concerned, she would be led to believe that Eric loves her, and this engenders expectations, desires, and beliefs in her. Soble puts the point well:

> creating all these beliefs in y on the basis of negligently false beliefs is a moral injury to y, since x will likely discover later that x's beliefs that y has S [the properties on which x's love for y is based] are false, and the love-related desires and concerns will dissipate. Indeed, it is plausible to claim that if x does want to be able to justify x's special, preferential concern for y, x is under an obligation to ascertain without negligence that y does have the S that grounds x's love. (1990, 284–85)

In terms of virtue, Eric's wisdom and his concern for Elizabeth—not just as a potential beloved but also as a human being worthy of decent treatment—would lead Eric to ascertain the truth of his beliefs about Elizabeth as much as is reasonably expected in such situations. This would allow Elizabeth to have the appropriate expectations, beliefs, and desires. In short, were Eric to be virtuous, then virtue would enable him to try to fulfill the obligation to find out whether Elizabeth does indeed have the properties that Eric believes she has.

Before discussing the second thesis, a few words are in order about the receptivity of romantic love. Receptivity or open-mindedness can be both action-oriented, as when the lover is receptive to the needs and the desires of his beloved and acts on these, or it can be non–action oriented, as when the lover is receptive to the qualities of his beloved and is led to appreciate them. Appreciation, moreover, is not an action, at least not in the usual way we understand the notion of "action," and that is why I claimed that receptivity is partly non–action oriented. Since receptivity in both of its forms is about desires and beliefs (appreciation necessarily includes beliefs about the beloved), I do not have much to add to the discussion above. I should note, however, that when a virtuous lover appreciates his beloved, he would do so by appreciating *her*, and not just her good qualities. Even though she might have some bad qualities, the virtuous lover, while not necessarily overlooking or ignoring these, would judge that overall they do not play a major role in terms of how worthy and good the beloved is. Of course, much depends on the nature of those bad qualities. But my assumption here is that the virtuous lover is already in a morally good romantic love relationship. If he is virtuous, and if all else is going well, then it would probably be the case that whatever bad qualities the beloved has are not so important as to lead the lover to abandon his love for her. The point is that the virtuous lover, just because he appreciates the beloved's good qualities, need not, and probably would not, appreciate some parts of the beloved while not appreciating others. Since in love we usually appreciate the whole person, the bad qualities, though they may be at times irritating or annoying, and so impossible to appreciate, would factor in an overall judgment of the beloved.

Let us now turn to the second thesis, and let us call it the "virtuous lover thesis." It states that as far as the nonbeloveds are concerned, for romantic love to be morally good, it needs to issue from a virtuous character. Like the virtuous love thesis, the virtuous lover thesis is also a thesis to be cashed out in terms of probability and not necessity and sufficiency. However, unlike the former thesis, the virtuous lover thesis branches out in its application to two types of people: the lover and all other human beings other than the beloved.

As far as the lover, x, is concerned, the general idea is that x's desires and beliefs in romantic love would be heeded in a virtuous way. That is to say, x's attending to her desires and beliefs would not be done at the expense of her own moral health. Eric would not, for example, attempt to satisfy his desire to be with Elizabeth at the expense of his own dignity. He would not try to make Elizabeth happy at the constant expense of his own well-being (I say "constant" because love is compatible with a certain amount of sacrifice; similarly for Eric's protecting and enhancing Elizabeth's well-being). Eric would not, finally, attempt to satisfy his desire that Elizabeth reciprocate his love if doing so would violate his integrity (if, for instance, Elizabeth's political views and actions are opposed to those of Eric).

Similar thoughts apply to the issue of beliefs about Elizabeth. Eric would attempt, given reasonable expectations, to make sure that his beliefs about Elizabeth are well grounded for the crucial reason that he would not want his romantic love to be mired in self-deception. Because Eric is one who desires his beliefs to be truthful or at least truth tracking, he would not want to love Elizabeth under false pretenses, so to speak. Moreover, Eric's self-respect would lead Eric to romantically love for the right reasons. He would not love Elizabeth simply because he is lonely or because he is desperate. Elizabeth's property of "ridding-me-of-loneliness" simply would not supply Eric with a good reason to love Elizabeth. As Soble puts it, due to self-respect "lovers are not able to think well of themselves if a strong need to be loved or to avoid solitude leads them to settle for anyone" (1990, 145).

But why should we believe this? Why believe that the virtues would lead the virtuous lover to tend to his own moral health? Why not, instead, claim that the preservation of the lover's moral integrity, self-respect, and well-being is an issue best left open, perhaps ultimately for the lover himself to decide? The reason this cannot be done is that it is inconsistent with being virtuous *and* with loving. It is inconsistent with the former because, and keeping in mind the discussion of integrity and care from the last chapter, the virtuous person is committed to moral ends, and, more importantly, recognizes that moral ends are important, if not overriding, ones (and he need not have any philosophical theory to back up this claim). If he were to allow his self-respect, his integrity, and his well-being to be sacrificed for the sake of romantic love, he would be allowing a serious blow to his moral character, and this would allow for the displacement of general moral ends, and, in their stead, the adoption of much narrower ones (such as the happiness of the beloved). And this is something that he could not allow, given his recognition of the importance of morality. Catherine Sloper, in Henry James's *Washington Square*, would not consent to even being friends with Morris Townsend, though she still loved him, precisely because he deceived her in pretending to love her and because he eventually left her upon realizing that, were he to marry her, he would not be able to get a penny of her money. Though she never married after he left her, she could not accept his friendship when he later came back into her life, and she could not accept it precisely because of her integrity.

Furthermore, sacrificing his (the agent's or lover's) own moral health is inconsistent with loving. For if the virtuous lover has any wisdom at all, he would realize that tending to the well-being of the beloved must be done carefully and morally. Otherwise, his romantic love might be defective and might seriously affect his beloved in negative ways. In this respect, the virtuous lover cannot accept such a sacrifice of his moral health, since it would lead to an insecure path on which to tend to his beloved morally.

Turning next to people other than x and y, the idea is simply that x's romantic love for y would not lead x to neglect to attend to other people's moral demands and claims on x. I should say at the outset that this claim is *not* that x would treat y in an entirely nonpreferential or nonpartial manner. The claim is much weaker: x would not neglect the fact that people other than y have legitimate expectations of a moral nature from x. This claim, it

should also be noted, is not a straw man. Love has the tendency—and not
just in its passionate phases—to push the lovers into a world of their own,
where they tend to believe that their beloveds always come first, morally
speaking. It is this claim that the virtuous lover thesis opposes.

Consider another example from literature. In *The Mill on the Floss* by
George Eliot, Maggie Tulliver, the main character, promises her love to
Philip Wakem, the son of her father's enemy. There is good reason to
believe that her love for him is based on the affections of friendship rather
than the usual passion of love. Also, because of the relationship between
their fathers, and because of the obstinancy of her brother, Tom, to preserve the honor of their father at any cost, Maggie and Philip could not see
each other in public, let alone marry. Moreover, while Maggie was visiting
her cousin Lucy for an extended stay, she meets Stephen Guest, a man who
is understood to be attached to Lucy, even though he has not made any
formal proposal. Maggie and Stephen fall in love with each other. Stephen
is insistent that she marry him. But Maggie would not agree:

> "Good God!" he burst out at last, "what a miserable thing is a woman's love
> to a man's! I could commit crimes for you—and you can balance and choose
> in that way. But you *don't* love me: if you had a tithe of the feeling for me that
> I have for you, it would be impossible to you to think for a moment of sacri-
> ficing me. But it weighs nothing with you that you are robbing me of *my* life's
> happiness."
>
> "No—I don't sacrifice you—I couldn't sacrifice you," she said . . . "but I
> can't believe in a good for you, that I feel—that we both feel is a wrong towards
> others. We can't choose happiness either for ourselves or for another: we can't
> tell where that will lie. We can only choose whether we will indulge ourselves
> in the present moment, or whether we will renounce that, for the sake of obey-
> ing the divine voice within us—for the sake of being true to all the motives that
> sanctify our lives. I know this belief is hard: it has slipped away from me again
> and again; but I have felt that if I let it go for ever, I should have no light
> through the darkness of this life." (477)

Under more pressure from Stephen, Maggie continues to resist, and she
invokes Philip, the fact that she does care for him, and the fact that he
expects her to be "the promise of his life." And she invokes Lucy and
Lucy's trust in her, concluding, "I cannot marry you: I cannot take a good
for myself that has been wrung out of their misery" (478).

I think that one can make a good case that Maggie Tulliver is reasonably virtuous (though I won't go into this here). If so, then this example
illustrates well how a virtuous person would refuse to justify and indulge
her love for another when such love is at the moral expense of others.

But the example illustrates only one aspect of the virtuous lover thesis, namely, how a virtuous person would not act on her romantic love. What the example does not illustrate is how the virtuous person would act towards others when already in a love relationship with another. In this regard, the reader should keep in mind that much of what has been said in the first chapter on partiality and care applies with equal force here, and I will not repeat the points and arguments. Suffice it to say that we should remember that most ethical theories allow for a good amount of room generally for moral agents to prefer their loved ones. However, it is also important to remember that such a preference and partiality is not always justified, and it is not always justified precisely because it comes at the expense of the moral claims of others. It is not morally permissible to violate just procedures in order to give one's beloved an advantage over others, for example. Nor is it morally justified to neglect the serious needs of strangers, especially when these can be met with a bit of effort, because the agent wants to attend to the needs of his beloved, when these needs can wait. This, I should add, holds in particular cases and in general, as a way of life, though I will not argue the point. Regarding the former, we should recall the case of the stranger who is in desperate need of attention as opposed to the beloved who is simply momentarily terrified. Regarding the latter, it is immoral to spend all of one's resources and energy on one's beloved (and circle of cared-fors) when some of these can be used, either by the agent herself or by others, to help distant others in need. To do so is simply to lack the virtue of charity in deep and pervasive ways, and this is—again simply—nonvirtuous.

The concept of romantic love is an essentially moral concept, given that it contains the notion of concern or care for the well-being of the beloved. If this is so, then romantic love can be morally good or morally defective. I have argued that the virtues enable romantic love in the deep sense that they provide it with a morally decent abode. When romantic love issues from a virtuous character, it is enabled because it is given in a truly moral form. And it is enabled in the best of ways, for its morality no longer concerns *just* the beloved and ensuring that the beloved is treated and loved rightly, but also concerns the lover and the people who are not part of the love, from friends and family members to strangers in distant lands. The tensions between romantic love and morality are done away with not just because we can see how romantic love can be moral as far as the beloved is concerned, but also how it can be moral as far as the lover and others are concerned. But now I turn to two objections against the virtuous love and the virtuous lover theses.

3.2.1. FIRST OBJECTION: THE LIMITED UNITY OF THE VIRTUES

The first objection needs some stage setting by way of some remarks about the issue of the unity of the virtues. The view regarding the unity of the virtues is one of the more difficult issues to come to grips with in virtue ethics. Aristotle famously—or notoriously—held that moral wisdom entails all of the virtues and that the virtues entail moral wisdom (1985, 1144b20 and 1145a1). This is a strong claim, for it stipulates that one virtue entails the rest. But the unity of the virtues doctrine need not be formulated in terms of the entailment claim. It can be formulated in terms of the weaker implication one: one virtue materially implies all the others. On another reading—and I am not sure where to put this in terms of weakness and strength of its claim—the unity of the virtues is the claim that all the virtues are identical with each other, even though one virtue might manifest itself differently in different situations (and so that is how virtues come to have different names). On still another weaker reading, we can construe the claim of the unity of the virtues as the claim that all the virtues are compatible with each other, that is, *if* all the virtues exist in one agent (and they need not, on this view), they would not, not even in practice, conflict with one another (kindness and honesty, on this view, would never conflict).[40]

Most writers on virtue ethics accept neither the entailment nor the implication construal of the unity of the virtues doctrine.[41] They tend to accept instead an account of the doctrine that limits the unity of the virtues in some way or other. For example, one can claim that wisdom enters all the virtues, and it is in this respect that the virtues are unified: wisdom is a controlling virtue in that it is the one that decides which virtue ought to issue in action in a given situation.[42] Or one can accept a position that claims that an agent can have one virtue in one domain (be kind towards friends) and yet lack it in another (be nonkind towards strangers), that the existence of virtue in one domain is incompatible with the existence of *vice* in any other domain, and that every virtue implies the existence of others in the same domain. Or one can vary this account: one can claim that because of practical wisdom, one would be virtuous in all domains but in different degrees and strengths.[43]

Before we can formulate the objection, we need to make an important point: it seems that any plausible account of the unity of the virtues must include two minimal claims. First, that moral wisdom is not discrete: one cannot have it in one area of one's life and lack it in another. For one to have moral wisdom, one must have an adequate intellectual and emotional grasp of certain basic ethical concepts, such as those of well-being, happiness, comfort, suffering, and pain. In this respect, one's having moral wisdom cannot be compartmentalized. At worst, what can happen is that one can lack "the emotional dispositions and fine-tuned perception and grasp of facts" that characterize one's having robust moral wisdom (Badhwar 1996, 320). Wisdom ranges over understanding, emotional motivation and reaction, and perception. If one has moral wisdom, one must have ethical understanding in all domains, though one may have the latter two components in some domains but not in others.

Second, and because one has moral wisdom in such a general way, one cannot have virtue in one domain and have vice and ignorance in another domain. This is the minimal claim one can make if one is to preserve some unity of the virtues. The more hopeful of us would make a slightly stronger claim: that one must have virtue in all domains, though one might have it in weaker ways in some domains rather than others, in precisely the sense that one might not be as apt to perceive the ethically relevant aspects of the situation in the domain in which one has virtue to a weak degree, and/or one might not be emotionally engaged, either motivationally or reactively, in the appropriate way in that domain. If, for example, one has kindness in weak degrees as far as strangers are concerned, then on this claim one cannot be callous to their needs, though one might not notice them or emotionally react to them as readily as one would in the domain in which one has kindness in strong degrees.

The objection now goes as follows: unless the discussion of the virtuous lover thesis was conducted in the context of an ideally virtuous agent—one who has all the virtues to the highest degree possible in all the domains of life—then the plausibility of the virtuous lover thesis is seriously suspect. For consider a virtuous agent x who has virtue in one domain—say, the domain of loved ones—but lacks it in another domain—say, the domain of strangers. It would then be plausible to claim that x loves y well—morally well—yet does not give a hoot about strangers' claims. If this is possible, then the virtuous lover thesis is implausible. Furthermore, given the implausibility of any strong view of the unity of the virtues, we must accept a limited view of such a doctrine, and this implies that the case of x just outlined is indeed not only possible but quite convincing. If so, then it would follow that the virtuous lover thesis is implausible.

I have never seen this objection in print. However, the thought underlying it is often enough found in popular beliefs to the effect that one can be a (morally) wonderful lover and yet nasty to boot when it comes to acquaintances, or colleagues, or strangers. This thought can be even found in one philosopher's claims about love. Robert Solomon seems to believe that one can be a bastard to people not close to one (public persona) and yet be a good person to the wife (private persona) (1991, 512). Of course, popular beliefs are not necessarily about *virtuous* people who are in love, but about people, period, and so for all we know, it might be the case that a nonvirtuous person might be a lamb to her beloved and yet be a Beelzebub to strangers (though I have doubts about the plausibility of such cases). What I have done is to capture this popular belief in an objection specifically tailored to the connections between romantic love and virtue. Moreover, it is an objection that would come readily to mind as soon as we have the virtuous lover thesis and the limited view of the unity of the virtues before our minds.

Contrary to the objection, however, it would not follow from the objection's premises that the virtuous lover thesis is implausible. First, the objection must shift the discussion from ideally virtuous agents to agents who are virtuous along realistic lines. There is nothing wrong with this move as such. But making it would take much force out of the objection. For the objection would be much more powerful if it were able to hit at the virtuous lover thesis in its pure theoretical formulation, namely, as a thesis about virtuous agents in ideal forms. (There is also nothing suspect about discussing ideal virtuous agents; all moral theories usually assume an ideal picture of their moral agents.)

Second, and more importantly, the objection, for it to succeed even at the realistic level at which it pitches itself, must assume that romantic or erotic love comprises its own domain. Otherwise, it must place romantic love under the domain of the ambiguous "loved ones" (as I intentionally formulated it). But if it does the latter, then it will not work: for it will only tell us what we already know, namely, that it is possible for the virtuous agent to be more virtuous in that domain than in the domain of strangers. But we can accept this claim, surely, without having to accept what the objection is really claiming, namely, that one can romantically love *y* and yet be nonvirtuous or minimally virtuous in other domains. For the objection to do this, however, it must assume that romantic love comprises its own domain. Would this be plausible?

The answer is "no." There are important differences, of course, between loving *y* romantically and loving *y* nonromantically. But whatever these differences are, they cannot be so basic so as to constitute a domain different from that of loving those who are near and dear to *x*, in general. The caring and concern, for example, that are essential to romantic love are also essential to friendships, sibling love, and parental love. And *x*'s desire for *y*'s company characterizes friendship, if not also parental love (and to some extent sibling love). The reason is simple: the very virtues—such as care, kindness, generosity, and compassion—that go into attending to the beloved *y* go into attending to those particular others who are close to us.

It is then extremely difficult to carve out a conceptual domain for romantic love separate from that of other types of loved ones.

The objection does, however, point to a potential worry. The very basis it uses to launch itself is the idea that the unity of the virtues doctrine can be accepted only if construed in a limited way. If this were right, wouldn't it cast doubt on the virtuous lover thesis? Yes, but only because it would cast doubt on many claims in virtue ethics and any other moral theory which takes the virtues seriously. Virtue ethics must come to grips with the fact that it might have to be able to offer a realistic picture of the virtuous agent, and in this respect, thinking of a plausible way of construing the unity of the virtues becomes crucial. But whatever negative implications this would have, they would not be confined only to the virtuous lover thesis, but to any claim that assumes an ideally virtuous agent. And this result is not theoretically dangerous, because any theory must be able to formulate its claims in ideal (theoretical) ways if it is to deliver its goods. Kantian ethics cannot, for example, propose the claim that an action is right, if and only if an agent motivated by good will would do it, if it were replied that such a claim applies only to ideal agents. For similar reasons, virtue ethics cannot propose that an action is right if and only if a virtuous agent would do it (nor can motive utilitarianism or expected-utility utilitarianism similarly advance *their* claims about right actions).

The first objection, then, does not succeed. It cannot make the case against romantic love as such. It can only make the case against love in general, but it would not then be telling us anything new. It does point to a possible worry, but I have argued that the worry is not serious if we keep in mind what the tasks of moral theories are.

3.2.2. SECOND OBJECTION: THE INCOMPATIBILITY OF ROMANTIC LOVE AND VIRTUE

Unlike the first objection, this second one has appeared in print. Martha Nussbaum develops it at some length as a form of a Stoic objection, inspired generally by the Stoic idea of extirpating the emotions, against the compatibility of leading a virtuous life (along the lines which Aristotelians advocate) and having the ability to love romantically (hence my earlier use of the label "Stoic-inspired"). She does so by using Seneca's *Medea* as the main and detailed example that a Stoic could use to press the objection. Very roughly, and acknowledging that I cannot here do justice to Nussbaum's detailed and complex use of the play, Medea was a virtuous woman, and the object of her romantic love, Jason, was a worthy one. Yet

due to the passion of romantic love, Medea committed some moral atroc-
ities. More generally, the issue is the following: "The Aristotelian holds
that we can have passionate love in our lives and still be people of virtue
and appropriate action: that the virtuous person can be relied upon to love
the right sort of person in the right way at the right time, in the right relation to other acts and obligations" (1994, 441). This is basically the virtuous love thesis and the virtuous lover thesis rolled into one. But enter the
Stoic: "Seneca sternly tells us that this distinction is empty. There is no
erotic passion that reliably stops short of its own excess. The very way of
caring about an external uncontrolled object yields uncontrol in the soul:
in Medea's soul, strong and heroic; in Jason's, split (as most souls are)
between love of passion and fear of morality" (1994, 442). I should here
note, and this will be clear in the discussion below, that the word "passion"
in this context does not refer to what I earlier spoke of as "falling in love,"
that is, the early passionate phases of romantic love. The word "passion,"
rather, refers simply to romantic love. It is important to mention this so as
to correct the reader's possible reaction that this objection is only forceful
against *falling* in love, and not to *being* in love.

From Nussbaum's presentation of the Stoic objection, we can actually
gather four different ways of formulating the objection, and depending on
which formulation we tackle, the objection may or may not succeed against
the virtuous love and the virtuous lover theses. All of these four ways rely
on the idea that being in love is in tension with being virtuous, and so all
of them assume that *x*, the agent, is virtuous and is in love. Moreover, since
all rely on the same assumption, I will not, for the sake of avoiding confu-
sion, repeat it; instead, I will merely mention it in the first formulation of
the objection, so as to give the reader an idea of how each objection should
be fully stated. I should also be explicit and mention that these ways of formulating the objection are mine, not Nussbaum's.

The first way to formulate the objection, then, is this: even if *x* is virtuous, and if *x* is in love, then there is no safe guarantee that *x*'s romantic
love would not lead *x* to commit immoral, and so unvirtuous, acts. (The
clause, "if *x* is virtuous and if *x* is in love" is the assumption that underlies
all four objections and the one that I will not repeat). Nussbaum puts the
objection in this way when she formulates the Stoic rejoinder to the
Aristotelian claim that the virtuous person is "mild and not prone to vindictiveness" (442). The second way to formulate the objection is stronger:
x's romantic love would in all likelihood lead *x* to commit immoral, and so
unvirtuous, acts. Nussbaum presents the Stoic objection in this way in the
course of responding to the sensible Aristotelian claim that not all romantic loves involve committing immoral acts because of love. The Stoic

rejoinder, as rendered by Nussbaum, is to list examples of bad actions as evidence of "the risks and uncertainties associated with erotic passion": divorce, abuse, betrayal, vindictive reprisals between lovers, manipulation of emotions, financial warfare, and excessive litigation (472). This response indicates that the Stoic believes that romantic love is almost always likely to lead to immoral action. Hence my second formulation of the objection.

The third way of formulating the objection is suggested by Nussbaum's reply (on behalf of the Stoic) to the Aristotelian claim that it is true that often enough harm to someone or other, due to romantic love, cannot be avoided. But, the Aristotelian continues, "a good person will do the harm with reluctance, without anger, as unfortunate necessity. He will do everything possible to promote the neglected good later on, to make reparations" (474). I do not think that the Aristotelian must be committed to the claim that the harm will be done without anger, given the Aristotelian's other claim that anger, like many other emotions, is justified in certain cases. But we can set this point aside. The point we should retain is the idea that harm is often necessary and unavoidable and what needs to be addressed is how it is to be dealt with; in this respect, a virtuous person would deal with it appropriately, to put the point generally.

Now the Stoic response is that this claim is "self-serving cant": the harm would have been avoided had the person not been in love and/or had he not valued romantic love (474). This leads to the third formulation of the objection, namely, that there is no guarantee that romantic love would not lead x to do harmful things (to himself, to his beloved, and/or to his children, if he has any). But given the examples of destruction mentioned above, we can formulate the objection in a fourth way: x's romantic love would in all likelihood lead x to do harmful things (to himself, to his beloved, and/or to his children, if he has any). I have not mentioned "virtue" or "virtuousness" in the last two formulations of the objection on purpose, of course. Because speaking of harms is different from speaking of immoral acts, what the Stoic considers to be self-serving cant might actually be an important distinction. Let us call these four formulations of the objection, respectively (and blandly), O1, O2, O3, and O4.

I want to dismiss, out of hand, O3 and O4 for two reasons. First, they reject the distinction between virtuous acts and harmful acts, and this is a distinction, it seems to me, that an Aristotelian cannot dispense with, without having her position on moral action succumb to a form of consequentialism, and a crass one at that. Virtuous actions could result in, or have as part of them, harms and hurts (and these are not identical) to one or more of the parties involved. Being honest can sometimes lead to hurt feelings and to some serious damage to the party one is being honest to and/or to other parties involved. Being courageous can lead the agent to being maimed or even killed. *All* virtues can issue in actions that contain an amount of harm, and there is no difficulty in constructing cases that show this.

Second, we must keep in mind that the objection Nussbaum raises on behalf of the Stoic against the Aristotelian has to do with the truth of either position regarding the place of the emotions—and romantic love in particular—in a good life. Now when it comes specifically to O3 and O4, the plausibility of these formulations of the objection pertains especially to the Stoic idea of the extirpation of the passions and the emotions. For without this idea, it is hard to see why anyone would want to advise that we can avoid harm by simply not being in love or by not valuing it. But if so, it is crucial to keep in mind that we are not here questioning the truth of Aristotelianism in light of the Stoic idea of extirpating the passions. In this respect, O3 and O4 are cases of overkill and pertain to issues that are outside the scope of the issues of this book. Also, once this is kept in mind, we can see that, and despite its Stoic rejection, there is no difficulty in accepting the distinction between virtuous acts and harmful acts maintained in the above paragraph.

So we are left with O1 and O2, objections that go beyond the specifically Stoic context that generated them. To remind the reader, the objections are as follows. O1: even if x is virtuous, there is no safe guarantee that x's romantic love would not lead x to commit immoral, and so unvirtuous, acts. O2: x's romantic love would in all likelihood lead x to commit immoral, and so unvirtuous, acts. It seems to me that O1 is pretty much innocuous, even though one or two things can be said by way of response to it, while O2 is unconvincing. I will start with the latter since handling it first makes handling O1 much easier.

Consider the examples given of acts of immorality and destruction by people in love and committed because of romantic love (Nussbaum 1994, 472). What would it require to make their use in the case against the Aristotelian convincing? One thing for certain: we need examples of couples who are *virtuous*. After all, the objection is offered against the Aristotelian, not against someone who claims that people, virtuous or non-virtuous, will commit bad acts due to romantic love. Yet Nussbaum's list of examples is silent on this; perhaps we are supposed to assume that the lovers are virtuous. But we cannot do this, because the whole point hinges on the lovers being virtuous; this is what needs to be offered convincingly if the examples are to do their job. Furthermore, it seems to me that most people are far from being virtuous. Here is how Rosalind Hursthouse, in a different context, nicely puts it: "Does anyone think that most human beings are good human beings? Does anyone think that, regarding ourselves as a collection of social groups or as one global one, we are flourishing, living well, as human beings? Surely not. We know that, ethically, many of us are rather poor ethical specimens, and when 'we' . . . think about how life is for the majority of other human beings, 'we' know that our . . . aspirations to live well even as healthy animals, let alone as human beings, are still, in general, but unrealized hopes" (1999b, 223).[44]

But what about those people who are indeed virtuous? Would love likely lead them to commit unvirtuous acts? It is extremely difficult to answer this question because it requires some serious empirical data. In my rejoinder to O1, I will offer one important nonempirical consideration to support the claim that the answer to the second question is "not likely." But for now, consider two examples from literature. First, here is Jane Eyre, a woman whose fault, if she has any, is that she is *too* virtuous, and who is in the throes of romantic love with Edward Rochester. Upon finding out that he has a wife—a mad one, but a wife nonetheless—Jane does the only thing she could morally do: leave him. She did not leave him out of vindictiveness, or to punish him; she left him because if she did not she would have to live with him as his mistress, and this she could not do, and rightly so, given the societal norms prevalent at the time. In leaving him, she hurt Rochester and herself, as any departure between two people in romantic love is bound to hurt them. But she did not do something unvirtuous; indeed, as far as we can tell, Jane Eyre, romantic love or no romantic love, has *never* done anything unvirtuous. She is a paradigm of virtue, and this is precisely the example we want in order to offer a case in which a virtuous person is not led to do something bad because she is in love.

Turn next to Ethan Frome. Here is sweet, virtuous Ethan, passionately in love with Mattie Silver (and she passionately in love with him), but who is nevertheless bound by obligation and law to his mean and vindictive (and also hypochondriac) wife Zenobia. He is thinking of making his getaway with Mattie to the West when he realizes that he does not even have the money for the train fare. After some thought, he considers going to his friends the Hales and borrowing money from them under the pretense that the sickness of his wife requires a servant. But after heading towards their house, he "pulled up sharply, the blood in his face. For the first time . . . he saw what he was about to do. He was planning to take advantage of the Hales' sympathy to obtain money from them on false pretenses. . . . With the sudden perception of the point to which his madness had carried him, the madness fell and he saw his life before him as it was. . . . He turned and walked slowly back to the farm" (Wharton 1970,

143). Ethan Frome could not even borrow money under false pretenses, let alone steal it, and let alone commit murder to get it. He is certainly no Medea. (But, the reader could object, in attempting to leave his wife, Ethan Frome might be seen as acting immorally towards her. However, this is at best a controversial claim, the reason being that Zenobia is convincingly portrayed as a vengeful, petty wife who does not seem to care about Ethan. If this is plausible, then another objection can be responded to, namely, that in committing joint suicide, both Ethan and Mattie were doing something wrong. The response to this, however, is that since neither of them has any obligations to others, and since the idea of living apart from each other is to them anathema, then they are not doing something wrong. Certainly, if each were to soldier on apart from the other, this would not be wrong either. But, I contend, neither would be their joint suicide.)

My point in offering these examples is not to show that a virtuous person would never commit an immoral act out of love, but rather to show that O2 is implausible. The examples of immoral acts need to be of ones done by virtuous people. But then again, examples of virtuous people could also convincingly tell us that such people might very well not do something unvirtuous. The likelihood objection, then, fails.

Turning to O1, and if we momentarily drop the word "safe" from its formulation for the sake of the argument, we end up with an innocuous objection: there are precious few guarantees we can offer by way of claiming that people will not commit bad acts. Incidentally, in this respect, we can also add that the objection would apply with equal force to someone who has tried and succeeded to a large extent to extirpate her emotions: Can we offer a guarantee that such a person would never commit a bad action due to a fit of emotion? I think not. If we now retain the word "safe," the objection would state that we can offer no safe guarantees that a virtuous person would commit immoral actions due to romantic love. But it seems to me that we can offer such a safe guarantee, and the reason why the objection might sound convincing is because it does not seem to take seriously the idea of a virtuous character.

Let us not worry about the idea that it is actually difficult for one to be virtuous, and let us focus on someone who is, indeed, virtuous. A crucial point to keep in mind is that a virtuous person is one who is well disposed with respect to both her actions *and* emotions. In other words, a virtuous person is one who is motivated to act and to react emotionally in appropriate ways. But this is a matter of *character*. One of the crucial ideas in Aristotelian ethics is that of someone who is morally *reliable*: someone who, because of her very character and traits that she has, can be relied upon not only to do the right thing in terms of thought and behavior, but also in terms of emotions. This is the reason for emphasizing the idea that virtues are deep and settled traits of character, that they are difficult to acquire but also difficult to shed, and that moral education should begin from infancy. In this respect, it is of course true that there are no guarantees that a virtuous person can never act out of character. But it is also true that, given these remarks, one can offer a *safe* picture of why a virtuous person would not likely commit immoral acts out of love. It is, indeed, hard to train the emotions and to be virtuous. But once one gets there, so to speak, one *is* morally reliable.

Perhaps one can argue that the emotions can never be trained in the way that an Aristotelian thinks they can. At one point in her discussion, Nussbaum offers the Stoic claim that Aristotelians do not really understand how the emotions function: "Aristotle has let the emotions into the good life without understanding how they operate, without understanding how little they are transparent—how much passivity, therefore, they bring to the life that lets them in" (1994, 455). But how are we to know the truth of the claim that the emotions are deep, passive, and "operate beneath the level of consciousness"? We have examples of people who *seem* to be virtuous and yet somehow manage to let their nasty passions take control. But we also have examples of people who seem to be virtuous and who are able to keep their emotions in check, and examples of virtuous people who do not need to keep their emotions in check and whose emotional responses are perfectly appropriate. It is because of such diversity of cases that the claim that the emotions are passive and function beneath the level of consciousness cannot be fully convincing. And when we keep in mind the perfectly obvious point that most people are not very virtuous, the contention that the emotions do not lend themselves in principle to harmonization with right thought and action becomes less convincing, because it will be seen to derive its force from the fact that most people are not virtuous. Moreover, that most people are not virtuous need not be attributed to the idea that emotions operate "beneath the surface." For it could be attributed to other causes, such as the far from ideal upbringing that most people have usually had.[45]

We should conclude, then, that we have yet no convincing reason to believe that passionate, romantic love is incompatible with a life of virtue. The reader should have noticed that the O1—O4 objections are all stated as contingent claims, not necessary ones, and Nussbaum herself shies away—rightly, I believe—from formulating the Stoic objection as a necessary claim. The reason is easy to see: if it were formulated as a necessity claim—that being in love necessarily leads to unvirtuous actions—then the objection would be implausible. For there is no plausible definition of "romantic love" that would entail such a claim; nor is there any good reason to think that even if we were to confine the claim to the passionate stages of being in love, the claim about immoral action would follow. The way to state the objection in its strongest light is to state it as a contingent claim. And, I have argued, such a claim is highly implausible.

4. The Value of Romantic Love

My concern in this section is with the importance of romantic love to a flourishing life. I will argue that while romantic love is indeed important for such a life, it is so because of those aspects it shares with other types of intimate relationships, such as friendship and parenting. In other words, the value that we place today on romantic love is due to contingent factors that have led to the devaluing of friendship relationships, among others, in comparison to relationships of romantic love.

Judging by what one hears and sees in popular culture, romantic love seems to be one of the most important values in life. Indeed, one often gets the impression that if one fails to be in love or to desire to be in love, then one is somehow defective in some way or other. But popular culture is not the only abode for such a view. Ethel Spector Person, a psychoanalyst, claims that romantic love is the primary mode of risk taking today, and that without risk taking there is no self-realization (1995, 112). Robert Ehman asserts that romantic love, "in its inescapable relevance to the human self, is as fundamental as morality, work, play, and death" (1989, 254). And Gabriele Taylor tells us that there "seems something sad or even sinister about the man who never loves at all" (1979, 179). Selfishness, meanness, arrogance, indolence, or cowardice may explain why Taylor's man never loves at all (179–80), and any, or all, of these point to, if not a sinister person, at least a morally defective one. Is romantic love as fundamental as morality and work? Is it the primary mode of risk taking? Most importantly, however, can there be a person who does not romantically love yet who is neither sinister nor unvirtuous? As an external good, how dispensable is romantic love to flourishing?

It should be noted that in the discussion of this section, romantic love is treated as an external good, the same way friendship is in Aristotle. This is important to note because even though I have argued that romantic love is not a virtue and so is, *in this respect*, dispensable to flourishing, romantic love's not being a virtue does not settle entirely the issue. For there is still the possibility that it might be a necessary or an important external good. Moreover, understanding romantic love as an external good need not in any way contradict the claim that it is an emotion, and this is so for two reasons. First, like other emotions such as hate and envy, romantic love need not be an emotion that one actually experiences in one's life, either by accident or by design. In addition to the Stoics, some Eastern traditions, for example, call on people to extinguish some or all of their emotions, and if this project is coherent at all, it tells us at least one thing, namely, that insofar as we can meaningfully inquire into whether some emotions are good to have, we are actually inquiring into whether these emotions are needed for a good life. In this respect, it is easy to see how these emotions can be treated as external goods and to ask whether they are necessary or dispensable for a flourishing life. I want to claim that in precisely these terms we can ask whether romantic love is necessary or dispensable for flourishing.

Second, that romantic love is an emotion does not, obviously enough, preclude it from manifesting itself in a relationship. But if we keep in mind that the value of romantic love ultimately rides on the idea of its being realized in a relationship (putting bizarre cases aside, it is hard to see why anyone would ultimately want to experience simply the emotion of romantic love without having it be requited), then it is easy to see how romantic love can be treated as an external good. The question would then be, "Is being in and having a romantic love relationship necessary for, or dispensable to, flourishing?"

I think one thing can be safely said at the start: romantic love is not a basic or fundamental good. Unlike having a minimal amount of political and social freedom, unlike having a minimal amount of economic means, of food, of health, not being in love does not as such deprive one of a minimally healthy and normal life.[46] Of course, to the extent that the concepts of health and normalcy are defined in terms of prevalent social standards, and to the extent that the standards of a society insist that being in love is an essential, or at least important, part of the picture of what a normal human being is, then whether romantic love is a basic value or not depends on how we are to define "health," "normalcy," and other related concepts. But there are philosophically good reasons as to why we should not define these concepts simply in terms of the societal norms under which they happen to operate, one being that we deprive ourselves of a good critical vantage point from which we can criticize such societal practices. With this in mind, the claim that romantic love is not necessary for a minimally decent life is plausible.

The issue then becomes how dispensable romantic love is to a well-lived life, to a flourishing one, rather than to a minimally decent one. Here, the claims often made on behalf of romantic love's indispensability do not seem to be very convincing. For example, there is the claim that romantic love is transformative, that it changes our boundaries and allows us to grow (Person 1995; Kupfer 1993; and, in somewhat modified form, White 2001, ch. 2, especially pp. 63–71). Now even if this claim is true, it does not seem to make romantic love indispensable, for it certainly is not the only way by which an agent can be transformed and can grow. This is not because there are ways of growing other than person-to-person (such as imbibing philosophy left and right); after all, there might be something especially crucial about transforming oneself and growing through another person. The reason is rather that there are other person-to-person modes that result in such growth and transformation. Examples readily come to mind: friendship and parenting are excellent candidates for performing this job, a job claimed on romantic love's behalf.

It is also claimed that in romantic love we experience *passion*, a stage of love through which we undergo unique—not in the sense of "unrepeatable" but in the sense of "not derived from another source"—experiences that hopefully culminate in being with the beloved, thus making the entire stage certainly worth having. The novel *Corelli's Mandolin* gives a description of the symptoms of such an experience. Dr. Iannis says to his daughter Pelagia about her newfound love:

> You blush in each other's presence, you both hover in places where you expect the other to pass, you are both a little tongue-tied, you both laugh inexplicably and too long, you become quite nauseatingly girlish, and he becomes quite ridiculously gallant. You have also grown a little stupid. He gave you a rose the other day, and you pressed it in my book of symptoms. If you had not been in love and had a little sense, you would have pressed it in some other book that I did not use every day. I think it is very fitting that the rose is to be found in the section that deals with erotomania. (De Bernieres 1994, 279–80)

We can quibble with some of the symptoms offered, but the general idea is quite familiar. Being in love, at least in the early stages, allows one to have a passionate experience such that one makes the beloved the focus of one's world and desires little other than to be with him. But despite the deliciousness of such an experience, it is obvious that it is dispensable. This is not because the experience often involves pain and frustration and so one is better off without it. The pain and frustration are often worth it and might well be part of the very deliciousness of the experience. The reason is that one can flourish, have a good and satisfying vocation, experience joys and sorrows, have close personal ties to others, and even be in love without having to have this experience.[47] This claim is thus not confined to people who live their lives in such a way that there is no room for romantic love in their lives, because, say, they are devoted to all-consuming projects. It applies equally to average people who can lead a good life without the passionate experience of romance.[48]

There are other claims, of course, given to defend the importance of romantic love. Plato, for example, claims in the *Symposium* and in the *Phaedrus* that love is crucial for wisdom and for doing good philosophy.[49] But such a claim is exaggerated, and, in the case of the latter work, moreover, it stems from a controversial reading of it. Since the *Phaedrus* seems to be really about the art of rhetoric and since it seems to *use* the subject of love as an *example* of rhetoric, this makes the truth-status of its claims about love suspect.[50] Another claim given on behalf of the importance of romantic love is that perhaps only in love can we experience deep, personal ties with someone else. It seems to me that it is this claim that has a good shot at giving romantic love its due indispensability, but it faces some obstacles, one of which I will mention now and elaborate on shortly: friendship seems to allow for the same value as the one just mentioned. Furthermore, whether friendship *does* allow for such a value seems to be a contingent, rather than, a conceptual matter. Consider Person's claim that it is primarily romantic love that gives us the chance to take some serious risks. Her claim is contingently true: because in our society friendship is not given the kind of intimacy and dependency that is allowed to romantic love, being in love is certainly riskier than having friendships. But were a society to allow friendship to have the same depth of intimacy and the same degree of dependency allowed to romantic love, then friendship would be as risky. This issue about the contingency of the societal stress laid on romantic love and friendship is central. I will return to it shortly.

But one might object: even if we grant that romantic love is dispensable to a flourishing life, not much follows from this. After all, eating and enjoying ice cream is dispensable to a flourishing life, but it does not follow from this that eating ice cream would not enrich life by making it more enjoyable. And a similar claim can be made about romantic love, namely, that its dispensability from a flourishing life does not show that having it would not greatly add to and enrich such a life. And if we look at people's lives, we do not need much acumen to see that most lovers' lives are indeed made better by being in love. True enough, romantic love can be painful, frustrating, and even destructive. But so can friendship, work, and a host of other aspects important to life.

The objection is in a sense correct: it is difficult and implausible to deny that romantic love certainly can, and often enough does, make one's life richer and better. But the objection is, in another sense, wrong: the point of claiming that romantic love is dispensable to a flourishing life is important not because we can invalidly derive from it the obviously false claim that it does not make life better or richer. The point is important, rather, in itself: it is quite a serious claim to deny that romantic love is indispensable to a flourishing life, given the pressure and importance which is laid upon the phenomenon of romantic love, both by popular opinion and academic opinion. This denial, in other words, goes against the usual ways of thinking about the importance of romantic love to a good life. To support this denial, I want to first offer a somewhat detailed case of a flourishing life that does not contain romantic love. The case is meant to illustrate and support the claim that one can flourish without romantic love. Next, I want to investigate the claim that the indispensability of romantic love to a well-lived life lies in its ability to forge strong and intimate ties between two people, and so return to the issue of the contingency of the societal emphasis given to romantic love.

Consider Yasser, a man in his forties, who is an accomplished, though not a world-famous, writer. Yasser is very much dedicated to his work: he spends about three to four hours writing in the morning, and, in the afternoon, he takes the book he is currently reading and goes to his local coffee shop where he reads and enjoys a cup of coffee. Yasser lives in a two bedroom apartment, with a spacious living room, kitchen, and bathroom. One bedroom is his own, and the other is a guest bedroom and study, the room where Yasser does his writing and where his out-of-town friends sleep when they visit. Yasser usually gets up very early in the morning, when he goes for a brisk jog and then spends some time exercising. In the evening, he often gets together with one or two of his local friends for a nice meal and maybe some other activity afterwords.

Yasser has published a few novels and has always managed to get his short stories printed in good journals and literary magazines. Yasser loves to teach, and he very much enjoys his college teaching job. His health is quite good, given his regimen of exercise and eating well. Quite crucially, Yasser, in addition to numerous acquaintances at his local coffee shop, gym, and other places, and in addition to his colleagues at the college where he teaches, has a few close friends with whom he shares his thoughts, feelings, and activities. They wish they could spend even more time together, but given how life works these days, they find it difficult to do so. And as for sex, Yasser every now and then goes out to a bar where he is able to meet someone to spend the night with. His sex drive is neither weak nor strong; these one-night stands are enough for him to go on merrily with his life.[51]

Yasser, it should be added, is subjectively quite happy and content with his life. The fact that it lacks romance and romantic love has not detracted from his subjective happiness. Moreover, he does not desire to have a romantic love relationship: he values his independence too much to want to be caught up in romantic love's emotional upheavals, and to want to have to subject his schedule, his apartment, and his work habits to the accommodation of someone else. His mother calls him up every now and then from back home to tell him that she found the "best" wife for him, but both he and she know that he will not marry any time soon (his mother does it because this is what is socially expected of her).

Granted that Yasser is subjectively happy, is he objectively so? That is, is he really flourishing? Is his life really going well, especially that he is not in love with anyone? I don't see how this can be denied: his work is going well, and it involves a pursuit that everyone would consider to be worthwhile; his health is fine; he has friends and acquaintances; and he himself is happy with his life. If one were to claim that his life is *not* going well precisely because it lacks romantic love, then one would beg the question. Furthermore, Yasser does not have any of those vices listed by Gabriele Taylor (1979) that might cause one not to love: he is neither selfish, nor mean, nor arrogant, nor lazy, nor a coward. But—one might object—perhaps he *is* a coward: Isn't Yasser a coward precisely because he is afraid to take the risks involved in romantic love? Given the case, the answer is negative. First, as part of the case, he is not, in general, a coward: he takes risks in his work, in his outspokenness, and so on. Second, and more importantly, he is not a coward when it comes to personal relationships: he has forged deep friendships, and these pose similar risks to those that romantic love does: losing one's friend, depending on one's friend, and loving one's friend are all risky businesses. But perhaps romantic love has the same kind of risks but these impact the lover more deeply than those of friendship. That may be true, but why should we be convinced that Yasser *is* a coward with respect to these? Why not, instead, respect his reasons for not wanting to be in a romantic relationship?

Does the fact that Yasser is male make the story more plausible? Perhaps women are more prone to be romantically involved given societal expectations. Perhaps they are more prone to be romantically involved because they are more caring than men. Or perhaps they need, more than men, to be in (heterosexual) relationships given the social power structure and its pressures on women. But I cannot see how these are more than general and contingent reasons as to why a woman in the position of Yasser is less likely to flourish. In other words, these reasons do not remove the plausibility of a case involving a female counterpart of Yasser.

No doubt, Yasser is not representative of everyone. He is not poor, for example. His job is not one he does not identify with, even if the job can bring in a good amount of money. But I have intentionally chosen a somewhat cushy life in order to illustrate the point of how a life can be good without romantic love. However, would Yasser's life be better and richer were he to be in love? Given Yasser's case, it is difficult to answer this question definitively one way or another. Being in love might enliven him, make him a better writer, allow him to see the world as a better place than he had thought, and so forth. But then again, being in love might take away his independence, might leave him with less time and energy for writing, and, in short, might change his life drastically. And it is difficult to make a case one way or the other and be able to pronounce Yasser's life better, period.

Perhaps Yasser will need romantic love in his old age, when he is mostly alone, in need of care and attention and companionship. There is much to be said for this suggestion, and I will come back to it shortly. But if Yasser's character is indeed independent, strong, and self-reliant, then Yasser might not feel the need for the companionship of romantic love in his old age. He might require someone to assist him in his physical chores, but this need not be done by his beloved. Moreover, it is certainly not plausible to make romantic love's necessity hinge on the beloved's ability to help move one to the bathroom in one's old age, especially, and for obvious reasons, if the "one" is male and the beloved is female. In any case, Yasser's example illustrates how one can have a well-lived life without romantic love. But now we should emphasize two points before moving on to the next step. First, had Yasser's life lacked friendships, it would have been a lot less convincing as a case of a well-lived life. Yasser would have emerged as either a lonely man, or a self-absorbed one, or one who is incapable, for one reason or another, including sheer bad luck, of forming a close relationship with someone else. On any one of these options, Yasser's life emerges as deeply lacking in important respects. I am not claiming that it is impossible to have a nondefective friendless life, but rather, that such a life would require a much more detailed defense. Second, there is much to be said for the suggestion that Yasser's life would be much better were he in his old age to have a companion. No matter how strong he is, how independent, and how self-reliant *now*, old age can render these things of the past. What both of these points have in common is the notion of a deep tie and closeness: whether in friendships or in romantic life companionships, it might well be indispensable to us human beings to be able to, and to actually, forge such deep ties. This means that the argument for the importance and even indispensability of romantic love can be made best on this basis. But if so, then we would be forced to think of romantic love on the model of friendship.

It is extremely difficult to find conceptual demarcating lines between friendship and romantic love. Every candidate for such demarcation lines falters either on the side of romantic love or on the side of friendship. For example, that lovers engage in sex with each other neglects the fact that friends sometimes have sex with each other, and the fact that lovers sometimes stop engaging in sexual activity with each other (say, in their old age, and, indeed, even sooner). Perhaps we can claim that lovers feel jealousy whereas friends do not. Again, however, some lovers are not prone to jealousy, and some friends do indeed feel jealous (anyone who thinks otherwise usually has in mind some type of loose acquaintance between two people). As Laurence Thomas puts it, "a person who appears to be a potential threat to a friendship will be a cause of concern and will generally occasion feelings of jealousy" (1989, 195).

Perhaps romantic love requires exclusivity whereas friendship does not. Again, romantic love does not seem to conceptually require exclusivity; at best, it requires that the number of beloveds be small. But then again, so does friendship, at least the type of friendship that is intimate. Maybe romantic love requires fidelity, a notion close to that of exclusivity, whereas friendship does not. But this also won't do. As Thomas argues (1989, 194), friends share things between them, be it time, activities, mementos, and so forth, and were one friend to share such items with a third party, it might plausibly be construed to be a breach in fidelity.

Passion—another demarcational candidate—does not seem to be necessary for romantic love. And constancy, reciprocity, and mutuality are as essential to friendships as they are to romantic love. Idealization does not work either: on the one hand, friends, just as lovers, can, in the throes and early stages of their friendships, idealize each other, and only later, just as in romantic love, come to see the error of their ways. On the other hand, romantic love does not require idealization; not all of its cases are ones in which one lover (or both) idealizes the beloved. In short, every candidate offered to conceptually separate romantic love from friendship seems to be subject to counterexamples.[52] Because such conceptual demarcational lines between romantic love and friendship are hard to come by, the claim that much that is important about romantic love is common to much that is important about friendship becomes highly plausible.

Today, we tend to think of romantic love as involving more intimacy, closeness, trust, vulnerability, and shared activity than does friendship, and this is probably true given the nature of our society. And it is thoughts such as these that perhaps lead philosophers such as Nozick to

essentially understand romantic love as the formation of a "*we*" and to
deny that friendship involves such a formation (1991). But that romantic
love is taken to involve more of the above-listed factors is not a conceptual
point. Aristotle, for example, required that friends live together (1985,
1171b32–35). This requirement has not been discussed extensively by
philosophers, probably because they understand it literally, and if one
understands it literally, then one is liable to dismiss it as archaic.[53] But
Aristotle could not have understood it as the requirement that the friends
literally cohabit, because Aristotle's discussion of friendship was primarily—though not exclusively—focused on two or more adult males, and this
means that both would probably have wives with whom they literally lived.
Rather, the living-together requirement amounts to the idea that the
friends, if the friendship is to be a good one, ought to share their activities
together: "Whatever someone [regards as] his being, or the end for which
he chooses to be alive, that is the activity he wishes to pursue in his friend's
company. . . . They spend their days together on whichever pursuit in life
they like most; for since they want to live with their friends, they share the
actions in which they find their common life" (1985, 1172a1–6). Notice
that while Aristotle understands living together to be sharing activities
together, this does not imply that they must share *all* of their activities
together, or that they must have more or less identical lifestyles. What is
crucial to Aristotle's notion of virtuous friendship is that the ends or goals
of the various activities are morally in the clear.[54] Also, this account implies
that the friends spend a good amount of time with each other, that they
will be intimate and close with each other, and that they will have to trust
each other. For notice what Aristotle says about the activities they engage
in: these are not things incidental to their lives, things they do because they
have to do *something* while they are together. Rather, these are the ends
and goals that each friend has chosen for him or herself. Insofar as these
are central to each friend's life (and they are), then when friends engage in
activities with each other they are opening up, or at least not hiding, what
is central to them. In this respect, friendship will imply trust and intimacy.

   Indeed, Aristotle's account emphasizes virtually every aspect considered essential to romantic love. In his discussion of virtuous friendships,
Aristotle emphasized the notions of constancy, wishing well for the other
for the other's sake, and the desire to spend time with one's friends.
Furthermore, he seems to intentionally de-emphasize the one criterion
most often taken to distinguish romantic love from friendship, namely, sexual desire and sexual activity. He sometimes speaks of it as one possible
basis for friendship (1157a11–14), and sometimes as one *form* of friendship (1164a4–14). In any case, whether the friendship starts in sexual

attraction and/or activity, and whether it has a sexual dimension to it are not emphasized by Aristotle: "For the emphasis of *philia* is less on intensely passionate longing than on disinterested benefit, sharing, and mutuality. . . ." (Nussbaum 1986, 354). Whether the relationship has erotic and sexual dimensions is not that important. What is important is its closeness, intimacy, shared activities, trust, and vulnerability. Romantic love is important insofar as it leads to friendship, hopefully of the virtuous kind. Or, to put the claim in less causal terms, romantic love is important insofar as it has those features that make friendship so morally desirable and good. As Anthony Price nicely puts it, "Aristotle envisages the emergence of that reciprocal concern and respect which constitute the best kind of friendship, linking individuals not merely as satisfiers of one another's incidental needs, but as partners in a life of personal self-realization. The moral end of love is to transcend itself in friendship" (1997, 249).[55]

How far are our conceptions from Aristotle's? It might seem that the answer to this question is obvious: "Very far," given the centuries that separate us from him and the changes in humanity's conception of romantic love. But this would be to exaggerate; we are actually not that far from Aristotle's views. Whether we are willing to admit it or not, we—philosophers and nonphilosophers—all know that the passion in romantic love dies. This is not to say that the lovers cease to feel love and desire for each other, but that those early stages of euphoria and elation do die out. We also all know that virtually every couple at some point down the road in its relationship discovers that the sex is not as exciting as it used to be. And couples know that to keep it exciting, new methods and techniques need to be explored. Furthermore, we all know that romantic love is not confined to the early passionate stages and to sexual activity. The more lovers in a couplehood clocks up years, the closer their relationship gets to be modeled on that of companionship and friendship, and this is, by the way, something that is *not* lamented by the couple's friends and relatives, but rather something that is celebrated. In other words, we do agree with Aristotle that the best of romantic loves are those that last. And if they last in the best of ways, then so much the better: in this respect we also agree with Aristotle that the best of loves are those that occur within close relationships of trust, affection, goodwill, and intimacy, to name a few aspects.

The strongest case to be made for romantic love's indispensability, then, rests on those features of romantic love that are shared with friendship. And in a society in which close and intimate friendships—those friendships that require time and privacy and effort to be deep and lasting—are rare, romantic love becomes all the more indispensable. As one philosopher recently put it, "If we look directly at the preoccupations of modern life, it simply is the case that friendship is no longer the exalted ideal that it once was. What concerns us . . . is the imperative of romantic love and the need to find someone with whom we might share the bliss of romantic union and the pleasures of domestic partnership" (White 2001, 14). When we look at Yasser's life and think that it is lacking because it has no romantic love in it, we are wrong because we are neglecting the fact that he has friends who can play the crucial roles played by love. Conceptually speaking, friendship is *not* just "the finest balm for the pangs of disappointed love," as the narrator ironically comments in Jane Austen's *Northanger Abbey*. Friendship constitutes those essential elements that make up what is crucial about romantic love, and, in this respect, can take the place of romantic love in a well-lived life. However, we are also right to think that something is amiss in Yasser's life, but only in a contingent sense: given our society, it is unlikely that those friendships of Yasser will play the role in those deep and lasting ways that romantic love, if success-ful, does.

Those, then, who view romantic love as indispensable to a good life are right, but only if their claim is understood in a contingent sense, given the way some societies de-emphasize friendship and emphasize romantic love. But they are wrong if their claim is taken to be necessary. For what is important about romantic love is also shared by friendship. This is why many instances of romantic love, when successful, end up being forms of friendship. Given this, let us all hope, along with Aristotle, that romantic love will indeed culminate in friendship, and let us also hope that when we do love, we love as virtuous people.[56]

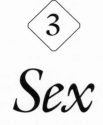

Sex

My aim in this chapter is to argue that certain ways of conducting one's sexual life are neither unvirtuous nor negatively consequential in any intrinsic way to one's flourishing. It is commonly and popularly believed, for example, that sexual promiscuity is not only wrong, but also inimical to its agent's living a good life. It is also commonly and popularly believed that being a sex worker, such as a prostitute or a stripper or a pornography actress, is also immoral and is also inimical to a good life. Lastly, it is believed that couples who are in open relationships or marriages are leading less desirable ways of life than their monogamous counterparts, and that, indeed, their way of life is a sign of trouble in their relationship and/or their individual psychologies.

These beliefs are no longer as ubiquitous as they used to be. Among the general, nonphilosophical (professionally, that is) population, for example, one can find an attitude of "live and let live" among the younger generations. Nevertheless, the beliefs are still prevalent. Turning to professional philosophers, a liberal attitude towards all sorts of practices can be easily found, such as Charles Fried's view that as long as justice and rights are not violated, and as long as one's practices do not harm others, one is morally free to do what one wants (1970, 227; 1978, 169–75). In specific regard to sex, one can find this attitude among a number of contemporary philosophers of sex, such as Alan Soble (1996) and Igor Primoratz (1999).

I do not wish to argue that the liberal position is wrong or that there are some wrong things in it. Rather, my aim is to vindicate the liberal position's attitude with respect to promiscuity, open marriages, and sex work from a neo-Aristotelian perspective. This has two advantages. First, it shows us the richness of the neo-Aristotelian perspective and the fruits it can offer us. Second, it allows us to feel more at ease with liberal conclusions, in the sense that we no longer have to worry that the agent, despite her harming no one and violating no one's rights, is nevertheless not leading a well-lived life. If we can show that promiscuity, sex work, and open marriages can be ways of life in full accordance with the virtues, then the agent who practices them, as long as she is virtuous, and as long as the usual list of external goods are within her life, should have no difficulty being described as leading a flourishing life. The conclusion, I should note, is not simply that it is logically and/or psychologically possible that these three ways of sexual life exist in a virtuous agent's life. The conclusion—with one exception regarding certain forms of open relationships—is stronger, namely, that there is nothing as such about a monogamous sexual way of life that enhances, or makes more probable, its agent's flourishing.

This project of vindicating the above liberal conclusions from a neo-Aristotelian perspective is all the more pressing given the following important observation. With the possible exception of Martha Nussbaum (I say "possible" because Nussbaum's views might not be an exception after all; see the introduction to section 2 and see section 4 below), almost all of the advocates of virtue ethics and closely related fields (such as Thomism) have been either silent with respect to sexual issues, or, what is worse, critical of nonconservative views. In the latter camp, for example, G. E. M. Anscombe, considered to be the philosopher who sensibly turned our attention to virtue ethics, is quite clear in her rejection of liberal sexual views (1976). Roger Scruton, who seems to think of his views as being inspired by Aristotle, rejects practically every sexual practice that deviates from heterosexual intercourse as perverse or immoral (1986). And John Finnis's views, which are Thomist, are well known for their rejection of nonmarital heterosexual sexual practices, including masturbation (1993, 1994). If my arguments in this chapter are convincing, then claims along the lines that reason leads us to accept monogamous heterosexual marriage as the only intrinsic good (Finnis 1994) would be false.

This is not to say that virtue ethicists who are silent about sex endorse the above conservative views. Nor is it to say that the above advocates of conservatism are legion. I think it was Alan Soble who once wrote—and I hope my memory serves me right here—"They stick out like a sore thumb" because they are so few in number. Nevertheless, it is important to be able to show that neo-Aristotelianism has the resources and the ability to accommodate nontraditional and nonconservative sexual beliefs and practices, and it is to this general aim that this chapter is devoted.

In the first section, I explore the virtue of temperance, how it is possible, and how it is different from continence. I also argue that we have two concepts of temperance, one having to do with amounts (too much, too little), and the other having to do with wrongdoing to others due to the agent's desire for sexual satisfaction. In this first section also, I offer a few remarks by way of indicating that these two notions of temperance are virtues because they satisfy the two criteria for what a virtue is. In section 2, I elaborate on the three ways of conducting one's sex life (promiscuity, open marriages, and sex work), and in section 3, I argue that none of these violate temperance in its sense of wrongdoing to others out of sexual desire. In sections 4, 5, and 6, I discuss promiscuity, open marriages, and sex work, respectively, in terms of their contravening the virtue of temperance understood as pertaining to amounts, and argue that they do not necessarily do so. In the final and brief section, I address some possible worries having to do with the plausibility of my conclusions, specifically in their application to women.

1. Two Virtues of Temperance

Temperance, as usually understood, is the virtue that moderates our desires for food, drink, and sex. A temperate person is supposed to be someone who satisfies such desires in morally good ways without, at the same time, having to struggle with himself to do this. On the other hand, a continent agent is someone who is able to refrain from indulging such desires when they should not be indulged, but who also feels an inner struggle in order to do this. In this section, I will primarily address the issue of what temperance and continence are with respect to sexual desires. In doing this, I argue that we should make a conceptual distinction between two types of temperance. Towards the end of the section, I also briefly argue that such traits—the two concepts of temperance—are indeed *virtues* because they satisfy the criteria for what a virtue is.

Recently, a few philosophers have held the position that sexual behavior is, in itself, morally neutral. That is, if a sexual act is morally wrong, it is so because of moral considerations that are general and that apply to sexual and nonsexual actions. The wrongness of adultery, for example, derives from the fact that adultery is typically an instance of promise breaking (or of deception), and promise breaking is, everything else being equal, wrong. Thus, Alan Goldman states, "There is no morality intrinsic to sex, although general moral rules apply to the treatment of others in sex acts as they apply to all human relations" (1997, 49). Goldman gives the example of rape: "The immorality of rape derives from its being an extreme violation of a person's body, of the right not to be humiliated, and of the general moral prohibition against using other persons against their wills, not from the fact that it is a sexual act" (1997, 50).[1]

I am certain that Goldman is wrong about rape; but I am also certain that rape is wrong not just because of the reasons mentioned by Goldman, but also because it is a *sexual* violation of another's body. However, even if Goldman is wrong about rape, he might be right about all other types of sexual acts, and this would mean that the view that there is no morality intrinsic to sexual behavior is left more or less intact. But is this view correct? We should immediately notice that if it were correct, it would yield a bizarre implication for a usual understanding of some virtues. For many hold that there are virtues whose domain is sexual behavior and feeling, but Goldman's view would seem to deny this; it seems to deny that there are *any* "virtues or vices of an essentially sexual nature," as David Carr puts it (1986, 363). What might such virtues be? Temperance (or moderation) is the virtue that regulates the bodily appetites in general. If we focus specifically on temperance in its regulation of sexual desire, then we would have one obvious candidate for a sexual virtue. Carr offers us chastity, a virtue "whose topic is sex," but which does not, in one of its senses at least, denote abstinence (Carr uses "temperance" to denote the virtue of the appetites for food and drink).[2] The questions that confront us, then, are the following: Is there a character trait whose domain of application is sexual desire? How is virtue in this area even possible? That is, how can one be *temperate*, rather than merely self-controlled, with respect to sexual desire? And, finally, would the existence of such a virtue render Goldman-like positions false? Once we have addressed these issues, we can move on to see whether certain types of sexual behavior are ruled out by temperance and why.

Carr argues that on first appearances chastity is a virtue of self-control; namely, that, like courage, which controls fear, chastity restrains the unruly sexual impulses. However, Carr thinks this is plausible when chastity is thought of as abstinence. But when it is thought of as being the virtue whose topic is sexual impulse, then it is not accurate to think of chastity as a virtue of self-control because "it is perfectly permissible for a man to express his sexual desires . . . just so long as the desires and their expressions occur within an appropriate context, one defined in terms of notions of fidelity, loyalty, love, responsibility, and so on" (1986, 366). I will (below) reject the above contexts mentioned by Carr as being the only appropriate ones for the expression of sexual desire (and his claims certainly do not imply that these are the only contexts). Nevertheless, his point seems correct: as long as sexual desire is expressed in the appropriate context, then there is no reason to withhold the virtue of chastity from the agent. If so, then chastity does not seem to be a virtue of self-control.

But things are not so simple. Sexual *expression* is not the only factor that enters into our assessment as to whether someone is temperate. As Carr rightly observes, there is something amiss with someone who is sexually faithful to his spouse but who is nevertheless constantly tempted to engage in sexual acts with other people. The problem becomes acute when we keep in mind that sexual attraction to other people is a general and bio-logical phenomenon difficult to eradicate precisely because it is rooted in our physiology. The problem then is this: if sexual attraction to others is more or less pervasive, and if a person who is sexually faithful to his spouse nevertheless feels sexual attraction towards others, it is difficult to see how he could be described as chaste. Indeed, if *un*chastity is not simply a mat-ter of sexual *expression* but also of experiencing sexual *urges*, in what, exactly, do the chaste differ from the unchaste?

Carr's solution, which I believe is essentially correct, is to locate the dif-ference between the chaste and the unchaste in the agent's values and atti-tudes. It is true that we all experience sexual urges, but the difference between the chaste person and the unchaste one, at least in the context of a discussion of sexual fidelity, is that the former does not invest the having and the expression of his sexual desires for other people with much, if any, value. The unchaste person is not one who is simply attracted to others; rather, he is one who *lusts* after others, and this means that such a person invests his sexual desires with value; he endorses them, at least to some extent: "To entertain lust or lechery in one's heart is to be already in the grip of certain values and attitudes of an inherently base and dishonourable nature and which are therefore quite incompatible with a state of genuine chastity as expressed in the desire to be, amongst other things, sexually loyal and faithful" (1986, 369).

While I think that Carr has given the essential outline of the correct way to approach this issue, there are some distinctions that need to be made. For one thing, Carr's condemnation of the lustful person is too quick precisely because he overlooks the distinction between two types of lustful characters (both of whom, we may suppose for the sake of the point, do not give expression to their desires). The first is that of an agent who experiences the lustful sexual desires but who does not *endorse* them, and the second is that of one who does endorse them. Carr may be right in that both would be correctly described as unchaste. But Carr would not be right to describe both as having a corrupt or dishonorable valuational sys-tem, and that is because the former agent might be one who rejects, or is actively struggling to reject, these desires as base, while the latter does not.

Second, we do not find in Carr's discussion a distinction between sexual appetites and sexual desires. The difference is that an appetite is a physiological state, whereas a sexual desire is a desire for the *pleasures* of sexual activity, and this latter desire need not always be rooted in the appetite for sex. Consider, by way of analogy, hunger. Hunger is a physiological appetite. Yet it is different in important respects from the desire for food, which is a desire for the pleasures of eating, and such desires need not be rooted in hunger at all, as when one desires to have a Mars chocolate bar even when one is not hungry. Similarly, one may desire sexual activity not because one is sexually frustrated, that is, physiologically motivated to engage in sex—whatever this means—but because one simply desires the pleasures of sex, be they orgasmic or not.[3] Of course, the fact that not every case of sexual desire is rooted in physiological appetite does not entail that sexual desire, in general, is not, and so does not entail that one can simply eradicate sexual desire, and it does not entail that the experiencing of sexual desire is not prevalent. Sexual desire, as Dent puts it, "is something to which human nature is naturally heir. Having once tasted such pleasures, we just do, as a matter of fact, very often wish to taste them again" (1984, 132). And the pleasures of sex, as Irving Singer reminds us (2001a, 72–78), need not be confined to the pleasures one derives from the sheer sensuousness of the sex act (such as the orgasm), but could also include the general enjoyment one derives from engaging in the activity of sex, much as one enjoys taking a walk without necessarily experiencing any specific hedonic state of pleasure. Aristotle, of course, and though he had little to say about sex as such, was aware of this distinction in general. In the following passage, he seems to precisely make the distinction between appetites and desires: "Some appetites seem to be shared [by everyone], while others seem to be additions that are special [to different people]. The appetite for nourishment, e.g., is natural. . . . On the other hand, not everyone has an appetite for a particular sort of food or drink or sex, or for the same things; hence, that sort of appetite seems to be special to [each of] us. Still, this also includes a natural element. . . ." (1985, 1118b10–15).

If we keep the above distinction in mind, we will realize that chastity or temperance is the virtue whose topic is not simply sexual appetites, but sexual *desire*, the desire for the pleasures of sex. This would make Carr's conclusion that temperance is a matter of the agent's valuational structure more plausible since it allows temperance to fall squarely within the inquiry of whether it is *good* or *noble* to endorse one's sexual desires, or, more correctly, particular types of them. And *this* inquiry would not make much sense if we thought of sexual desires as merely physiological appetites. More importantly, if it is impossible, or extremely difficult, to regulate one's sexual appetites, and if a discussion of temperance is confined to these, then temperance would turn out to be a phantom virtue, a virtue that is rarely applicable to our lives. But if it is possible to regulate one's sexual *desires*, then temperance does indeed have a place in our ethical discourse.

What then is temperance? We know that it has something to do with the agent's endorsement of her sexual desires, her desires for certain sexual *pleasures*. But more can be said. It is obvious that whether an agent endorses a particular type of sexual desire (for example, desire for sex with people who are not the agent's spouse) is a matter dependent upon the agent's believing such desires to be good or bad. An agent who does endorse such desires believes them to be good (or at least not bad, and this is going to be an important issue below; I am shelving it for now), and an agent who rejects such desires believes them to be bad. Let us, then, call "P" those sexual pleasures that an agent *rightly* decides not to enjoy, that, indeed, it would be wrong to enjoy. A temperate person, then, would be one who (i) either does not feel the desire for P or one who does feel the desire for P but who gives this desire no weight in her practical deliberations, and (ii) is pleased, for the right reasons, at either not feeling the desire or at not giving it any weight.[4] These two characterizations require some elaboration.

For purposes of clarity, let us assume that the agent *rightly* rejects a type of sexual desire. Furthermore, let us use an uncontroversial example of a wrong sexual desire, that is, an example of a desire that ought not to be endorsed by an agent: the desire for sexual contact with children. To make the case as uncontroversial and yet as realistic as possible, let us further assume that the children who are the objects of desire are neither infants (so as not to convert the agent into what many would consider to be subhuman or beastly) nor pubescent and older (so as not to convert the child into what many would consider to be a preadult and so capable of genuine choice).

The above characterization of a temperate person tells us that, first, the agent does not feel the desire for the pleasure obtained from having sex with children. But this should immediately occasion some reservations. For while some people grow up to find that they are attracted to children, many are morally lucky enough to grow up to find themselves not having this sexual disposition. Are we to believe that we are temperate in this respect? How can this be when this is due to luck? The short answer to this objection is that if part of what it is to be temperate or chaste is to *not* desire and enjoy sexual pleasures inappropriately, then those who are not pedophiles are, to that extent, temperate, and bringing in a causal account (luck) of how one got to be this way is simply irrelevant. Someone, for example, who grows up to find herself fearing important dangers and yet is able to overcome her fear and fight for her goods is brave, even if she did not have to undergo rigorous moral training. I see no reason why nonpedophiles should not be called "temperate" with respect to the absence of sexual desires for children.

However, we should keep in mind that the temperate person is pleased at not having such desires, and is pleased for the right reasons. Someone who is pleased at not being a pedophile *only* for the reason(s) that he does not have to deal with society's prohibitions, that he does not have to go through difficult and risky ways to satisfy his sexual desires, and/or that he does not have to worry about being sexually unfulfilled were he to refrain from acting on his pedophiliac desires, would *not* be pleased for the right reasons. The right reasons are that having sex with children is wrong, that such an activity is liable to harm the child, that it is a form of coerced sex given children's general inability to consent to sexual acts, and that not having such sexual desires is good precisely because of not having to be in a position whereby one is tempted to do what is wrong.

We must not forget, however, that a temperate person need not be one who does not feel sexual desires for children; he could be one who *does* feel such desires but who does not give them any weight. What this means is, roughly, that the agent does not give such desires any role in his life; he would not act in such a way to satisfy them on any given occasion, and, more grandiosely, he would not structure his plans, his schedules, his career, his recreations, and so forth, around them in any way. Indeed, if the agent is virtuous, he would be repelled by such desires, and his disgust at having them might be sufficient to motivate the agent to not act on such desires and to not plan his life around them in any way.[5] Here, clearly, reason or practical wisdom has an important role to play in the rejection of such desires. This should not be surprising, if only for the simple reason that temperance, in being a virtue, is supposed to be suffused with reason. Moreover, all of the remarks offered above in connection with the agent's being pleased at not having such sexual desires apply to this variation of the case. Here, of course, the agent would be pleased at not giving such desires any weight. But the rest of the remarks hold.

It is even possible that were the agent to undergo rigorous training, he might be able to expunge them more or less entirely, but whether this is successful will depend on the kind of sexual desires at issue, and this is important. It is important because of the following possible objection: Why call such a person temperate to begin with? If we were to consider a parallel case of honesty—the objection continues—we would not be tempted to call a person who has desires to lie or steal but who does not give them any weight "honest." Rather, he would be a kind of a continent agent, an agent who feels the desire to steal or to lie, but who is able to control her actions and so refrain from stealing or lying.

This objection is interesting because it forces us to think about continence. It seems, for instance, possible to make a case for two types of continent agents. Both have desires to steal, and both refrain from doing so. One, however, does not give much or any weight to such desires, while the other does. I am not sure whether the latter possibility is coherent. What does it mean to claim that an agent gives weight (or some weight) to her desires to steal but yet refrains from doing so? What would this weight consist of? Presumably, she, to some extent, structures her life around such desires. But then why do so if the agent, by definition, is able to refrain from stealing? While it makes sense to speak of the first agent as not giving weight to such desires and as refraining from stealing, the same is difficult to hold with respect to the second. But if so, would this not indicate that the above temperate person, the one who has sexual desires for children but who does not give them any weight, is also continent? If the possibility of a continent agent who gives some weight to her bad desires is ruled out because of its seeming incoherence, then the above so-called temperate person seems more and more continent.

This would be true if it were not for one crucial thing: the desires at issue are *sexual* in nature. The thought is this: since these desires are sexual (and I am now speaking of sexual desires generally, and not just of sexual desires for children), then they are present in most, if not all, human beings, especially after a certain age. One expects that human beings would naturally—so to speak—have such desires. Hence, they have an existence which is somewhat independent of our control (in Dent's terminology, they are "good-independent," that is, they, as such, seek pleasure and are devoid of considerations of what is good and bad). I say "somewhat" because the extent, duration, and depth to which they can come under rational control is controversial. There is no doubt that they can be controlled to some, and even large, extent, and so they are not entirely and hopelessly independent. But whether they can come to be *fully* controlled *is* a matter of speculation.[6] The point is this: if our sexual desires have some measure of independence from reason, then we should, if we are to be realistic, allow that chastity is compatible with a certain amount of sexual desire. Consider, before going back to pedophilia, someone who is in a committed monogamous relationship. Such a person may very well feel sexual desire for people other than her spouse, but she may not give such desire any weight. She does not, for example, feel tempted to hire an employee because—assuming our agent to be heterosexual—he is "cute," even if the potential employee's record is enough on its own to justify hiring him. The fact that she is able to deny such desires any voice is sufficient for her character to possess temperance.

This conclusion can be supported by the fact that we can make a coherent case for a *continent* agent who nevertheless gives his bad sexual desires some weight; unlike the desires-for-stealing case, such a case is plausible. Let us return to the pedophilia case. Our pedophile is now a continent agent, and so he does not act on his desires; he does not engage in sex with children. But he does structure his day so that he can spend a couple of hours browsing through the internet for pictures of children; or he is willing to spend a few hours each day fantasizing about what he would "like to do" to the neighbor's kid. Such an agent refrains from actual pedophiliac sex because he knows it is wrong, but he nevertheless indulges in what he might consider to be harmless daydreaming, resulting (sometimes or often) in masturbatory sexual release. It seems to me that we have a perfectly plausible case of a continent agent who gives a good measure of weight to his sexual desires, desires which he deems to be bad. This, I contend, cannot be done with respect to the stealing example, without undermining the agent's sanity (and on the assumption that the agent is not hard up for money). Moreover, even if one were to claim that we can imagine our continent thief spending hours fantasizing about the best way to rob the neighborhood bank, and that we can do so without undermining his sanity, the fact that his desires are nonsexual should give us pause in attributing to him virtue. If he were virtuous he would not have such thoughts because he could have changed himself; and he could have changed himself precisely because desires to steal are not, in general, desires rooted in our biology. But the sex case is not analogous in this respect: it is extremely difficult to be able to eradicate one's sexual desires, and so our best hope is to give them little or no weight. This might be the best we can hope for if we are to allow people the virtue of chastity. Furthermore, by giving them little weight, and by undertaking particular training regimens, one may hope to lower the affective intensity and frequency of such desires, if not eradicate them entirely.

There is, however, one caveat. I had mentioned above that whether expunging a sexual desire is possible depends on the kind of sexual desire. This has repercussions for our discussion. For whether one who has bad sexual desires but gives them no weight is chaste will depend on the type of sexual desire felt. For example, in the adultery case, we have no difficulty in claiming that the woman who feels sexual desire for people other than her spouse but who does not give the desire any weight is chaste. The main reason is, I think, because we recognize how pervasive and natural such sexual desires are. Is this the same also with respect to the man who feels sexual desire for children? Consider, as a quick aside, homosexuality. Many of the people who thought that a person can change from being gay to being straight believed this *precisely* because they thought that homosexual tendencies were somehow unnatural. If they were unnatural, then, they thought, it should not be *that* difficult to change back to one's natural state. On this point, these optimists were severely disappointed. But the general question remains: Are certain sexual dispositions less natural than others, *in the sense that* their very existence is more controllable? I do not have the answer to this question, and I don't think that many do either (this is an understatement). But the point is that whether our agent who has sexual desires for children but who gives them no weight is temperate will depend, to a large degree, on how much the very existence of these desires are under the agent's control.

I have, in effect, answered the first two questions posed earlier. By way of summary, the questions and the answers are as follows: the first question is whether there is a character trait whose domain of application is sexual desire. The second question is whether virtue in this domain is possible. The answers to both questions are affirmative. Regarding the first, given the distinction between sexual appetites (or drives) and sexual desires, it makes perfect sense for an agent to ask herself the question of what place, weight, and value she is to give the latter in her life. Given the variety of sexual desires and given the different ways sexual desires can be exercised, such questions become crucial for a moral life. I have given examples of two types of sexual desires—desires for children and desires for adults— that differ from each other precisely because they differ in their objects. But one can give other examples. For instance, one can raise the question of the *extent* to which one should act on one's (morally healthy) sexual desires: Is it okay (for me) to be sexually promiscuous? Should I be in a monogamous sexual relationship?

Regarding the second question—whether virtue in the domain of sexual desire is possible—the affirmative answer to it is based on the fact that we can distinguish different types of responses to certain sexual desires. One can merely control them and refrain from acting on them. This seems to indicate continence. But one can also try to give them no weight whatsoever, and in this case, even if the desires are present in the agent to some extent, the agent would be temperate. I have argued that since desires are not entirely insulated from reason, then temperance with respect to sexual desires is certainly possible.[7] One should notice, then, that temperance and continence with respect to sexual desire are not so much a matter of low and high affective intensity and frequency of sexual desires, respectively. Indeed, it seems that the thought behind denying the possibility of virtue relies on the fact that we have sexual urges and desires and that there is little we can do to eradicate them. But one need not deny the pull of sexual desires in order to admit of sexual virtue. Sexual virtue is more a matter of how much weight such desires are assigned by the agent and the agent's emotional reaction to such a weight assignment. A continent agent is one who assigns bad desires *some* weight or one who assigns them no weight but is extremely distressed at having to do so (an agent who claims to assign them no weight but acts on them would, of course, be incontinent).

It is worth emphasizing two points. First, this account of temperance and continence departs from a common picture of temperance as being lack of temptation in the face of certain goods. For example, Vincent Punzo characterizes the temperate man as one who has "so determined his appetite for food, drink, and sex that it responds with *ease*, consistency, and pleasure to the proper use of these goods" (1969, 154). What I am pointing out is that the picture might be more complicated than Punzo seems to think. Second, it is a good thing that temperance and continence are not a matter of intensity. For if they were, then we would run into the problem of trying to prove that a person who has low sexual desires (e.g., for children) is so "by nature" (and so does not deserve praise) or is so by moral training (and so deserves the term of praise "temperate").

But the reader should also have noticed by now that temperance does not turn out to be *just* an issue of excess and deficiency as far as *amounts* are concerned. Consider, to approach this point somewhat differently, Aristotle's doctrine of the mean. If we were to interpret it as being about how much or how little one engages in an activity, chastity seems to be an aberration in this respect. For we have been discussing it as being more about types of sexual desires to avoid having or giving weight to, and this does not seem to be an issue of how much. For example, it is not intemperate to have sex with one's spouse twice a day, seven days a week. But if one thinks about it, having sex fourteen times per week is a *lot* (and I hope I am not unwittingly revealing any personal information here). Yet it does not seem to be intemperate, and it is time to delve a bit more into what intemperance is, since, in addition to helping us understand the virtue of temperance better, this also allows us to answer the question as to whether Goldman-like accounts of sex are wrong.

Let us consider what Aristotle says about temperance and intemperance. On a number of occasions, Aristotle seems to think of intemperance as being not so much a matter of excess or deficiency of desire, that is, not so much a matter of too much lust or too little sexual drive, but more a matter of desiring the *wrong* objects. For example, he states that the "intemperate person . . . has an *appetite* for all pleasant things, or rather for the pleasantest of them, and his appetite leads him to choose these at *the cost of everything else*" (1985, 1119a1–4; my italics). At 1118b25, Aristotle tells us that intemperate people enjoy hateful and so wrong things, and that this is *why* they go to excess. At 1119a15, Aristotle states that the temperate person does not find *pleasure* in the wrong things, and, at 1119a19, that he desires what does not deviate from what is *fine*. It seems to me that this sample of evidence indicates that Aristotle thought of temperance and intemperance as being a matter of desiring the right and wrong things, respectively, *because* the agent finds these to be pleasurable. This is made clear in Aristotle's remarks about adultery. He tells us that adultery does not admit of a mean (1985, 1107a15) and that it has nothing to do with amounts—how many times one commits adultery—because the act itself is "wicked" (*Eudemian Ethics* 1984, 1221b20). Once we keep in mind that "adultery" to Aristotle (and to popular Greek morality of the time) did not mean "extramarital sex" but something along the lines of "sexual seduction of someone who should not be seduced" (such as the wife, widow, or daughter of an Athenian citizen), we realize that understanding intemperance to apply to engaging in wrongful acts for the sake of pleasure is a plausible interpretation of Aristotle's views.

However, there are places, some of which are the same as the above, in which Aristotle seems to think of temperance and intemperance as being connected to health, and so as being a matter of excess and deficiency in terms of amounts. For example, Aristotle states, "If something is pleasant and conducive to health or fitness, [the temperate person] will desire this moderately and in the right way; and he will desire in the same way anything else that is pleasant if it is no obstacle to health and fitness, does not deviate from what is fine, and does not exceed his means" (1985, 1119a16–20). Here, in addition to relying on the notion of the fine, Aristotle seems to tell us that temperance is connected to health in important ways, and these ways are those of moderation. The only way I can understand this is in terms of amounts and occasions. Earlier (1119a15), Aristotle stated that moderation means having an appetite for pleasant things to the right degree and the right time. Presumably, this means that a temperate person would not, for example, eat too much on a certain occasion, and he would not eat at all if the occasion does not call for it (for example, during church service, communion aside).

At 1118b (1985), Aristotle claims that "[e]ating indiscriminately or drinking until we are too full is exceeding the quantity that suits nature, since [the object of] natural appetite is the filling of a lack." Aristotle calls these people "gluttons" and claims that they are slaves to their appetites.[8] Since gluttony is a form of intemperance, here we have a conception of the latter as being mainly in terms of amounts. In the *Eudemian Ethics*, Aristotle considers "drunkenness, gluttony, lecherousness, gormandizing, and all such things" to be forms of intemperance (1984, 1231a20). And all of these are primarily understood, by Aristotle and by us, as being about amounts. Here, excess and deficiency *do* apply to how much and when.

I have dwelt on this issue not only because Aristotle's doctrine of the mean has been understood as being primarily about desiring the wrong objects (and not primarily about amounts),[9] but also because it yields an interesting account of temperance and intemperance. For it seems that we can uncover in Aristotle *two* concepts of temperance, both of which are conceptually independent of, but perhaps causally related to, each other. The first is temperance regarding amounts of food, drink, and sexual pleasure. Temperance here means not eating, drinking, and having sex excessively or deficiently (too much or too little). Temperance here is supposed to be *good for the agent*, first and foremost. This is so not simply for physical health–related reasons (sexual diseases aside, it is doubtful that too much sex can somehow make one sick), but also for flourishing-related reasons. Overeating can lead one to forego many other activities in life, activities important for the agent's flourishing. In this connection, certain types and amounts of sexual practices could be considered harmful for the agent, such as the idea that too much sex (promiscuity) is not good for the agent (whether this is true is an issue I will look into below; for now, I am offering it only as an example of how too much sex is thought to be harmful to the agent). Call this concept of temperance "T1."

The other concept of temperance governs not excess and deficiency of amounts, but *wrongful acts the agent does to others*, such as eating someone else's portion of food when one should not do so, or having sex with a friend's spouse.[10] Here temperance would imply that the agent would not engage in such not-fine actions. Call this temperance "T2." The two concepts can, of course, be causally connected. One's love for too much eating could very well lead one to guzzle someone else's food ration. Perhaps we can even venture a psychological law–like claim to the effect that the more one is intemperate in the first sense (IT1), the more one is likely to become intemperate in the second sense (IT2). Perhaps this is what Aristotle had in mind and perhaps this is why he failed to distinguish clearly between these two concepts.

Nevertheless, the two are conceptually distinct, and this is quite easy to see, because the conditions under which they hold are distinct. We could conceive of an agent who, for instance, would not hesitate to pursue the pleasures of eating, drinking, and sex, at the expense of others, *even if one did this in moderate amounts.* To give a more specific example, he might not hesitate in raping a woman to obtain his sexual gratification were the woman to refuse him sex. Such a man need not be a sex-crazed maniac who simply *must* have sex a large number of times per week. Rather, this is a man who knows the pleasures of sex, enjoys sex in moderate amounts (by plan or by accident does not really matter), yet is perfectly willing to trample on women's rights and rape them were they to refuse his sexual advances.[11] Furthermore, it need not be the case that this man *entirely* lacks the virtue of justice for this example to make sense. To suppose this is to suppose—I think—that the doctrine of the unity of the virtues is true.[12] But without getting into this difficult topic, imagine someone who lies, due to greed, about a certain amount of money ("Excuse me, sir, but have you found a five-dollar bill around here?" "Who me? No. Of course not. If I had found it I would have taken it up to the front desk," the man replies, while his hand gently caresses the bill tucked safely away in his pocket). I do not think that we would be quick to infer that this man does not have the virtue of honesty to some degree or extent. He might not have it to the highest degree, or he may have it but be able to exhibit it only in domains in which money is not involved. Similarly, the claim applies to T2.

Here, however, we must tread carefully. For one might object that, in the rape example just given, it is hard to accept the claim that one can have the virtue of justice in nonsexual domains if one is willing to rape others. Rape, the objection continues, is a serious moral crime, and a person who is willing to commit it is a person who does not respect the autonomy of others and is one to whom we ought to be hesitant in ascribing the virtue of justice, even in minimal ways or domain-specific ways.[13] The objection is plausible for three reasons. First, when confronted with such an agent, we find it difficult to believe that he can nevertheless be just in other domains, and this is precisely because rape is a serious immoral act. Second, we may surmise, without implausibility, that a person prone to rape is not usually the kind of person who is liable to be just in general. Third, even if a person who is prone to rape can be just with respect to other nonsexual issues (for example, giving others their due), we might plausibly think that the justice he possesses pales in comparison to the justice he lacks when it comes to sex.

But we ought to keep a tight grip on the conceptual point, namely, that a case involving such an agent is not incoherent. Men like this agent might be rare, and his having justice with respect to other domains might, indeed, pale in comparison. Nevertheless, these points do not show that the agent lacks justice entirely. Furthermore, we should keep in mind that the conceptual point about T2 is supported by other examples, such as a spouse who can rarely, if ever, resist the temptation to commit adultery when the opportunity arises, even when he knows that he is deceiving his spouse. Such a case, it seems to me, entails neither that the agent lacks honesty nor that he lacks justice in other domains. So the objection is correct in its pointing out how we usually tend to react to such people as the man in the example, but it does not defeat the conceptual point at hand.

Turning next to T1, one can imagine cases of people intemperate in the first sense, who are IT1 (e.g., spend too much time in adult bookstores, spend yet another afternoon watching yet another pornography movie rather than writing the philosophy paper they had been planning on writing, and spending half the day asleep because they just had to go out *again* the night before to find yet another one-night stand) but who are not intemperate in the second sense, who are not IT2 (e.g., they would not even *dream* of having sex with their best friends' spouses, they would not tolerate even fantasizing about having sex with children, and they cannot entertain even the idea of peeping at their neighbor undressing, let alone committing any of these actions). It is, I think, clear that we seem to have two concepts of temperance (and intemperance) at work.

This should not be a very surprising result, once we keep in mind that each concept is organized around a different good. In other words, each type of temperance responds to a different type of value. The first notion of temperance is organized around the agent's health, be it physical, psychic, or ethical. The second notion of temperance, however, is organized around respecting the goods and rights of others. It is, nevertheless, a notion of *temperance* because the agent gladly refrains from satisfying her *bodily pleasures* at the expense of others. Other virtues are similarly organized around specific values. Benevolence, for example, revolves around the value of minimizing the suffering of others. Justice revolves around upholding others' rights. (Courage might seem to be a split virtue. After all, one can be courageous with respect to one's own goods *or* with respect to the goods of others. But this is slightly misleading. The organizing concept underlying courage is that of overcoming fear in order to defend important goods, be they of the agent or of others.) And this is the reason why we have two types of temperance; each type is a trait of character that has its own field of experience, so to speak.

Furthermore, any attempt to find a unitary account of temperance faces difficulties. For example, one can propose that the organizing good of temperance is, simply, bodily pleasures. But this will not do. Bodily pleasures do constitute a crucial area of human concern, of course, but simply proposing these as the central notion of temperance fails to distinguish between temperance and intemperance, for both of these have to do with bodily pleasures (that is why in the above paragraph I did not simply state that benevolence is organized around the suffering of others, but around the minimizing of this suffering). One can, however, propose that the organizing good of temperance is the regulation (or some other related concept) of bodily pleasure. This attempt fails because it takes us back to the question of what is meant by regulation. And *this* issue leads to the distinction between "regulation" as referring to *amounts* and "regulation" as referring to refraining from coveting the goods of others, and these are very different terrains. I have, of course, not exhausted the ways in which one might attempt to offer a unitary account of temperance. I have merely indicated why I think it is difficult to give a unitary account of temperance that is plausible, interesting, and not too unwieldy.

I began this section by raising the question as to whether Goldman-like accounts of sexual behavior are true, that is, whether claims to the effect that sexual behavior has no morality intrinsic to it are true. I now want to briefly return to this issue because its treatment allows us to bridge the gap between actions and virtues, and because it gives us a good segue into the next section.

Whether Goldman and Goldman-like accounts are correct depends on how narrowly or broadly we understand "action." An action is right in virtue ethics if, and only if, it is what a virtuous person, acting in character, would do in the circumstances.[14] To say that an action is wrong is to say that it is an action that a virtuous person would not commit, and she would not commit it because doing so would be contrary to a virtue. So, for example, a virtuous person would not seduce a friend's spouse because the action is intemperate (under either or both types of temperance). A virtuous person would not spend excessive time engaging in sexual behavior and thinking because it is intemperate (under the health type of temperance). And a virtuous person would not rape a child because it is intemperate (let this case fall under the disrespect type of temperance). If we construe the actions broadly enough to include in them not just their effects on the victim and not just those aspects related to the victim, but also the reasons and the motives behind committing the actions, then these behaviors are wrong *precisely* because they contravene a virtue whose domain is the sexual. One can seduce a friend's spouse in order to take revenge on the friend, and one can do so in order to satisfy one's sexual desire.[15] The first is wrong, not because it is contrary to a *sexual* virtue, but because (and this is a nonexhaustive "because") it is contrary to a nonsexual one (for example, loyalty). The second is wrong precisely because (again, nonexhaustively) it is contrary to a sexual virtue (temperance).[16]

Goldman would be right were we to restrict our understanding of "action" only to those aspects related to the moral patient. For now we can speak of rape as wrong because of its harm to the victim; we can speak of adultery as wrong because of its deception of the nonadulterous spouse. And these concepts (for instance, harm and deception) are concepts not exclusive to the sexual domain of life. However, even here we must be careful. For there is that type of temperance that is primarily related to the health of the agent, and there is nothing in what Goldman says that indicates his being aware that this area might constitute a legitimate ethical field for the sexual. His discussion is in terms of moral rules. Moral rules govern the interaction between people. This is why, I think, Goldman does not pay enough attention to the idea that in conducting one's sexual life in a certain way, one may not be living a decent life, one may not be flourishing. Since flourishing is an ethical issue, then it might turn out to be the case, contra Goldman, that there are questions and issues surrounding sex that are ethical but that are not governed by general moral rules (or at least not the ones he seems to have in mind).[17]

Igor Primoratz, while aware of the notion that people can lead different sexual lives, nevertheless seems to think that there is nothing specifically moral about this. He claims that these are better thought of as ideals and so fall within the domain of the prudential rather than the moral. Whether one lives one's life by having sex only with people one is in love with, or whether one lives one's life by having sex with people one is not in love with (for example, sex with strangers) is a matter of personal ideals. Furthermore, according to Primoratz, even if ideals "have moral significance," they cannot be prescribed for everybody, because they exhibit diversity in their contents and can even be incompatible with each other (1999, 171). Indeed, "A person who adopts such a moral ideal and lives up to it may be appreciated, admired, praised for it. But a person who does not is not properly subjected to moral condemnation on that account. Such a person may be said to be failing to realize something morally valuable, but not to be doing something morally wrong" (171).

Primoratz *might* be right about all of this. But his discussion is still defective. It is defective because he does not take seriously the question as to whether certain sexual ideals *do* constitute moral failures of a sort, the moral failure to live an ethically good life. In the above quotation, Primoratz agrees that one might, in adopting one set of ideals rather than another, fail to realize something morally valuable. But failing to realize something morally valuable is not the same as adopting morally flawed ideals. One can fail to realize something morally valuable and yet incur no negative moral judgment. One who adopts ideals that are morally flawed, however, would incur negative moral judgments. Now it *might* be the case that there are no sexual ideals the adoption of which would constitute such an ethical failure (and it is because of this that Primoratz may be right). But Primoratz should have at least recognized this issue as an issue. Thus, in the sections that follow, I will address this very issue by addressing three examples of ideals that have been traditionally claimed to constitute moral failures, namely, living one's life by opting for promiscuous sex and by foregoing a sexual relationship; living one's life within a sexually nonmonogamous relationship; and living one's life by choosing the vocation of sex work. The discussion of all three will benefit from data from the experiences of gay people, especially men, and of sex workers. I use these data not due to the mistaken impression that everyone can imitate such lives, but because they furnish us with realistic examples that can be used to argue for the rationality of the three ideals.

However, there is one important question we have not yet settled. If these two types of temperance are virtues, they should satisfy the two general criteria of enabling their possessor to live well and of enabling her to live a good human life *qua* being human. Now we know that it is possible to moderate sexual desires, and so we know that it is possible to have such character traits. But *do* they satisfy these two neo-Aristotelian criteria of a trait being a virtue? Perhaps we can avoid answering this question since it is a traditional thought in the history of philosophy that temperance is a virtue, and uncovering *two* concepts of temperance need not weaken such a thought. Still, it would be good to answer this question, at least in outline. I will do so along the lines familiar to us from the previous chapters, affirmatively, and I will do so now since we need their answers for the next section. (However, out of respect for the traditional thought that temperance is a virtue, what I will not do is explain how both concepts of temperance fit the definition of "virtue." This can be done easily and the reader can do it on his or her own.)

Consider first T1. Does the possession of this trait benefit its agent? The answer is affirmative. It is especially clear with respect to food and drink: given the connections of T1 with the health of the agent, over- or underconsumption of food and drink puts the agent's health at risk. This is obvious with respect to physical health, but it is also true with respect to mental health, not in the sense that the agent becomes crazy or insane, but in the sense that the agent might very well become preoccupied with an activity (eating and/or drinking) at the expense of other activities. In other words, lack of T1 might render the agent's practical reasoning and deliberation about ends defective (though not necessarily in any detrimental sense), and they are defective because the agent loses sight of what is worthy about life. As Charles Young puts it, Aristotle "regularly associates profligacy with a view about the *worth* of the pleasures of eating and drinking in human life" (1988, 536). If we add sex to eating and drinking, the point that intemperate people get things wrong by assigning to them the incorrect value would apply to it as well. This should not conjure in the reader's mind a comic picture of an agent who is running around hunting and sniffing for food and drink. Rather, the picture to be conjured is of someone who simply has his priorities wrong.

But what about lack of T1 with respect to sex? As far as physical health is concerned, it is difficult to see how the lack of T1 could endanger the agent's health. Sexually transmitted diseases enter the picture only marginally, since T1 is about *amounts*, and so for all we know the agent could be having *lots* of sex but with just one partner. Moreover, even if the agent is having lots of sex with different people, the agent may be taking precautions, and this, again, renders the problem of disease marginal. Aside from diseases, does having too much (and let's not forget "too little") sex endanger the agent physically? I cannot see how it can do so. The old and traditional folk wisdoms ("Too much sex can make your penis melt away," or "Don't masturbate too much or else you'll develop hairy palms [or a nasty hump, à la Quasimodo]") turned out, happily, to be nuggets of ignorance.[18]

The only case to be made would be, as far as I can see, about mental and psychic health (again, not in the sense of being crazy or stricken with dementia). It could be argued that too much sex can lead to, or simply be a manifestation of, an overvaluation of sexual activities over other types of activities, and this could undermine the agent's entire ability to deliberate correctly about ends in a human life. And *this*, simply, cannot be good for the agent. It turns the agent's head—to borrow and slightly change a phrase from George Eliot—into a mere satellite of the agent's body. (A similar argument cannot be made for too little sex in an agent's life; the argument against this has to be made either along the lines that too little sex makes the agent's life difficult to lead, given the naturalness of the sexual urges, or along the lines that too little sex or no sex at all betrays a lack of the correct ordering of life's goods on the agent's part.) This argument is, no doubt, very sketchy. But it seems to me that someone who does spend too much time thinking about, searching for, and/or engaging in sex, and does so not out of frustration, but due to a strong libido, is certainly on his way to undermining his ability to be a good practical reasoner. And undermining this ability will eventually land him in a lot of trouble (for example, no publications, no tenure, and so forth). Underlying this reasoning are two crucial ideas. First, that while sex as an activity is important to our lives, it is not so important as to allow for an agent to—to some extent at least—organize his life around it. Second, there is a rough way of ordering the activities in our lives such that some are worthier than others, and such that those which are worthier make room for an agent organizing her life around them. Thus pursuing science is a worthier activity than drinking alcohol, and an agent who organizes her life around the former does not, normally, undermine her practical reasoning. I will return to these issues in a bit more detail in the following sections.

One crucial question, of course, is, What is too much sex? This is the question that I wish to indirectly tackle. I say "indirectly" because I will do so by asking whether the three ideals sketched above are examples of too much sex. And one good way of answering this question is by seeing how they could possibly undermine an agent's ability to deliberate about his life and/or by seeing how they could possibly deter the agent from having other important goods in life. But more on this below.

Does T1 allow the agent to become a better human being, *qua* being human? The answer is "Yes." When Aristotle rejected the life of gratification as being a good candidate for the *eudaimon* life (1985, 1095b19), he did so on the grounds that those who lead it are "slavish *since* the life they decide on is a life fit for grazing animals" (my emphasis). The "since" is important: it tells us that Aristotle is not giving us *two* reasons for rejecting such a life, but *one* reason: the slavishness of the life of gratification. The problem with this life is that the agent's rationality is entirely undermined. It is undermined not in the sense that the agent will no longer use her reason (she might, after all, use her reason to secure yet another night of steamy sex), but in the sense that reason becomes the tool of her desires; it is no longer the leader, the arbitrator, in her life. And to undermine reason in *this* way is surely to lead a defective human life, because, as the above quotation from Young points out, it reflects an incorrect valuational system on the part of the agent, given the understanding that we are social *rational* animals.[19]

A similar thought applies to those people who are insensible with respect to sex. We should keep in mind that to Aristotle, the pleasures of eating, drinking, and sexual activity are not just pleasures that we do, as a matter of fact, enjoy. They are also ones that it is *proper* or *right* that we enjoy, given that we are human *animals*, so long as we do so as reason enjoins. Thus, insensible people are not ones who do not eat and drink and have sex, but are ones who simply do not take pleasure in such activities. Since the pleasures of such activities are proper for us to enjoy, insensible people show themselves in this respect to be defective.

Of course, someone who is IT1 need not be leading his life in such a way that she does nothing *but* seek sexual pleasure. So in this respect, our IT1 agent might not perfectly fit Aristotle's characterization of someone who decides to lead a life of gratification, that is, someone whose life is *entirely* ruled by sexual passion. However, the point remains basically the same: our IT1 agent has neither rational control, nor, more importantly, rational regulation over how much sex she has and desires to have. To the extent that her sexual desires undermine her rationality, she is leading a defective human life.

Let us turn to T2. An agent who is intemperate in this sense is one who is willing to lie, steal, deceive, rape, behave unjustly, unkindly, and/or with cowardice in order to achieve sexual gratification. Such an agent, in other words, is willing to do what is base because he is unable to infuse his sexual desires with reason. But it should be clear that such an agent opens himself up to being caught, treated badly, punished, shunned by others, and so on, and such risks cannot constitute a bene-fit to the agent. IT2 is ruled out here as allowing the agent to live well for basically the same reasons dishonesty, cowardice, and other vices are ruled out (Hursthouse 1986 and 1999b, part 3). Thus, IT2 does not benefit its agent.

Moreover, such an agent leads a defective human life because he goes against the social and rational parts of our essence. T2 plays an extremely crucial role in human life. Without it, it is difficult for human beings to trust and rely on each other, because of the danger that we are willing to wrong each other simply to attain the gratification of sexual desires. In other words, having T2 allows for a good functioning of our social inter-actions. In addition, one who is intemperate in this sense is one who sub-ordinates his reason to his desires, and to that extent leads a defective human life. Thus, IT2 positively hinders its agent from being a good human being *qua* being human.

I have conducted the discussion about whether T1 and T2 are virtues mostly by envisioning what it means to lack them. But in doing this, I open myself up to the charge that I have only argued against viciousness, since a continent agent could avoid the pitfalls I have mentioned. In response, it is indeed plausible that from an Aristotelian perspective a continent life is higher up on the scale of good lives than that of viciousness, and to this extent the charge is correct. However, it does not follow that a continent life is as good as a virtuous one. A continent life is characterized mainly by a disharmony and so a struggle between the agent's reason and her desires. To the extent that such a life is characterized by internal struggle, a life of virtue (and hence of T1 and T2) is more beneficial to the agent in the straightforward sense that it is less painful, if not also more pleasurable, to lead.

Furthermore, to the extent that a life of continence is characterized by disharmony between reason and desire, a life of virtue (and hence of T1 and T2) instantiates a better human life *qua* being human. If rationality is our hallmark, and if our desires and emotions can be infused with reason, as an Aristotelian claims, then the more the former are shot through and through with reason the more we will lead a *human* life, and it would be, for that reason, a better life. In addition, when reason regulates desires, acting morally in normal cases will be done gladly and not grudgingly. That is why on most construals of virtue ethics the virtuous agent is portrayed as one who not only is disposed to do what is right, but who also desires to act in that way. To this extent, being virtuous allows human beings to rely on each other better and to trust each other quite a bit more than being continent. And so to this extent, continence goes against the social aspect of our nature.[20]

I conclude, then, that both T1 and T2 do indeed satisfy the two criteria for a character trait being a virtue.

2. Three Sexual Ways of Life

People sometimes decide to live their lives in such a way that, as far as sexual practices are concerned, they engage in sexual promiscuity, or they are part of a relationship that is "open" (the parties to it agree to have sex with people who are not their spouses), or they have as their main line of work "sex work" (prostitution, acting in pornography, working in phone sex, and so on). More importantly, such people are often—and at best—the objects of pity, while at worst they are the objects of moral condemnation. It is thus important to investigate whether such moral condemnation is justified. Since this is a book inspired by virtue ethics, I will specifically investigate whether such moral condemnation has any justification from within this moral theory. In this section, I will be concerned mainly with spelling out why I have chosen these three ways of life and not others to discuss, why I designate them as "ideals" and "ways of life," and how we go about, from within virtue ethics, finding out whether they deserve moral condemnation.

In the first section, I stated that I will discuss the three ideals of leading a life of promiscuous sex and foregoing a sexual relationship, leading a life of a nonmonogamous sexual relationship, and having sex work as one's primary job. But why these three ideals? Why not others? My main reason is simple: they seem to me, given the general way in which they are stated, to be pretty much exhaustive of the possibilities. Consider the first two. All human beings can lead their lives by either being in a sexual relationship or not. If the former, they can either be in the relationship monogamously or not. Of course, there are people who decide to lead their lives by being sexually inactive, by abstaining from sex altogether, such as—ideally—priests and some other types of religious devotees. But this is not a sexual ideal. It is sexual only in the sense that abstaining from sex is a choice made in regard to the sexual domain; but it is not a sexual ideal in the sense I am interested in, which is the way that human beings can conduct their lives sexually.

But, one might ask, what about people who commit adultery but do so not because they have entered into a nonmonogamous relationship, but, say, due to a weak will in the face of temptation? My answer is that such people—the majority of adulterers out there—do not commit adultery out of an ideal they hold (exactly as the hypothetical objection claims),[21] and so they are not examples of people who have ideals not covered by my terrain. These are people who are in monogamous relationships (but who slip every now and then, so to speak) and so do not fall under another type of ideal. One issue concerning them is how we are to morally evaluate their *acts* of adultery.[22] However, my concern with them in this chapter is at best indirect, since I am more concerned with those people who are in long-term relationships but who are also nonmonogamous (these relationships are often called "open marriages").

Consider next sex work. There are many people (mostly women) who have vocations that have come to be called "sex work,"[23] such as prostitution, stripping, nude modeling for sex magazines, pornography, and phone sex work. It is true that such people seem to be covered by the first two ideals, in that they are either in relationships or not, and on either possibility they will be covered by one of the two ideals. However, sex work adds an important element to the discussion because it introduces the element of vocation, a life-affecting and person-affecting dimension that cannot be ignored. And if our issue, as I will momentarily explain, is the flourishing of human lives, the question whether sex work detracts, enhances, or leaves unaffected human flourishing becomes a central topic.

More importantly, however, I have chosen these three ideals and not their main counterpart (a life of being in a monogamous relationship) because all three have been frowned upon by traditional morality. All three, moreover, have been frowned upon by many philosophers, although nowadays there is more being written to favor a liberal sexual ethic. But, as far as I know, none of these philosophers—I mean those who have championed a liberal sexual morality—have done so from a neo-Aristotelian perspective; they have approached the issue from the usual discussion of moral rules, from Kantian ethics, and from consequentialism.[24] (There is also nothing strange in juxtaposing "liberal" and "Aristotelian" in one sentence, because one might arrive at the same, or very similar, conclusions of a liberal philosophy of sex by starting with neo-Aristotelian premises.) Furthermore, with the possible exception of Martha Nussbaum (but see next paragraph and further discussion below), those philosophers who are neo-Aristotelian or who are linked to Aristotelianism via another closely related school of thought, such as Thomism, have proven to be extremely prudish about sexual issues (I have in mind Anscombe, Finnis, Scruton, and other less famous figures). Must one be conservative about sexual issues if one is an Aristotelian? It is, it seems to me, quite important to see how rich Aristotelianism can be on these matters, and that is why I have undertaken the project of proving that sexual liberalism is quite compatible with—and perhaps recommended by—Aristotelianism.

Even Martha Nussbaum, a liberal Aristotelian, often falls short—for no good reason it seems to me—of defending such sexual practices. Her case is complicated because she often writes as if sexual practices such as casual sex, sex work, and so forth are morally in the clear. Consider the following quotation from "Taking Money For Bodily Services" which, though about sex work, applies equally well to casual sex in general:

> What seems to be the real issue is that the woman is not attended to as an individual, not considered a special, unique being. But that . . . may not even be immoral, for surely we cannot deeply know all the people with whom we have dealings in life, and many of those dealings are just fine without deep knowledge. So our moral question boils down to the question, Is sex without deep personal knowledge always immoral? It seems to me officious and presuming to use one's own experience to give an affirmative answer to this question, given that people have such varied experiences of sexuality. (1999, 292)

However, in her essay "Objectification" Nussbaum defends a view regarding casual sex at odds with the sentiments just quoted. She argues that sex acts are wrong when they "do not take place in a larger context of regard for humanity" because otherwise they would be tantamount to using human beings as tools for the sexual purposes of others (1999, 238). This sounds correct. But when we look at how she applies this to casual sex, we find the conclusion that casual sex involves such objectionable treatment: "For in the absence of any narrative history with the person, how can desire attend to anything else but the incidental, and how can one do more than use the body of the other as a tool of one's own states?" (1999, 237).

I do not know whether attending to the sexual body parts of others is "incidental" (one good casual sexual experience can provide its participants with intense pleasure and future fond memories), and I do not know why attending to the incidental entails a morally vicious form of using another. But the answer to the second question is clear: one can also provide the other with pleasure. In short, unless Nussbaum simply wants to dismiss casual sex out of the moral hand, her arguments against it are not impressive (I will return to the issue of objectification below). So even Nussbaum's views fall short of vindicating practices that to many seem immoral and unvirtuous.

It is important to note that the above three ideals are *ideals*, not ways of life that the agent is *forced* to lead. Otherwise, much of the ground of speaking in terms of virtues and vices would be undercut. For if force (or, more generally, difficult circumstance) is what drives our agents to engage in the sex they engage in, then we would not be able to study our agents as they are themselves, so to speak; we would see them in their not-so-normal situations, and this would strongly qualify any discussion of their virtues and vices. So we will stick with ideals. And by "ideals" I do not mean something along the lines of "aspiring to lofty principles," or "unrealizable states of affairs," but rather "ways of life that the agent desires to lead" (and "way of life" does not entail permanence, of course). Thus (and I will go into these ideals in more detail in section 3), the first ideal is not to be understood as applying to an agent who is, and has been, hopping from one person's bed into another's in order to find someone with whom he can be in a relationship. Rather, the agent has more or less decided that he does not want to be in a relationship, and that he will get his sexual satisfactions from one-night stands, or by seeking it with sex workers, or by some other means. (So the agent I have in mind is also not one with a low sex drive or one who is disgusted by sex, etc.)

The second ideal is also not to be understood as being about a relationship that has gone sour and whose parties, unable to solve their problems, start seeing other people on the side. Rather, the ideal I have in mind involves a couple who have decided that their lives would be much enriched were they to have sex with other people. Other than a bad relationship, the *how and why* they do this is somewhat unimportant. What is important is that they both willingly decide and agree to this arrangement and see it as desirable. Similarly, the way of life I have in mind when it comes to sex work is one that the worker has, more or less, chosen. I do not have in mind sex workers who are forced into the profession by a pimp (as often happens in streetwalking prostitution) or their family (as frequently happens in some third world countries). I say "more or less" because it is difficult to have many clear-cut cases here. A woman, for example, who decides to go into stripping in order to make ends meet could—in some sense of "could"—have chosen another job. So she was not forced into it. But sex work is highly stigmatized work and whoever "chooses" it must, in some way, be under much duress, and wouldn't this make it a case of coercion? I am not convinced by this reasoning. After all, sex work often pays a lot more than working as a cashier at Wal-Mart. But I mention it simply in order to explain to the reader why I say "more or less," namely, that there are plausible reasons for the claim that sex work is, at least somewhat, coerced.

I have been speaking of ideals, ways of life, and not of acts. I have also just mentioned flourishing. My concerns, in this chapter, are with these two, namely, these ideals and flourishing. My central question is this: Do any of these three ideals detract from a flourishing life? Do any enhance it? And how do we go about answering these questions? The strategy to answer these questions from a neo-Aristotelian perspective is to rely on ethical naturalism, the project of basing ethics in human nature. Since a number of capable philosophers have done a fine job of defending such a project, I will only retain those elements relevant to my task without defending them.[25]

Under a neo-Aristotelian ethical naturalism, in order to argue that a certain type of human life, such as that of a gangster, is defective (vicious), one does not start with that particular type of life and then argue that there is something wrong with it. Rather, one starts by validating certain character traits as virtues (those traits that benefit their possessors and that enable them to be good human beings *qua* being human), and then one claims that defective human lives lack such traits. If, for example, justice, charity, and honesty are virtues, and if your average gangster lacks these virtues, then, to that extent, your average gangster is a vicious, that is, a defective, human being.[26] In our case, we want to find out whether people leading a promiscuous, no-relationship life, a nonmonogamous life, or a life of sex work are defective human beings. How are we to go about doing this?

According to ethical naturalism, we need to ask whether such lives lack the relevant virtues. Suppose we plausibly take temperance as our locus of discussion. We have seen that there are two types of temperance, T1 (moderation) and T2 (not wronging others). We also know from the last section that both T1 and T2 are virtues. Do the above mentioned ways of life lack T1 or T2 (or both)? Or, to put it more accurately, do they contravene T1, T2, or both? I will start with T2 since its treatment is easier and more direct than that of T1. My next task will be the extended one of discussing the three ways of life with respect to T1.

3. The Three Ideals and T2

This section addresses whether the three ways of life are necessary indicators of the presence of intemperance in the second sense (IT2—wrongs
done to others due to desire for pleasure) in the agent. I will argue that
neither promiscuity nor open relationships entails IT2, and that both are
compatible with T2. Furthermore, I will argue that sex work is also compatible with T2, and also that it is compatible with a host of other virtues.
It is important to bring up other virtues in a discussion of sex work because
sex work, unlike promiscuity and open relationships, is not about—or primarily about—the sexual desires of the sex worker.

It should be obvious that *neither* of the first two mentioned ways of
life—promiscuity and open marriages—need lack T2. And if any of them
do, indeed, lack it, and even have the vice of intemperance in this sense
(IT2), they will do so not because of anything intrinsic to them as ways of
life. They will do so because of a myriad of other factors, the very same factors that explain why many people have the vices of dishonesty, cruelty,
and/or greed, for example.

Consider the second way of life. Here is a person who is in an open
relationship with another and who every now and then (or often; frequency here is irrelevant) engages in sex with someone other than his
spouse. It should be obvious that he could very well do so and be T2: he
would never desire to engage in sex, let alone actually do so, with someone else *at the expense* of his spouse, that is, by deceiving, lying to, or ignoring his spouse. Furthermore, even if no deception or lying to the spouse
occurs, our agent would never desire to engage in sex, let alone actually do
so, with someone other than his spouse if engaging in sex meant deceiving
or lying to that person, or forcing sex on that person, or if that person were
a child, and so forth. In short, open relationships do not preclude their
members from being T2. Indeed, just as a person in a traditional, monogamous relationship can be T2 or IT2, so can a person in a nontraditional,
nonmonogamous relationship.

Similar remarks apply to the first type of ideal. A person who is not in a
relationship and who is happy having sex with multiple partners (not necessarily at the same time) need not be IT2. Such an agent might very well
be virtuous and have T2. In this respect, he would not desire to have sex
with the wrong person (e.g., a minor, his friend's spouse); he would not
desire to have sex in the wrong way (e.g., by forcing himself on another, or
without using appropriate protection); he would not desire to have sex for
the wrong end (e.g., have sex with X to take revenge on Y); and he would
not desire to have sex at the wrong times (e.g., while attending a funeral or

a wedding). In short, there is nothing about leading the first way of life that necessitates lacking T2. One can glimpse this fact by considering people who are in monogamous marriages. Some of them have sex with their spouses in ways that indicate that they lack T2 (forcing sex on their spouses, not paying heed to the pleasure and pain of their spouses, pushing for sex even when their spouses are not particularly desirous to engage in sex, and so on). Having or lacking T2 is not a matter of monogamy or a matter of being in a relationship. It is a matter of character.

There are, however, two possible difficulties. First, one might object that I am somehow being extremely wrongheaded about this. Here is how the hypothetical objection goes: surely flourishing requires that we lead monogamous lives and surely flourishing requires that promiscuity, if promiscuity is indeed entailed by the first ideal or way of life, not be practiced. But if so, then none of the conclusions given above can be sustained. In setting out this possible objection, I have not done so by making it part of an argument. The reason is simple: I do not know how one can go about making an *argument* to support this objection. Below—and to modify the thought in the last sentence—I will discuss and reject a few positions that have indeed claimed that adultery, promiscuity, and so forth, are inhibitors of flourishing. Since the above-mentioned objection seems to be merely an assertion, I will offer below cases that serve, among other functions, as counterexamples to it.

Second, one might object that while I have shown that there is no logical or psychological incompatibility between the first two ways of sexual life, on the one hand, and T2, on the other, I have not shown that the former do not threaten T2 or render it less likely. For example, consider the first sexual way of life. Someone who enjoys one-night stands and casual sex might be led, out of spiraling lust due to the very way he conducts his sexual life, to desire more and more sexual encounters. And this excessive sexual desire would surely endanger his T2. Are there any considerations that one can bring forth to at least alleviate this worry?

There are two such considerations. First, I am not convinced by the hypothesis of spiraling lust in the above objection. Surely there are, or could be, people whose taste for sexual pleasures leads them to be more and more lustful. But I wonder to what extent this is true of the majority of people. My worry is that while this example might describe *some* people, it might not offer a realistic picture of how the majority of people conduct their sexual lives. Second, the first point I just raised becomes more plausible when we keep in mind that we are speaking about virtuous people. To briefly repeat a point from the last chapter, a virtuous person is morally reliable. Should he conduct his sexual life along the lines of the first sexual type of life, then in order to make the objection plausible, a case needs to be made that his desire for sexual pleasure would indeed become so consuming as to threaten his T2. Moreover, a case needs to be made that when such a threat is present, the agent in question is not likely to take steps to ensure that his virtuousness is intact. And this seems difficult, in the sense that it does not render the probability claim in the objection—the claim that the first two sexual ways of life threaten T2—plausible.

If my reasoning is correct so far, then not only are the first two ways of sexual life logically and psychologically possible within a virtuous life, they are also not likely to threaten virtue. In other words, there does not seem to be anything about the first two ways of life, as such, that makes for a tense existence with virtue, in this case T2.

The treatment of the ideal of sex work is similar to the above treatments, but is also different in important respects. A sex worker need not cheat her clients; she does not force sex on them; she is usually very cautious about using protection; and though she often engages in a variety of sexual acts to satisfy the myriad desires of her clients, it is a tall order to claim that these sexual acts (such as bondage and dominance, role playing, and threesomes) are ways of having sex in the "wrong ways," for it seems to me that as long as the parties are genuinely consenting to the acts and are not harming anyone, their actions are not contravening any virtues. Of course, I am being a bit quick here, and it might be the case that some types of sexual acts do go against some virtues. But my point is that unless an argument is made to the effect that one or more of what a sex worker does contravenes a virtue, then sex work, as such, need not involve the vice of IT2 or the lack of T2. Indeed, it need not lack any of the other virtues, and this brings me to the important differences between sex work as a way of life and the first two ones.

Most of the women (and men) in the sex industry emphasize the claim that they consider their work to be, simply, *work*. Most of them claim that it is not about *them* deriving *sexual* pleasure from their work, but that, as far sexual pleasure is concerned, it is the client's that is of importance. *They* are in it for the money and for a host of other reasons (for example, a flexible work schedule, or a sense of being desired).[27] This is not to deny that *some* sexual encounters are sexually enjoyable for sex workers, nor is it to deny that a general liking of sexual activity might help. It is rather to put the issue of the sex worker's sexual pleasure as far as her work is concerned in the right perspective. And when this is done, we should be able to see that we are very far, indeed, from T2, for we are no longer talking about sexual pleasure, and temperance is precisely about sexual (and bodily) pleasure.

In this crucial respect, then, sex work marks an important difference from the other two ideals. However, what this point indicates is that it becomes important now to see whether sex work *necessarily* goes against virtues other than temperance, virtues such as justice, courage, kindness, benevolence, and so forth. Does it? Again, it is I think pretty clear that it does not necessarily do so. Whether a sex worker is unfair, deceptive, or cruel has nothing to do with the sex work as such, but more to do with the character of the person herself.[28]

But let us not be too hasty. For it is true that sex workers often engage in what seems to be unvirtuous behavior, and, more importantly, such behavior seems to be required by the very work they engage in. For example, it is well known that sex workers often lie to their clients about how desirable they (the sex workers) find them (the clients). This is important because it is crucial for the sex worker to put the client at his ease, to make him feel good about himself, and, most importantly, to make him think that she finds him desirable. So remarks such as, "I love your hairy chest," "What a gorgeous smile you have," "What muscular arms!" and "You're exactly my type" often come with the very territory of sex work (and the examples have to be varied depending on the kind of sex work one is speaking about).

Consider another type of seemingly unvirtuous behavior. Sex workers often have to pretend that they are sexually enjoying what they are doing. If they are prostitutes, they pretend that they are sexually enjoying the sexual act. If they are strippers, they pretend that dancing naked for clients is something that turns them on. If they are phone sex workers, they pretend to be masturbating on the other end of the line. And so on. But most of this is, as I kept mentioning, pretense. Sex workers engage in it so as to make their clients comfortable and happy. And they engage in it so as to act on one of the oldest sexual psychological observations: when a person perceives his sexual partner to be enjoying the sex, the former gets more excited (this is, of course, not an invariable law). By simulating sexual pleasure, they help their clients get more sexually excited and achieve orgasm faster. In doing this, they are able to see more clients per day and so make more money.

Both of these types of behavior *seem* to involve deception and lying. And both seem to be essential to sex work if one is to be successful at it. But they are not forms of unvirtuous behavior, for the simple reason that they are either not really instances of lying and deception, or they are expected, innocent lies. A client has to be stupid or out of touch with reality to believe that the woman feigning orgasm at the other end of the phone line is *actually* having an orgasm. No pornography viewer in his right mind is going to believe that those screams and spasmodic head turns are the screams and turns of the ecstasy of orgasm. This is not to say that no sex worker ever achieves an actual orgasm or ever sexually enjoys her (or his) work. The point is simply that much that sex workers say and do as part of their sex work has to be taken with a lump of salt, and any client who believes otherwise does so of his own fault. The oohs and aahs of sex work are rarely true, but they are not dishonest, either. (It is important to add here that it is not only sex workers who engage in this pretense; husbands, wives, and lovers in general often engage in the same pretense. Unless one is ready to believe that such relationships contain a good amount of deception and lying due to this feigning of pleasure and flattery, then one must be ready to accept that this is a pretense that fools no one.)

This of course takes us into some deep questions about how fantasy works in such situations. For obviously the feigning and pretense *does* its job. Equally obvious, however, is the fact that most viewers of pornography and clients of sex workers *know* about the pretense that the former engage in. So we seem to have some sort of a paradox, perhaps a paradox parallel to that found in the problem of "fearing fictions" in the philosophy of art. I do not want to go into this issue because I do not need to, although my hunch is that human psychology is complex enough to accommodate both sets of observations. And I do not need to go into this issue because what is important for my point is the reader's assent that clients of sex workers—except for the ones who are *really* living in a fantasy world—*know*, at some level, that sex workers engage in a large amount of pretense.

I will also not go into some of the other accusations given against sex work. Here is a sample: sex workers cannot consent to their work; sex work leads to drug use; sex workers are victims; sex workers were (and are) victims of child abuse; sex work is dangerous; sex work is degrading; sex work is a form of slavery. These are all criticisms given of sex work and they have been adequately dealt with.[29] I am also not confident that all of them, even if true, contravene a virtue or virtues. While lack of consent and degradation might contravene the virtue of integrity, for example, some go deeper and others are barely serious charges. For instance, *if* (and this is one big "if") sex work is indeed a form of slavery, then sex work will deprive the worker of her autonomy, and this undercuts the very possibility of leading a flourishing life (I will address the argument that sex work is a form of slavery in section 6 below). On the other hand, that sex work can lead to drug use is not, as such, a charge against sex work.

However, there is one accusation that I will briefly delve into for the reason that it has been pervasive in the recent literature. It makes the sex worker complicit in evil and so highly unvirtuous. This is none other than the charge, coming from some feminist quarters, that sex work enhances patriarchy. Let us suppose for a moment that the sex industry does indeed enhance and support a male-dominated society. If so, then women who, willingly or unwillingly, enter the sex industry are engaging in the oppression of other women, even if they themselves do not directly oppress any women, let alone intend to. It is important to note that this argument need not claim that the sex industry is essentially an oppressive system. It need only assert the weaker claim that the sex industry supports oppression contingently, and that this is nevertheless sufficient for the plausibility of the charge that a sex worker is supporting oppression by being a sex worker. Someone, for example, who does not own slaves but who works in an institution that supports slavery (the institution is not that of slavery itself; otherwise, it would be an essentially oppressive institution) is, regardless of his intentions, supporting slavery. He cannot claim that his actions and his work are morally neutral. A similar charge can be brought against women sex workers, if indeed it is true that the sex industry supports the oppression of women. And if oppression is what results, then being a sex worker contravenes the virtue of justice. This is more than sufficient to make sex work quite an immoral vocation. Furthermore, in this day and age of feminist discourse about sex work few female sex workers can justifiably claim ignorance of these basic issues, especially those in the West. With what has been discussed and written on the subject by feminists, including sex workers themselves, most sex workers must have a good idea about what is at stake; and if a sex worker claims ignorance, then her ignorance is culpable, unless we have an extreme case on our hands.[30]

But how does one go about arguing that the sex industry oppresses *all* women? ("All" here is not meant to convey the idea that each and every single woman is oppressed, but that it is not only women sex workers who are oppressed; sex work has oppressive repercussions beyond the industry itself and on women *in general*.) The argument I will sketch gives the main structure of a family of arguments designed to achieve the same type of conclusion, namely, that sex work oppresses women in general.[31] The argument goes as follows: (1) Historically and traditionally, women have been viewed as being, first and foremost, bodies (and not minds), be it via their procreative, nurturing, emotional, and/or sexual capacities. (2) This view of women has been the major, if not the only, contributor to women's inferior status, and hence oppression, in society. (3) The sex industry enhances the image of women as being, first and foremost, bodies, through its projection of women as primarily sexual entities (whether as objects or subjects is irrelevant).[32] (4) Hence, the sex industry contributes to the oppression of women by enhancing the image of women as primarily sexual entities (note that one need not deny that the sex industry is also an *effect* of sexism in order to accept that it is a cause of it). (5) Hence, women who work in the sex industry are, irrespective of their avowed and explicit intentions, contributing to the oppression of women in general.

What are we to make of this argument? Advocates of such an argument have no problem accepting the idea that sex work is primarily about sex. In other words, they are not aligning themselves with traditional objections to sex outside of a love and/or marriage context; they are not, that is, supporting a prudish argument against sex as such. Rather, the problem the advocates of the argument have is with sex work being primarily about sex in a historically and traditionally oppressive *context*. It is the fact that sex work occurs within a history of oppression that the argument takes issue with. And it is this insistence on context that is a strength and a weakness of the argument. It is a strength because—to give one reason—it tells us that the argument is not antisex as such. It is a weakness because it makes us realize that once the contingent feature of sexism—and, hopefully, sexism *is* a contingent feature of our world—is removed, the argument will have no force against sex work. In other words, once sexism and sex oppression are eradicated, sex work cannot be objected to on these grounds.[33]

The real difficulty with the argument, however, is simply the falsehood of the third and crucial premise. It is no doubt true to claim that sex work—like many other cultural activities and practices, such as modeling, watching TV commercials, watching Hollywood movies, and going to shopping malls—affects *some* people by way of making them believe that women are, first and foremost, sexual beings. But the problem with the third premise is that it says much more than this; it is a general claim to the effect that sex work does this (and it needs to be general if the argument is to have hope of success). But surely this premise needs to be queried. For cultural images come to exist not by divine intervention, but via people's beliefs and practices. And once this is kept firmly in mind, we must insist that unless we think of people as being passive and permanent retainers of ideas, we ought to reject the third premise as being too ambitious and hence false.

Consider, as an illustration, applying the third premise to male teenagers.[34] By doing this, we catch men, so to speak, at a sensitive and formative part of their growth. We can then say that by being exposed to pornography, by going to have sex with prostitutes, by attending strip clubs, at that tender age, our young men are imbibing beliefs to the effect that women are primarily sexual entities, and that these beliefs affect their future behavior and attitudes towards women. But this would be at best a highly tenuous psychological claim. It neglects other conflicting beliefs that teenagers might hold; it neglects the fact that teenagers are not passive and stupid recipients of images; it neglects the fact that teenagers interact with women all the time in nonsexual ways and contexts; and, most importantly, it neglects the possibility that even if teenagers passively receive ideas at that age, they need not continue to hold these beliefs as they grow up, nor need these beliefs continue to implicitly affect their actions from behind the scenes, as puppet masters. My point in this illustration is not to claim that the argument has usually been given with teenagers specifically in mind; my point is to illustrate, by giving one seemingly plausible application of it, the type of problems it must face.[35]

The argument contains more than a grain of truth. It relies on the extremely compelling idea that given the way society has thought of, and continues to think of, women, we expect, to some extent, sex work to contain and to play on such views of women for it to succeed. And because of this, we expect that sex work will to some extent help maintain sexist views about women. But it remains difficult to sustain the thought that sex work is bad or evil because it aids in the oppression of women, and to state such a thought in blanket, general ways. How, when, under what conditions, and with whom it does help oppress women are open questions. Because of this, the argument is not rationally compelling. A sex worker is not being irrational if she were to reject such an argument on these grounds. More importantly, she would not be acting in ways that go against the virtue of justice (acting unjustly) by being a sex worker.

Granted that sex work is not logically incompatible with virtue, specifically T2, one might wonder, however, whether it is in tension with it. That is, one might wonder, given possible cases of virtuous sex workers, whether such cases negate the claim that sex work and virtue, especially T2, are nevertheless inimical to each other. By way of response, we must not confuse two things with each other. First, the sex industry, as it exists today and most likely in the future, is a huge and a highly varied one. That some, and perhaps even many, women and men sex workers are led due to numerous contingent factors to lie, cheat, and engage in all sorts of immoral behavior is not surprising. And in this respect, such behavior does go against a myriad of virtues. But, second, there is the further issue whether sex work as such leads to such behavior. In other words, are these cases of immoral behavior due to the fact that we are, as human beings, in general far from being good people? Or are they due to sex work itself? Comparing such behavior in the sex industry with the behavior of people in other types of jobs leads one to speculate that the answer is the former, namely, that it is because of the fact that most people are far from being virtuous.

With this point in mind, our question is more focused: Is there anything about sex work that is inimical to virtue? My answer is negative. Sex
work is in many important ways similar to other business transactions. It
basically involves the selling of sexual services on the part of the sex worker
to clients. Unless one shows that there is something specific about sex
work that makes it essentially different from other types of work (I will
examine a few arguments of this sort in section 6 below), then it does not
seem to be the case that there is anything about sex work that is inimical
to virtue. With the exception of the few innocuous lies I mentioned above,
sex work as such does not raise the probability of a sex worker being unfair,
dishonest, cruel, and cowardly, to mention a few vicious types of acts.
Hence, sex work, as such, does not sit in tension with virtue.

I have, in my treatment of these three ways of life, neglected two crucial issues. The first has to do with pregnancy, abortion, and contraception. To state the obvious, the most usual way for pregnancy to occur is
as a result of sexual intercourse. Were women (and men) who are promiscuous, were women (and men) who are in open relationships, and were
female sex workers (and male sex workers who have women as their
clients) to be careless about contraception, then they would be, to put it
simply, intemperate (not to mention selfish, reckless, and shortsighted).
For they would be willing to engage in sexual behavior that might very
well lead to an unwanted pregnancy, which disregards the importance and
value of human life. Of course, not all sexual behavior is in the form of
intercourse, and so not all sexual behavior is of the type that could lead to
pregnancy. But when we are speaking about sexual *intercourse*, then carelessness about contraception, including use of such methods as *coitus inter-
ruptus*, would indicate a disregard for human life. In this respect, women
and men who are promiscuous and/or in open relationships would be
intemperate, since they would be willing to risk unwanted pregnancy. In
either case, there is a certain attitude towards human life that falls short of
what is morally acceptable, an attitude held simply for the desire to engage
in sexual pleasure. In the case of sex workers, especially prostitutes, and
given that their work is not so much about sexual pleasure but about
money, then their carelessness about contraception would contravene
virtues other than temperance, virtues such as justice (in its aspect of
respect for human life), nonselfishness, and being responsible. (Of course,
most sex workers are not careless about contraception because they cannot
afford to be.)

With these remarks about contraception on record, I will set aside these
issues, while also reminding the reader that for this chapter especially, but
also throughout the book, I have assumed that the people I discuss

(promiscuous people, people in open relationships, and sex workers) are, when the issue is relevant, *not* careless about contraception.

The second crucial issue I have so far neglected is that of objectification. A number of important thinkers have argued to the effect that casual sex objectifies its participants. Kant, for instance, condemns sexual activity outside the confines of marriage as debasing our humanity, with "human nature [being] thereby sacrificed to sex" (1963, 164). A cluster of arguments have emerged with the general, common theme that promiscuous sex, casual sex, sex with a prostitute, and even masturbation, are wrong in that they somehow reduce the parties involved to mere objects or means to sexual pleasure (and not all of these have Kantian bases.[36]) I will designate these sexual activities appropriately enough with the label "casual sex." For it is obvious that all of the three ways of life under discussion involve casual sex. Promiscuity necessarily entails casual sex, since one of the hallmarks of promiscuous sex is sex for the sake of sex without commitments. (Casual sex, however, does not entail promiscuity, because the latter has a built-in repeatedness to it that the former does not.) Sex between sex workers and their clients is also necessarily casual, and much sexual activity on the part of spouses with those who are not their spouses is also casual sex, although this is not a necessary element to it (consider, for example, having affairs with others). If the argument that casual sex objectifies its parties is sound, then all three of our ideals—a promiscuous life, a life whose agent is in an open relationship, and a life whose main vocation is sex work—will surely involve treating others as mere objects, and this one behavior that contravenes the virtue of justice, given that justice is a virtue that commands us to, among other things, treat others with respect.

The reader will excuse my somewhat sketchy treatment of this issue because it has been adequately dealt with in the literature. Almost any book or article on sex and sexual ethics has addressed one or another version of this argument.[37] We can begin by stating that when two parties (or more) agree to engage in sex for the sake of the sex itself, and not as part of expressing love or as a preamble to a relationship or what have you, they, simply, need not be treating each other as means or as objects. They are engaging in an activity together, enjoying it together, and heeding each other's needs and desires as they do so. Unless we believe that to enjoy sexual pleasure we must do so only within certain contexts (such as that of marriage), then it is difficult to deny the moral permissibility of the act of two people providing each other with sexual pleasure while also respecting each other's agency, desires, and autonomy. No doubt, there are ruthless people out there who, even if they secure another's consent, go on to treat them quite shabbily during the sex act, paying attention only to their own pleasures. Such cases can be plausibly maintained to involve treating the other as a means only. But, surely, not all cases of casual sex are like this.

The above argument can be put in a specifically Kantian way, and this is important, given that most arguments accusing casual sex of objectification are Kantian or Kant-inspired. Especially relevant here is Kant's second categorical imperative: "Act in such a way that you treat humanity, whether in your own person or in the person of another, always at the same time as an end and never simply as a means" (1993, 36). It seems to me that casual sex typically does not violate this principle at all. Consider the following nonsexual example (borrowed from Hill 1980). Suppose one hires carpenters to build an opera house. In a sense, the person who hires them is using them as a means. But as long as the carpenters are *able to* (they need not actually do so) adopt, according to Thomas Hill, Jr., the end or the goal of the person hiring them, then they are not used *merely* as a means. And this satisfies Kant's formula. In a typical case of casual sex, the partners are not only *able to* adopt each other's goals, but they actually do share them, and this fact makes the case satisfy Kant's formula in even stronger ways than that of the opera house. While similar things can be said about open relationships, in a typical case of sex work, the wording must be in terms of the ability of the parties to adopt each other's goals. In any case, it does not seem that promiscuity, open relationships, and sex work violate the Kantian formula.[38]

But more can be said about this issue of objectification. Martha Nussbaum has done us all a great service in distinguishing between seven senses of the term "objectification" ("Objectification" 1999, 218). It would be extremely useful to go through this list and demonstrate that, first, casual sex need not, and typically does not, characterize some of these senses, and, second, that those senses which it does characterize, it does so in a morally innocuous way.[39] If we can do so, then we can show that the case against casual sex as necessarily involving immoral objectification is simply wrong. At the very least, the burden of proof shifts to those who wish to maintain this claim.

The first item on Nussbaum's list is instrumentality: "The objectifier treats the object as a tool of his or her purposes." We have seen in the discussion of Kant's Categorical Imperative that this is true, but that it can also characterize most of our transactions with people. As long as the parties to the transaction do not treat each other *only* as tools, then this sense of objectification is morally innocent. And while this sense of "objectification" generally characterizes cases of casual sex, it is morally innocuous.

The second sense of "objectification" is denial of autonomy: "The objectifier treats the object as lacking in autonomy and self-determination." This obviously is not a necessary characterization of casual sex. Indeed, it is highly atypical of cases of casual sex. Clients of sex workers, for example, typically respect the limits that the sex worker sets for what she is willing to sexually engage in. Moreover, in other forms of casual sex, such as one-night stands, the parties typically take into consideration the fact that their partners are autonomous beings who can determine for themselves whether they wish to engage in sex, when, with whom, under what conditions, and in what forms of sexual activity they wish to engage. That some sexual partners treat their partners as lacking in autonomy does not characterize casual sex, let alone constitute an essential attribute of it.

The third sense is that of inertness: "The objectifier treats the object as lacking in agency, and perhaps also in activity." Of all of the senses listed by Nussbaum, this is one of the ones that is the least true of casual sex. The reason is simple. In casual sex, the partners typically desire to have sex with other *human beings*, not with inert objects.

The fourth meaning of "objectification" is that of fungibility: "The objectifier treats the object as interchangeable (a) with other objects of the same type and/or (b) with objects of other types." This is a usual way of describing promiscuous people, and Nussbaum herself finds this sense of "objectification" to be morally lacking (see section 4 below). As we will see (section 4), promiscuous people are often thought of as indiscriminate in their sexual desires. If a gay man, for example, goes out cruising in a bar, then any man will do (after all, a man is an object that is interchangeable with other objects of the same type, that is, other men). But this claim is false. Promiscuous people, clients of sex workers, and spouses in open relationships often look for something specific. A gay man, for example, might desire to have sex with men of certain other types, such as Asian men or young men. To give another example, in a recent article in the *Chicago Reader* ("Did I Say That?" June 28, 2002), an anonymous phone-sex worker documents the large number of specific fantasies that the clients on the phone wished her to indulge in. Indeed, this is a common observation among sex workers about their clients. So a person seeking casual sex need not objectify his partners in the above two senses of "fungibility."

Still, one might object, the man in the above example seeks a certain type of man, and this would be a case of treating this type of man—for example, Asian or young—as fungible. And the phone-sex clients do not really care who is on the other end of the line, as long as she is able to play the role convincingly. This is true, but it would not render objectification as fungibility morally wrong. After all, when we want a car fixed, we look for car mechanics that fit a certain type (for example, those who can fix German cars). That car mechanics are fungible in this way does not render our seeking them out morally wrong. And this, by the way, is a pervasive feature of our dealings with people. Unless an argument can be produced to show why fungibility is wrong in the context of sex, we have no reason to believe it differs in its moral aspects from other ways of treating people as fungible in this respect.

The fifth sense of "objectification" on Nussbaum's list is violability: "The objectifier treats the object as lacking in boundary integrity, as something that it is permissible to break up, smash, break into." Like inertness, this is obviously not true of casual sex. Rare psychopaths notwithstanding, people seeking casual sex do not typically seek to break into, smash, and/or break up their partners. The same thing can be said about the sixth sense of "objectification," ownership: "The objectifier treats the object as something that is owned by another, can be bought or sold, etc."

The seventh and last meaning is denial of subjectivity: "The objectifier treats the object as something whose experiences and feelings (if any) need not be taken into account." No doubt, there are some people who do not take into account the feelings and experiences of their sexual partners, and this is sometimes true in cases where the sex is between two people in a love relationship. Outside the context of sex with sex workers—because clients are neither expected nor required to take into account the sexual feelings of sex workers—this is morally wrong. But even in the case of sex workers, the client is morally required to take into account the nonsexual feelings of the sex worker. He should not, for example, insult her. He should morally treat her within the same parameters that human beings should generally treat each other. That some people do not abide by these moral requirements, however, does not by any means characterize casual sex. Typically, partners in a casual sex encounter take into account the desires and decisions of each other. Moreover, this is not often done begrudgingly, as if it is something one had to do. Rather, it is considered part of the pleasure of the sexual experience, namely, knowing that your sexual partner is enjoying him or herself can be extremely satisfying. Of course, often times we hear the claim that in many cases women consent to sex acts but that their consent is not genuine (see, for example, West 1997). This is no doubt true. But admitting this does not amount to the claim that casual sex objectifies women in this sense. That there are cases of nongenuine consent does not establish the claim that casual sex necessarily amounts to not heeding one's partner's sexual desires and feelings.

I have argued that the three sexual ways of life do not necessarily involve any morally wrong objectification and so do not necessarily involve violating the virtues of justice and respect. I have also argued that they do not, as such, render virtue less likely or that they are somehow in tension with virtue. In addition to the other arguments offered at the beginning of this section, we can conclude that none of the three ways of life necessarily contravene T2, and that an agent might instantiate one or more of these ideals and yet also be T2. Whether an agent, in short, has T2 depends on the agent, not on these sex ideals.

4. The First Ideal and T1

The topic of concern in this section is whether leading a life of sexual promiscuity contravenes or is incompatible with temperance in the first sense (T1)—temperance regarding how much sex an agent has and its repercussions on the agent's flourishing. Does, in other words, living one's life by not being in a committed relationship and by having casual sex necessarily entail the absence of T1 in the life of the agent? I will argue that the answer is "no," and that not only can one be fully virtuous *and* sexually promiscuous, but also that there is nothing about promiscuity as a way of life that renders virtue less likely.

Minimal support for a negative answer to the above question can be used from the last chapter: we have seen that a deliberate abandonment of a loving marriage or marriagelike relationship (not that love and marriage are always wedded to each other) need not necessarily detract from an agent's flourishing. However, we can begin to build on this point by discussing the sexual aspect of it, namely, the desire of the agent to engage in nonloving sex with others. Here, we can introduce two different variations of the type of sex. The first would be found in the agent having sex with *one* person only; this would not deny that the agent is not in a loving relationship, because the relationship envisaged here is only sexual. The other variation would not contain just one person with whom the agent is having sex; rather, it would contain multiple partners. And this variation has some interesting different contingent features. Some of the multiple partners could be *repeat* sexual partners (that is, sexual partners that the agent has had sex with more than once) or nonrepeat ones. Another different contingent feature could be the *frequency* of the sex acts: the number of times the agent engages in sex, say, per week.

In order to build the strongest case, I am going to set aside the first variation: I am not going to discuss the case in which the agent has sex with only one person. I am also going to set the case up in such a way that the agent can be plausibly described as promiscuous. It should be obvious that a way of life in which the agent decides to forgo love relationships and marriage need not entail promiscuity. If the agent, for example, had sex twice a year, even with two different people, we would be hard pressed to describe him as promiscuous. It is of course difficult to define "promiscuity,"[40] but we do not need a definition to realize that the frequency of the sexual act and the fact that the sexual partners of the agent are not the same person have something important to do with our understanding of promiscuity. The less frequently the agent has sex, the less promiscuous he is, for example. So let us imagine that our agent has sex once a week with a new person; at least, he *seeks to* have sex once a week with a new person, a person with whom he desires no relationship. Surely we should have no difficulty in describing his behavior as promiscuous if he is, generally at least, successful in his endeavors. And when we keep in mind that he *wants* to do this, that this is the way of life he has chosen, that he is not doing this due to his belief that this is a good way to find himself a life partner, then we would surely have no difficulty in calling *him* "promiscuous." He would also be promiscuous in the worst way from a traditional point of view, since he has no causes that could excuse his behavior and desires, such as loneliness, frustration, depression, and so on (even though, as I will briefly argue towards the end of this section, these are fully compatible with virtuous promiscuity). Just note, in this connection, how sexual wantonness is often included in the way people describe others as promiscuous.

In giving some detail to one instance of the first ideal and making its agent a promiscuous person, I am building the strongest case for my argument. Promiscuity is often seen in a highly negative light, and the term "promiscuity" itself is usually negative in its connotations.[41] Indeed, philosophers sometimes take this fact for granted (for example, one philosopher begins a sentence as follows: "While wanton promiscuity is surely a vice . . ." [Scoccia, 2000, 70]). If a promiscuous person turns out to be not necessarily IT1, and if a promiscuous person might indeed very well be T1, then other ways of instantiating the first ideal would follow suit as far as these conclusions are concerned. If, in other words, a promiscuous person can be T1, then an agent who is not promiscuous but who leads his life along the lines of the first ideal can also be T1. Of course, there are different ways of being promiscuous: one can be promiscuous in ways that relegate every other aspect of one's life to practical nonexistence, and one can be promiscuous in more moderate ways. But once we see how an account of deliberation can accommodate promiscuity, then my claim that promiscuity gives us the strongest case will be vindicated.

But how do we go about proving that promiscuity is compatible with T1? One indirect way is to show that it is not incompatible with T1. And we go about doing *this* in two ways. First, we can show that being promiscuous does not undermine the agent's psychic and moral health. Second, we can show that being promiscuous does not undermine something else (an activity, a practice, a value) that the agent needs for a flourishing life. One account has it that promiscuity undermines one important value that the agent needs in order to flourish. It is this account that I will address next.

In a recent paper, Kristjan Kristjansson argues that casual, promiscuous sex can lead its practitioner to be incapable of forming a meaningful and loving relationship with another, and this—he indicates—is in strong tension with adopting a naturalistic view of human beings, a view which Kristjansson thinks moral philosophers ought to adopt with respect to their subject (1998, 106). Kristjansson has in mind the kind of casual sex that is "serial (diachronic or synchronic) liaisons with different sexual partners over a period of time (a few months or years), without any psychological or moral commitment" (98–99). I mention this in order to assure the reader that both Kristjansson and I rely on a similar picture of a promiscuous person. Once we delve into his argument and see its mistakes, we will be able to take an important step towards seeing how casual sex and promiscuity can be part of a meaningful and as naturalistic a human life as Kristjansson would want it to be (the "can" in this sentence does not just refer to logical possibility, but also to pyschological likelihood).

Kristjansson relies on an observation made by G. E. M. Anscombe to the effect that promiscuous people become shallow (Anscombe 1976, 148).[42] He offers, by way of a rough analogy, the image of a mushroom picker. Such a person does not discriminate between the mushrooms she picks, as long as the mushrooms fall within rough and general criteria, because the picker does not really care about—is not after—the individuality of each particular mushroom (101).[43] This picture is meant to illustrate the behavior and attitude of the promiscuous person. Of course, it relies on a mistaken view of promiscuous people. The promiscuous person, unlike the mushroom picker, does not go and pick tens of people during an hour or so (while the mushroom picker does just this)—not unless he is having an orgy and he is out shopping for participants, a possible but rare enough phenomenon. Nor does the promiscuous person necessarily confine himself to rough and general criteria in his choices of sex partners. Indeed, some are quite picky: to them, only people of a particular type (slim blondes under the age of thirty, for example) will do. Some, of course, are also not picky, and it is not clear which of these types predominates. But the point is that it is wrong for Kristjansson to characterize promiscuous people as not picky.

It is important to note that this picture of the promiscuous person underlies the views of other philosophers. Consider, for example, those of Martha Nussbaum. In her essay "Objectification," she cites a passage from the novel *The Swimming-Pool Library* by the British author Alan Hollinghurst and goes on to characterize the attitude of the narrator as involving a sexually indiscriminate way of looking at human beings, *despite* the fact that the passage Nussbaum cites contains evidence to the contrary. In the passage, the narrator is in the shower room of a health club frequented by gay men: "And how difficult social distinctions are in the shower. How could I now smile at my enormous African neighbour [showering neighbor, that is], who was responding in elephantine manner to my own erection, and yet scowl at the disastrous nearly-boy smirking under the next jet along?" ("Objectification" 1999, 216). Nussbaum comments on this by stating, "Hollinghurst's hero represents himself as able to see his fellow Londoners as *equal interchangeable bodies or even body parts*, under the sexual gaze of the shower room, a gaze allegedly independent of warping considerations of class or rank" (217, my emphasis). But Nussbaum here seems to unwittingly fall for the popular view of promiscuous people as indiscriminate, and her claim that the bodies and body parts are interchangeable is simply unsupported by the passage she quotes. Indeed, if anything, it supports the claim that they are not indiscriminate. That the narrator describes one erection as "elephantine" and the other as "nearly-boy" is—never mind the racial stereotype in the former description—evidence of discrimination.

Be that as it may, let us move on with Kristjansson's argument. Kristjansson continues, "Now, given that he picks his bedfellows as indiscriminately as his mushrooms, he will also cease to view sex with 'the individual person P' differently from sex with any other mushroom—sorry *person!*—whatsoever. Thereby, however, he forfeits his chance of a deep, serious sexual relationship with another individual" (101).

Now one important basis of Kristjansson's argument, according to Kristjansson, is found in some deeply held views about romantic love. According to these, romantic love has three important features. First, it is aimed at persons and not just their qualities; one loves Omar, not (just?) Omar's dark eyes, and so one cannot just replace Omar with anyone who has his properties. Second, romantic love is characterized by some sort of interpersonal unification between the lovers: they aim or desire to become one.[44] And third, romantic love is time consuming: knowing and trusting another—let alone becoming one with him or her—take time, and both knowledge and trust are staples of romantic love, and perhaps even defining features of it (102–3). The point now is that if these are correct features of romantic love, then we "do not need to think hard to realize that promiscuous sexual relationships fall short of all these three requirements" (104). Promiscuous sex treats sexual partners as replaceable, it does not aim at a relationship, let alone union, and it does not take much time. Whether promiscuous sex "falls short" of these three features of romantic love is a valuational issue; but it certainly is *different* from them, and this much we knew all along. What we did not know—and hopefully Kristjansson's argument will illuminate the point for us—is that promiscuous sex can lead one to forfeit the above three features in one's life.

So Kristjansson brings in the notion of *habit*: "There is no need to be a die-hard Aristotelian, let alone a behaviorist, to appreciate the importance of *habituation* in our upbringing. . . . Promiscuity, i.e., non-committal sex, gradually inures us to a deep loving relationship with a single other" (104). The promiscuous person "learns" to enjoy sex without romantic love, and this "may preclude the possibility of the ideal [of commitment] ever being realized" (104). Once we add to this the idea that romantic love "is one of the fundamental values—if not *the* fundamental value—in human life" (105), we get the argument that promiscuous sex can lead to the forfeiture of a deeply important aspect of our lives. Thus, Kristjansson's argument (though Kristjansson himself does not put it this way) is an example of one of the ways sketched above of arguing that promiscuous sex can lead to a nonflourishing life. If such sexual activity can lead to a forfeiture of a fundamental value—indeed, perhaps *the* fundamental value—then one can certainly see how a promiscuous person is not flourishing. Who can flourish when a fundamental value is missing from her life? And if the value is *the* fundamental one, then we can certainly kiss flourishing good-bye.

Kristjansson's conclusion, however, is that promiscuous sex *can* lead to giving up on romantic love. But *does* it? Or, at least, what is the likelihood of it doing so? After all, "can" indicates possibility, and possibilities can be weak, depending on how close or far the possible worlds we have in mind are to the actual one. Now whether promiscuity does lead to forfeiting romantic love is a factual issue, and Kristjansson is aware of this and so of the fact that he needs evidence. The evidence he gives is the testimony of his students, "more than half of whom seem to come down every year on Anscombe's side" (105). The majority of his students, year after year, tell him of friends and relatives who have "rendered themselves *forever* unable to form a shared identity with another person" by becoming "slaves" of their sexual, promiscuous habits (105; my emphasis).

It is, I believe, important to dwell a bit on this offered evidence, since doing so would inform us about what kind of evidence it would take to vindicate a claim such as Kristjansson's. First, Kristjansson's evidence is testimonial, and secondhand at that. While testimonials are appropriate forms of evidence in certain contexts (eyewitness reports, for example, in genocides and other less dramatic accidents and events), in the context of this argument they are defective. They are Kristjansson's students' interpretations of their friends' and relatives' lives, and with this comes suspicion about how accurately they have understood and analyzed these lives. How do his students know, or even strongly believe, for example, that the people who appear in their stories have *forever* become unable to form a shared identity with another? Indeed, they seem to also assume that being unable to form a shared identity is a bad thing. But this is not so obviously true. If having a shared identity is a bad thing or is neither good nor bad, then being unable to share one's identity with another need not be a bad thing.

Second, the evidential base is too narrow and possibly biased. What we have is a sample of students from roughly the same age group being taught by the same teacher. We need more samples from across a spectrum of the population. Third, there is contrary evidence. There are plenty of promiscuous people who eventually get—simply—bored with their lives and who decide to be with one person. This indicates the content of the fourth point: what Kristjansson needs is not simply evidence to the effect that there are promiscuous people who are doomed to a romantically loveless life, but evidence that would tell us the percentages of such people over a period of time. Once this kind of evidence is given, then we can begin to make headway. Otherwise, the argument remains weak: all we know is that promiscuity *can* lead to a loveless life, and that it has done so with *some* people (much as we know that knives *can* be used to kill people, and that they have been so used by *some* people). However, if we can come to know that it has done so in the majority of cases over a period of, say, 50 years, preferably covering diverse economic and political eras (in order to rule out external causes), then we have a meaty claim on our hands, a claim that deserves to be taken highly seriously.

Fifth, what we also need is evidence that would show that the habit of promiscuity is the *cause*, or at least one major cause, of the forfeiture of a romantic love life. Otherwise, the possibility remains that promiscuity and lovelessness are symptoms of a deeper problem, such as severe depression or a deep-seated inability to form intimate relationships, or of a certain type of character trait (which need not be a bad character trait). This is none other than the problem of proving that X is a cause of, rather than a mere correlation with, Y. Perhaps the fourth point above can take care of this worry, if the evidence is large and deep enough to rule out such non-promiscuity causes from the study. But one can see, I hope, how difficult the gathering and interpreting of such evidence is likely to be.

But there is a deeply troubling aspect of Kristjansson's argument that I have not yet attended to and that goes beyond any difficulties having to do with evidence, namely, the ease with which he assimilates romantic love and sex. A number of philosophers have recently pointed out how romantic love and sex are different in their aims, origins, and phenomenal feel.[45] Consider, very briefly, the last. There is a world of difference between how sexual arousal feels to one and how falling (and being) in love does. The former is primarily focused on the body, or body parts, of another person, while the latter is not. The former primarily seeks bodily *pleasure*, whereas the latter need not. Indeed, when two people who are in love engage in sex, no matter how expressively and affectionately they start and end the sex act, there is bound to be a point—if the sex is good—at which the lovers become simply immersed in the *sexual* act, paying attention primarily to each other's bodies and/or the sensual pleasures they derive thereof. The point of this excursion is that it is hard to see, à la Kristjansson, why being habituated to an activity such as sex can, and sometimes does, lead to giving up on being able to be in love, *when these two are very different phenomena*. I do not mean to exaggerate the point. Sex is often associated with romantic love, and, as Bonnie Steinbock once claimed, people see adultery as wrong precisely because it indicates a form of intimacy and affection which usually comes with sexual activity.[46] Nevertheless, the two are different.

Indeed, we can see this point through the three features of romantic love that Kristjansson himself emphasizes. Even if one were not sexually promiscuous, how would having *sex* with one's own spouse conform to the three features of romantic love given above? Is sex time consuming like romantic love? Is it aimed at the person rather than their body parts? Do lovers use it to (try to) achieve union? My hunch is that "It depends" would be the answer to all three questions, whereas there is a general agreement, at least from within the tradition that Kristjansson advances his claims, that there is no such contingency were we to be speaking about romantic love. So how is it that two such different things can be seen to stand in such intimate connections? How is it that sexual promiscuity can be seen to be so intimately causally connected to romantic love? What is the link between them?

The only answer I can think of is monogamy. It is this which best explains Kristjansson's remark (quoted above) that the promiscuous person will cease to view having sex with an *individual person* differently from having it with myriad others. Otherwise, and if romantic love is indeed different from sex in important respects, it is hard to see how this comment by Kristjansson is plausible. For if the "individual person" is one's lover, then surely having sex with one's lover is different from having casual sex. The animality is there; the attention to bodily parts is there; the heat is there. But the fact that one is having sex with another whom one knows, has spent good times with, has shared trust, intimacy, and affection with, would render the sex act also importantly different from casual sex.

What seems to be lurking behind Kristjansson's argument is the following thought: promiscuity, once habitual, instills in its practitioner a desire for novelty in sex. One becomes, so to speak, addicted[47] to sex with strangers and to novel bodies, and this makes it difficult for the agent, if not also impossible, to be monogamous. And monogamy is crucial for a loving relationship (this would be a necessary assumption for this argument). So the link between promiscuity and forfeiting romantic love comes via monogamy: by being promiscuous one forfeits monogamy, and this leads to forfeiting romantic love. (This chain of causes, by the way, does not fit a run-of-the-mill adulterer, for he does not engage in promiscuous sex.)

This argument is faulty on a number of grounds, such as its reliance on the assumption that promiscuity undermines later monogamy. But perhaps the most important is the assumption that monogamy is crucial for a loving relationship. Of course, the assumption can be strong or weak, depending on whether we interpret "crucial" to mean "necessary" or "gives one a very good way of maintaining a loving relationship." The latter sense would make the conclusion of the argument much more plausible, although much depends on what kind of nonmonogamous sex one is having, a topic with which I engage in the next section. This version of the argument also faces evidential problems similar to those that faced the original argument. How many promiscuous people *do* actually become incapable of leading monogamous lives? And whatever happened to the old nugget of wisdom that one should experiment sexually before one sexually commits to another? The thought contained in this adage seems to run counter to the thought contained in the new version of Kristjansson's argument, for sexual promiscuity now counts towards the fulfillment of a sexual drive that would otherwise lurk dangerously beneath the calm surface of monogamy. (I am not, of course, endorsing this prescription; I bring it up to indicate the diversity of beliefs on this issue of the connection between promiscuity and monogamy.)

I have dwelt on Kristjansson's position for two main reasons. First, it provides an excellent example of arguing that promiscuity detracts from flourishing because it (promiscuity) leads to the neglect or lack of possession of something that one needs in order to flourish. In Kristjansson's case, this something is romantic love (and I have not questioned the claim that love is necessary or at least important for flourishing, because I have already done this in the second chapter). Second, investigating Kristjansson's position allows us to see how tenuous it is: there seems to be no good reason to think that promiscuity renders its practitioner unlikely to form romantic love relationships. At best, it renders its practitioner unlikely to form *monogamous* love relationships, but this claim, obviously enough, does not mean that the agent has forfeited romantic love. Investigating Kristjansson's argument also puts us in a position to raise the following question: What other kind of good could promiscuity lead to forfeiting, such that without that good one does not, or one finds it difficult to, flourish? Romantic love is the most obvious and plausible candidate, and we have seen how difficult it is to make such a claim, given the important differences between sex and romantic love.[48] What remains? Health (vis-à-vis sexual diseases) is another important consideration, but the few fatal sexual diseases, such as syphilis and AIDS, either can be treated or can be avoided by using protection. I do not, by any means, wish to minimize the importance of sexual diseases, nor to make light of the ethical issues that can surround them, especially HIV and AIDS. I do, however, mean to indicate that sexual diseases are not, nor have they been, the sole reason that a moral tradition would indict sexual promiscuity. It is not as if, were sexual diseases to vanish tomorrow, my parents, with Anscombian-like support, would say, "Go bed hopping, make the best of it, and may God be with you."

I think that at this point it is reasonable to conclude that the burden of proof falls on whoever wants to pursue the strategy that promiscuity leads to forfeiting X, where X is a good that is necessary, or at least important, for flourishing.[49] I turn to the second strategy: showing that promiscuity directly undermines the agent's moral and psychic health. The argument I have in mind is familiar, powerful, and straightforward: promiscuity indicates that the agent is ruled by his sexual desires, and this, in the most direct ways possible, undermines the agent's flourishing by undermining his rational control over his life. The agent plans his life around sexual pleasure, allows his reason to carry out, so to speak, the dictates of his sexual desires, and this is precisely what Aristotle had in mind in calling a life of pleasure "slavish."[50] It is in this direction, perhaps, where one should develop, in a non-Catholic and secular way, Anscombe's suggestion that casual sex makes people "shallow": they become shallow in the sense that their reason plays a role subservient to their desires. And *this* is the most basic, important, and dangerous sense of "shallow" we could fasten upon. In many respects, it also fits a popular image of promiscuous people, who are typically seen as immature, desire-driven, and desire-controlled simulacra of human beings. In responding to this argument, I will sketch a way in which promiscuity can have a place in a rational, virtuous life.[51] Doing so allows us to see that this strategy against promiscuity is plausible yet limited in application.

Let us begin with a simple example of peanut eating. One might, on a certain occasion, desire to have honey roasted peanuts, but also desire to keep his figure trim. The fact that a desire pulls an agent in a certain direction does not entail that the agent will act on the desire. Whether he does so depends on his deliberation to that effect. Does the agent have a reason for pursuing the course of action of eating the peanuts? Whether he has such a reason depends on what roles or place he considers peanut eating to have in his overall conception of his life and the way he wants his life to go. Now of course the agent might think that peanut eating has no bearing on his life at all. If this is the case, in eating or not eating the peanuts he might just simply follow his inclinations. But if he thinks that it is important for him to have a nice and trim figure (he is, say, a model), then whether he decides to eat these peanuts will figure importantly in his conception of what life he wants to have. But the decisions might differ. If, for example, he has not eaten peanuts for a long time, and if he has been quite good at maintaining his diet, then eating these peanuts now, in such-and-such a quantity, might be acted upon. If, however, the agent has been having a stormy and erratic relationship to his diet, then he might decide not to have these peanuts. In either case, deciding to pursue that course of action will depend on how it fits in his overall view of his life plan. One can put this by saying that desires are given by the agent different weights depending on how they fit into the agent's idea of how he should lead his life. In this way, practical reason determines which desires are to be effective and which desires are not to be. Those desires which are given most weight in the process of deliberation can be called, following Dent, "rational desires," for they are the desires endorsed by the agent's reason.

The example of the peanuts is not meant to be analogous to the issue of promiscuity. Its point is to highlight one crucial feature of deliberation about action: that often deliberation is called for when the potential course of action has relevance to the agent's life plan. Indeed, it is very rare to find actions that have no relevance to life plans, but not all such actions can simply be embarked upon, without deliberation. Whether a desire should be effective, that is, lead to action, is often an issue that requires thinking. Furthermore, there is nothing especially difficult about the notion of a life plan; specifically, it need not be understood as involving a robust, detailed, comprehensive, and even consistent view of how one's life should go (doing so would make it difficult to see how many people can have such plans). The notion needs to simply be "a conception which embraces some set of considerations in some sort of order, which provides at least a partial picture of the proper way in which one should live, as one thinks" (Dent 1984, 109).

Promiscuity, of course, is a practice, a way of life, and in this respect, its discussion cannot simply be couched in terms of individual actions. The question is not so much whether one may engage in *this* sexual act at *this* time, but rather whether one may lead one's life in such a way that, rationally, it contains significant room for promiscuity. To put it differently, the issue is whether one's sexual desires should become effective along particular lines (outside the confines of a relationship, with multiple partners, and so on). The way to go about addressing this issue is to situate sexual desires within the larger context of a life plan.

In the peanuts case, whether the agent may eat the peanuts depended primarily on the ways in which dieting is relevant to the agent's life. If the agent, for example, is a model, or simply wants to look a certain way, then eating or not eating these peanuts gets to be an issue. Even if the agent does not deliberate prior to a particular act of peanut eating, how much to eat, when, and how, and under what conditions become highly pertinent questions for the agent given his life plans. Indeed, peanuts are just one tip of the food-berg. If the agent is a model, then he has to negotiate food consumption in general, not just peanuts. The idea is, simply, that the agent needs to find a place for food consumption in a life governed by reason. Let us now transfer this picture to sexual activity, and in so doing we shall see that we will emerge with a picture that is very much akin to what Aristotle had in mind in describing the temperate person.

Sex, without a doubt, is an issue with which we must all negotiate. Even those who decide to lead a life of celibacy must deal with sexual issues, at least in the sense that they have to decide *not* to engage in sexual activity anymore. If we want to be married, legally or substantively, we have to make decisions about monogamy (an issue that many couples, it seems, simply do not think about seriously enough). If we want to be parents, we have to decide what sort of exemplars we want to be for our children, and this is bound to have implications for what sex lives we are to lead. And if we desire not to be parents, or even not to be in any serious romantic and/or marriagelike relationship, we have to decide what role sex is to have in our lives. If we want it to have a role, then we must figure out how, when, and under what conditions we are to obtain it. More importantly, we have to decide how much room to give it.

Consider the following hypothetical, yet realistic, example involving a deliberation process about promiscuity in an agent's life. Firas is a generally

virtuous man in his mid-twenties. He has just finished obtaining his Ph.D.
degree in social work from a good university, and has just obtained a nice
job at an academic institution that expects him to be a good and effective
teacher but that also expects him to do good research in his field. More
importantly, Firas is quite excited about his new job and life. He has no
desire to be seriously involved with anyone romantically, because he—for
the time being at least—would like to be independent from the cares and
woes of romantic love so as to pursue a rich academic life, with plenty of
room left for other activities he enjoys, such as watching movies, reading
literature, and traveling. This is not to say that he is an apathetic individual when it comes to human relationships. He has, indeed, a number of
close friends with whom he shares intimate thoughts, worries, emotions,
and joyous and sad times. It is just that Firas does not desire to be romantically involved. And from what he has seen of other romantic couples, to
be honest, there was not much to whet his appetite.

But Firas also has a healthy sex drive. He is not obsessed with sex; but
he likes sex, he enjoys it, though he does not—and in this respect he is similar to many other people—consider it to be the focal point of his life. So
he reasons that his best bet to obtain sexual pleasure is by having one-night
stands, or casual sex in general. Why not have a relationship with just (or
primarily) one other person which is purely sexual? Because, Firas worries,
it might transform into something else. This is not because he thinks *other*
people (but not him!) are needy and always end up being emotionally
dependent. Indeed, he might not trust himself; he might worry that he
himself might become too attached, and if this happens, then his entire life
plan is undermined. True, he might have a new life with different but as
exciting values in it (for example, romantic love)—and he agrees with this
sentiment—but he does not want this life as of yet. So for now, sexual
promiscuity it will have to be. And it is important to see that this is *not a
grim option* for Firas. He fully endorses and prefers this life to other alter-
natives. He is, more specifically, not saddened by the fact that he is sexually promiscuous; he has not chosen promiscuity simply because it is the
only way to have a sex life without the commitment or the risk of commitment (this is just one reason for his choice). He also likes sex; and he
has no problem—to put it mildly—with having sex with multiple partners.

There are five more points worth mentioning. First, Firas could be
either gay or straight (or have some other orientation; I restrict the options
to gay and straight for simplicity's sake), and not much, conceptually,
hinges on which sexual orientation he has (practically, however, it might be
easier for Firas if he were gay, given that gay bars and nightclubs often offer
better sexual venues than straight establishments, unless he does not mind

paying for sex). Second, if Firas were a woman, then he might have a harder time realizing his ideal, given certain social double standards about the sexual behavior of men and women, even though the times are changing. Again, however, there is no conceptual difference to be registered (I will, however, address the gender issue at the end of this chapter). Third, Firas is not reckless. He uses protection in his sexual escapades and does not irresponsibly engage in sexual acts that have a high degree of transmitting dangerous diseases. Fourth, Firas does not deceive, lie, or mislead his potential sex partners about his intentions in having sex with them. He does not, for example, mislead them into thinking that the one-night stand they are about to have stands a good chance of being a precursor to a long-term relationship. Fifth, this way of life that Firas has adopted is not necessarily permanent; he might want, at some future point, to revise the role that sex, romantic love, and attachment play in his life. However, his way of life is not necessarily temporary either; he might just stick to it till his deathbed.

It seems to me that the above example contains a perfectly rational way of life in which there is quite a bit of room for promiscuity. And this should tell us something important, if the case given is at all plausible, namely, that the main moral issue with promiscuity should not be just an issue of *amounts*—how much and how often and with how many—but should be, first and foremost, an issue of what *place* promiscuity has in an agent's life. The issue of amounts is important because of what it *tells* us about the issue of *place*. We balk at someone who is extremely promiscuous (spends night after night at bars, is obsessed with having sex with others, and so forth) not simply because he is spending too much time on it and because he is having too much of it. We balk at this person because the extent to which sex takes up of his life is a good *indicator* that this agent is not leading his life according to a life governed by reason. His life is slavish.

Firas is not like this at all. He is, no doubt, promiscuous. But his promiscuity is, to put it simply (and seemingly paradoxically), temperate. To see this, consider the following passage from Aristotle. In describing the temperate man, Aristotle states, "If something is pleasant and conducive to health or fitness, he will desire this moderately and in the right way; and he will desire in the same way anything else that is pleasant if it is no obstacle to health and fitness, does not deviate from what is fine, and does not exceed his means" (1985, 1119a16–20). Sex is pleasant and Firas desires it. Sex is not an obstacle to health and fitness (indeed, it might even be conducive to these). In seeking it, Firas does not do so by deviating from what is fine: he does not lie to get it; he does not force himself on another; but more importantly, his sex life does not come at the expense of reason, and since *ex hypothesi* Firas is virtuous, his sex life will not come at the expense of what is fine, in general. Lastly, we can happily claim that Firas does not seek sex beyond his means. Indeed, it would be difficult to see how this could be possible in his deliberated life plan.

Someone will no doubt object that the sticky point between Aristotle and myself is the "moderate" business, for wouldn't "desire this moderately" (from the above quotation) indicate amounts and wouldn't this *not* fit the description of the Firas case? Indeed, I have offered a number of quotations early on in this chapter to support the idea that one concept of temperance that Aristotle held is that of amounts. But now we seem to be back to square one: Wouldn't such a concept of temperance rule out promiscuity? How can Firas be T1 and yet be promiscuous? The *general* picture that this objection is trying to force upon us is of an agent who is a *rational* deliberator and yet who somehow decides to give sex and sexual activity the organizing role in his life. The objection wants to further claim that the Firas case is one instance, albeit a moderate one, of this picture, which is not one of someone who is virtuous, though it is one of a rational deliberator. If Firas were virtuous, he would not be promiscuous, precisely because T1 is about amounts and is thus incompatible with promiscuity.

But the issue of amounts, as I have said above, is crucial in what it tells us: someone who partakes in sex intemperately, in terms of amounts (in the sense of IT1), is someone whose life is not ruled by reason; he is ruled, rather, by his appetites. But the Firas case is not like this at all. Firas is not someone who lives for the moment, the moment being yet another sexual conquest and, hopefully, satisfaction. If that were so, then Firas would not be planning his future and his life, because he would be, as I said, living for the moment (nor would he be *able* to plan his future, given the role and structure of his desires). But the case I gave was premised precisely on someone who plans his life. Furthermore, Firas is not a sophisticated hedonist; he does not plan his life in such a way so that he can secure *future* sexual encounters and satisfactions, even at the expense of foregoing present ones. He has not gone into the field of social work because he thinks this is where he can meet—to quote Hobbes (the cartoon character, not the philosopher)—a lot of "hot babes." His life, simply put, does not revolve around the aim of achieving sexual satisfaction, no matter how clever one can be at planning such a life. He has neither deliberated for such a conclusion nor is there any reason to see that, in the end, he must be seen as a hedonist, albeit a sophisticated one.

Furthermore, the general picture that the objection entertains is incoherent. It envisages an agent who rationally deliberates to make sex the organizing goal of his life. But the question is this: How is this picture different from that of the sophisticated hedonist? The only difference that I can see is in terms of how each agent possibly came to be the way he is. The hedonist perhaps came to be so because, from the very beginning, he was raised in a bad way. From the start, the dark horse of desires has been in command of his chariot, to use Plato's nice metaphor. The other agent, however, need not have been like this. Rather, at some cool moment in his life he sat down and thought, "I have come to realize that sex is the most important thing in life; at least, it is way up there. If so, why not make it my goal in life? So from now on, I will plan my life in such a way that I try to have as much sex as possible."

Perhaps we do have different types of agents here *as far as their origins* are concerned. But once we put their origins on the side, it becomes difficult to see in what other ways they differ. Both have sex as their overarching goal in life. Both use their reason to secure sexual encounters. Both consider almost everything else in life instrumental to their sexual goals. Both will have to be nonvirtuous agents, since they both believe that sex is the most, or one of the most, worthwhile thing in life. Connected to this last point, both agents simply have the wrong conception regarding the value and importance of sex in general. Of the two, it is the rational agent who would be most guilty of this charge, since he is the one who reasoned his way to this conclusion. Sex is, of course, both pleasurable and an important aspect of life that needs to be negotiated. But its pleasures are brief and do not, as such, confer meaning on our lives. Sex is valuable, but its value is similar to that of a host of other activities we engage in, such as eating, playing tennis, spending time at the beach, and going to the zoo. To transform this value into an overarching one is to make a mistake of placement. Sexual activity, to be sure, is not on a par with blades-of-grass counting or bottle-cap collecting. But it is also not on a par with spending your life working with refugees or producing works of art. To think that its value is on the same level with that of any of these activities is to make a mistake.[52]

I have spent space and time discussing this hypothetical objection for one main reason: I needed to strengthen and support my claim that the issue of amounts is important for what amounts *signal*. Those agents who do engage in promiscuous sex in inordinate amounts tell us that their desires lead their reason. By rejecting the above objection, I reject the probability—not the mere possibility—of a rationally led life that contains a large amount of promiscuous sex. This is, of course, not a prudish conclusion. It steers a midway course between ethically censoring human lives whose agents are promiscuous, on the one hand, and ethically allowing any type of a human life whose agent is promiscuous. Promiscuity is perfectly compatible with T1 as long as it is part of a rationally constructed life plan, a life plan which gives the value and importance of sex its proper place in a well-lived life.[53]

Before finishing this discussion, there is one point that should be kept in mind. To claim that there is room for promiscuity in a virtuous life does not mean that once this room is secured, then the agent will engage in a sexual act as long as the opportunity is there and as long as the sex act does not go against T2. The point is perhaps obvious but needs to be said. Firas need not have sex with Nadia just because she is available and willing. He need not have sex with Bilal just because Bilal is good looking and desirous. Indeed, Firas might refuse to have sex with Bilal on the grounds that *this* sexual act, at *this* time, would be wrong or unacceptable. Just as I might refuse to eat *those* peanuts even though my diet allows me to have peanuts in general, Firas might decline having sex with Bilal because, say, he has already had his "fill" this week and having sex again would be time spent at the expense of other things that Firas should do. The point is simply this: Firas's life has room for promiscuity. But Firas might still need to negotiate and think about whether to engage in *individual* sexual acts.

Promiscuous people are so for a number of different reasons and/or causes, such as loneliness, depression, the love of sex and sexual pleasure, the love of sexual variety, vanity, the need for constant affirmation of one's desirability, overvaluation of the place of sex in one's life, the refusal to be in a monogamous relationship, and the psychological inability to be in such a relationship because, say, they are overly possessive and so too jealous to be happy in such a relationship. In some cases, more than one of these are operative. And some of these causes, even when operative, need not rule out a rational way of incorporating promiscuity within the agent's life. For example, even if Firas gets to feel loneliness, the solution to this need not be a monogamous relationship. If promiscuity can get rid of it, then so be it. In this respect, loneliness, sexual frustration, and other causes are compatible with a virtuous life of promiscuity. But other causes might not, and even cannot, be part of a virtuous and rational life plan (for example, vanity, and the need for constant reaffirmation that one is physically desirable). But that some causes of promiscuity cannot be part of a virtuous life need not entail that all causes of it are so. What is crucial is that it be part of a thought-out plan for one's life, a plan that gives sexual activity its proper role and place.

But, one might wonder, why promiscuity to begin with? We know that sex is valuable, but what we want to know is why promiscuity is valuable. Does it have any value other than, say, relieving sexual frustration or getting rid of loneliness? The answer is affirmative. People tend to sexually desire an indefinitely large number of (other) people. Sometimes, when other things are at stake, we leave this desire unfulfilled, and even give it no weight, for the sake of these other things (for instance, being with another person and realizing that the only way to keep the relationship going is to abstain from sex with others; or when we know that we are too weak to resist the eventual decline into a life controlled by our sexual desires were we to take the initial step of being promiscuous). But when there is not much else at stake, there is no reason to withhold from engaging in sexual activity promiscuously. The thrills of being with a new person whom we find sexually attractive, of hooking up with someone we find interesting and cute, and of even being in a dark room with lots of people having sex (as happens in many bars and discos) provide us with tremendous pleasure. As Richard Mohr puts it, "In intensity and in kind it [sexual pleasure] is unique among human pleasures; it has no passable substitute from other realms of life. For ordinary persons—not mystics or adolescent poets—orgasmic sex is the only access they have to ecstasy" (1988, 113).[54] Mohr might be exaggerating here, for as Soble correctly points out, there are people who enjoy sex but who would also "*die* for their pots, or dances, or stamps, or drugs, for the ecstatic pleasure these things, not sex, make possible" (1996, 19). But Mohr does not need to exaggerate. Sex is highly enjoyable, and as long as no moral requirements are violated, there is no reason why one should not see its pleasures. We do not ordinarily require justifications for "promiscuous" mountain climbing, comic-book reading, and movie-watching, to give a few examples. Why should things be different for sex? In promiscuous sex, the intensity and ecstasy are experienced always in heightened ways simply because they occur with new human beings perceived to be exciting.[55] In saying this, I have in effect answered a question posed earlier in this chapter: Does the first ideal enhance its agent's life? My answer is "Yes," as long as the reasons behind it are compatible with virtue, and, which amounts to the same thing, as long as the sex is given its proper objective place.

We can safely conclude that promiscuity can be perfectly compatible with T1. An agent can be virtuous and promiscuous, as long as the conditions set out above are in place. Furthermore, the case of promiscuity sheds light on what it takes to be a sexually active person who is not in a meaningful relationship and who is also virtuous. The general idea is that moderation in sexual matters, having T1, is accommodating of various forms of sexual activities as long as these are part of a rational life plan that accords sex its proper role and place. But the discussion in this section will also take us a long way into examining the other two ideals to which I now turn.

5. The Second Ideal and T1

What does the way of life of being in an open relationship amount to? And how is it connected to temperance in the first sense? In this section, I will elaborate on open relationships as a way of life, explaining them, enumerating some of their varieties, and distinguishing them from a life of promiscuity, especially as far as moral aspects are concerned. I will then indicate how open relationships can endanger flourishing by undermining romantic love, a value that parties in open relationships are committed to. By investigating this potential danger, I will round off the dicussion by offering two hypothetical cases of open relationships, discussing their differences, and arguing that neither is incompatible with temperance and hence neither need undermine their agents' flourishing.

What does the second ideal, more or less, amount to? I say "more or less" because this ideal, much like the first, can involve quite a number of variations. I will start by sketching a picture of one form this ideal can take, and then indicate some possible variations. I will then move on to note some of the important differences between this way of life and the first, differences that can dictate crucial further variations in their treatment.

Imagine a couple (it does not matter at this point whether the couple is heterosexual or homosexual) who have decided to make their relationship an open one. Whether they do so initially or later in the relationship depends on their reasons. But suppose the reasons they give are that each of them desires to have sex with other people, that each one of them thinks (and feels) that monogamy is too stifling, and that it is good that they indulge these sexual desires. They need not think that being monogamous will lead to the eventual ruin of their relationship because it is, they think, too stifling. They might realize that, if they wanted, they could be monogamous; it would involve some serious sacrifice on their part, for sure, but they can do it.[56] Rather, what they do think is that they do not need to make this sacrifice, and that, since they do not need to, they might as well enjoy the pleasures of sexual transactions with others.

All such relationships are adulterous; they all involve at least one spouse engaging in sexual activity with someone other than his or her spouse, and this, no matter how difficult it is to define "sexual activity," is adultery.[57] Now this might cause some eyebrows to be raised in suspicion. Isn't adultery just plain wrong, in virtue of the very meaning of the word? But if so, then wouldn't this rule such open relationships out, given that they all involve adultery? These questions are understandable; but they are misguided. Adultery is not wrong by definition, even if the word has negative connotations, and to claim that it is so is to rule out the interesting questions surrounding its morality. Of course, when adultery involves deception and lying and other such moral failings, we have on our hand paradigm cases of wrongful adultery (although even in these cases adultery can be sometimes justified).[58] The point is simply that we should not settle by fiat highly interesting philosophical and moral questions due to dogmatism, and that there is, therefore, nothing paradoxical about claiming that adultery can be quite in accordance with virtue.

The open relationships under discussion can and do exhibit some extraordinary variety, some of which signal important conceptual issues. Open relationships, for example, can, conceptually even though not frequently in practice, allow for each, or at least one, spouse to have a long-term lover on the side. In more common jargon, open relationships can allow for each spouse to have an *affair*. But they also, and more usually, allow for less temporally extended forms of sexual encounters. A recent television media report, for example, claimed that there are a number of heterosexual swingers "clubs" in the Chicago area. These "clubs" are the meeting places (sometimes the houses) of the members of the group, and admission is highly selective (no noncoupled individuals or drugs, for example, are allowed). What is interesting about this form of sexual outlet is that it is midway between having an affair and having a one-night stand, in that the couples know each other (they are at least acquainted and familiar with each other, if only by face) and see each other more or less regularly at these sex meetings.

But of course open marriages allow for the usual one-night stand, which could consist of a pick up at a bar or sex with a sex worker (one-night stands do not have to involve a whole night, literally). They also allow for more anonymous sexual encounters, such as gay cruisings in parks and bathhouses, group sex in sex clubs and discos, sex in orgy or dark rooms (places where people—mostly gay men—can have anonymous sex), and so forth. These distinctions are made not just to indicate the kind of variety that exists or could exist. The distinctions are conceptually important: the more anonymous the sexual encounter is, the less room there is for emotional involvement. And the less room there is for emotional involvement, the less risk there is for seriously harming the open relationships. I will, however, return to this issue below.

The variations found in the second ideal are not only confined to types of adulterous sex. Variations are found in the *reasons* for having an open relationship. The reasons could be that the couple thinks that having sex with others is, simply, a good thing to have, or that being sexually diverse is *one* good way of alleviating the sexual boredom that the couple experiences. Another reason could be that being sexually diverse is the *only* way to get rid of the boredom in their sexual lives (they have tried watching pornography together; they have tried role-playing; and they have licked whipped cream off of each other). Yet another reason could be more political than personal: the couple believes that being sexually monogamous is a way of conforming to socially oppressive norms, and so the spouses attempt to lead their relationship in nonconformist ways. And what better way is there than nonmonogamy?

Variations can also be found along temporal dimensions. Two spouses might make it a *condition* of being in a relationship that they be non-monogamous. Another couple might find out, later in the relationship, that monogamy has taken its sexual toll on them, and that it is now time for a change. And here we can register another type of variation: those couples who do opt for nonmonogamy after being together for a while might become nonmonogamous either quickly, like simply jumping into a pool of water; or they might do so slowly, like going into the pool gradually, first by getting wet up to the knees, and so on. So such a gradual opening up of the relationship might first take the form of three-way erotic massages, then hiring a sex worker for a three-way. Sex workers are professional, so there is less danger for emotional entanglement and future stalking or harassment by the third party, or, as a friend of mine said, "the microwaving of our dear pets" (in reference to the movie *Fatal Attraction*).

But this is enough of variations. I have stated these in order to give the reader a good idea of how open relationships can differ. At this point, we should register two important differences between the first two ways of life or ideals. First, the second ideal, unlike the first, directly involves another person whose nonsexual (and, of course, sexual) interests and well-being are important for the agent. The agent (and I use "agent" to refer to either party in the relationship) is involved in deep and meaningful ways with another person. And so her actions cannot be looked at as issuing from a life plan that primarily only includes her. More importantly, whatever room for sexual activities the agent's life plan has, it is bound to have direct implications for her spouse. So we cannot morally assess such a life plan without reference to the agent's spouse.

Second, given that we are speaking about the agent being in a relationship with another, the issue of romantic love comes up in crucial ways. The agent under the first ideal has no romantic love in his life. The agent under the second ideal, however, does, and he or she does so in virtue of the very way we are construing this second ideal. In other words, this ideal essentially involves a romantic *love* relationship between the two spouses, and so any discussion of adultery and promiscuity here requires paying important attention to this feature. Indeed, Kristjansson's argument boiled down to the idea that a promiscuous agent forfeits romantic love precisely because he cannot be monogamous. And so we are led to the question of whether a life of nonmonogamy is incompatible with romantic love. If it is, then this agent will be well on his way to a nonflourishing life. The reason is not because romantic love is *the* fundamental value, but simply because it is *one* important value, and because the agent, as this second ideal has it, *wants* to have romantic love in his life. If his nonmonogamous way of life leads to the ruin of his love life, then he cannot live by his own truth-tracking conception of his life ("truth-tracking" because he believes romantic love is important, and this belief is true). If he cannot do so, then he cannot plausibly be said to flourish. Flourishing is an objective phenomenon, of course, but it refers to a subjective element, in that it is necessary that the agent's life go along the lines of the agent's conception of it. For if the agent were not, subjectively, content with his life, if he believes that his desires and beliefs about his life were not, respectively, satisfied and true, then he would not to a large degree be happy. And if he himself—subjectively—were not happy, then we would be hard pressed to claim that his life is flourishing.[59] Let us then begin by seeing whether nonmonogamy is incompatible with romantic love.

Bonnie Steinbock, in her essay "Adultery," bases her argument against adultery on the plausible general claim that whatever views we have about adultery, they are bound to be connected in important ways to our views about romantic love, marriage, the family, fidelity, jealousy, and exclusivity (1991, 188). In regard to open marriages, she goes through a number of dialectical steps to reach her conclusion that sexual fidelity should be the ideal in relationships. First, Steinbock makes the case for the desirability and attractiveness of extramarital affairs (they are exciting, and so make our lives richer). Second, she gives the counterresponse: sex is an expression of affection and intimacy and so "should be reserved for people who love each other." Next, Steinbock gives the reply to this counterresponse: Why can't we divorce sex from romantic love? Sex is a pleasurable activity in its own right, much as some meals are enjoyable in their own right also. Finally, Steinbock gives her own response: to divorce sex from romantic love in this way is simplistic. Here I will quote her at some length:

> Feelings of love occur between people enjoying sexual intercourse, not out of a sense that sexual pleasure must be purified, but precisely because of the mutual pleasure they give one another. People naturally have feelings of affection for those who make them happy, and sex is a very good way of making someone extraordinarily happy. At the same time, sex is by its nature intimate, involving both physical and psychological exposure. This both requires and creates trust, which is closely allied to feelings of affection and love. (190)

There are two things happening here. First, sex is connected to affection via a chain which starts with sex, goes through pleasure and happiness (and, one hopes, Steinbock is not using these two interchangeably), and ends with affection. Because sex gives us pleasure, this makes us happy. The idea is that we tend to develop affectionate feelings for those who sexually please us because they make us happy in (and by?) having sex with us. Second, due to the intimacy of sex and the exposure it often requires as part and parcel of it as an activity, sexual partners develop trust between each other. And both trust and being made happy by x, though Steinbock does not explicitly say it, lead to loving x by way of feeling affection for x. This is not to say, nor does Steinbock do so, that affection is sufficient for romantic love. The claim is rather a more general one: feelings of affection and trust are usual components of and/or causal lead-ins to romantic love. I say "and/or" because Steinbock's position is unclear as far as the exact nature of the connections between affection and trust (and pleasure and happiness), on the one hand, and romantic love, on the other. But this unclearness does not seriously affect the discussion. Her claim is intuitive and plausible enough for us to be able to tolerate the ambiguity.

Steinbock concludes that open relationships are not immoral, but that they "deviate from a valued ideal of what marriage should be" (191). Since marriage is ideally about romantic love, and since adultery is generally inimical to romantic love, then open marriages are inimical to romantic love. This conclusion needs to be modified to read "*some* open marriages are inimical to romantic love," namely, those that do actually lead to its demise or endangerment. For surely some couples could have open relationships and yet still love each other. But since couples cannot know how sexual openness will affect their love beforehand, then we can take the first, more general, conclusion to simply be a prudential one, namely, that it is best not to enter an open relationship since there is a (good) chance that it will endanger the romantic love between the couple. Furthermore, Steinbock rejects the idea that one can love more than one person at a time: "exclusivity seems to be an intrinsic part of 'true love.' Imagine Romeo pouring out his heart to both Juliet *and* Rosalind!" (191).[60] In doing so, she rejects the reply that x can be in an open relationship with y, have an affair with z, and yet love *both* y and z at the same time. And she must reject this as a (viable) possibility; otherwise her argument against adultery would lose much of its force, since having an affair with z need no longer be a sign of an emotional "betrayal" of y (192).

I have explained Steinbock's argument and claims because they seem to me to illustrate a type of argument that tries to show how open relationships could seriously endanger romantic love. Their general strategy is to rely on the idea that adultery and sex with someone other than one's spouse are somehow inimical to the love between the two spouses. In discussing Steinbock's version, we can see clearly the pitfalls and the victories of such arguments. Let us begin with the pitfalls, so that we can get the nasty business of criticism out of the way first. My main point of contention with Steinbock's essay is the conception of adultery it relies upon. It is obvious that Steinbock has in mind *affairs* when she discusses adultery. She uses the word "affair" often enough and, when she does not, the context makes it clear that she has in mind more or less long-term sexual liaisons (187–92). The problem is that when we consider types of adultery other than affairs, Steinbock's argument weakens considerably. I should add that Steinbock is not the only philosopher who makes the mistake of thinking mainly of affairs when discussing adultery. The mistake is a common one, but it almost always leads to some serious defects in the conclusions of whatever argument is employed.[61] Nor do philosophers have an excuse for this mishap. True enough, many of us have the classic image of the business man having an affair with his secretary glued in our minds. But many also have other firmly stuck images (and I do not deny that all of these might very well be crass generalizations), such as the man who has sex with a prostitute, the college kids who copulate for one night with no strings attached, and the gay man who goes cruising in a park. Surely these also deserve to be classic images!

When x has an *affair* with y, x and y are engaging in a more or less long-term sexual escapade, of which time, energy, planning, and money are almost always part. More importantly, it is in affairs that the emotional vulnerability, the trust, and the affection due to pleasure most strongly come in. For affairs typically involve more than quick sexual encounters. They usually involve talking (prior to and after the sex, and sometimes during it), petting, kissing, undressing and dressing in front of each other, and having sex in a room, on a bed or something comparably comfortable and/or enhancing of the sexual experience (for example, on the floor, on the kitchen counter, in some department store's dressing room). Furthermore, the longer the affair, the more serious the talk gets, the more intimate the things that are exchanged, be they objects or personal information. The physical and psychological exposures that Steinbock mentions are at their height.

But compare this to a sexual one-night stand. True, it involves talking, but the talking is generally more of a chitchat than anything serious. True, a bed is often used for sexual purposes, but both parties understand that one of them (in case they are at one or the other's residence) or both of them (in case they are in a room that belongs to neither) will most likely not see this bed again *because* they will most likely not have sex with each other again. True, they might have to undress and dress in front of each other, but the psychological dynamics that accompany these are much more casual, given the knowledge that this is a one-shot sexual act (even if it takes all night). Even if one of the parties feels awkward about his body, for example, and thus feels exposure at having to take his clothes off in front of the other, the feeling is vastly different from that of affairs. The former is more along the lines of shyness and awkwardness, with hopes that the other party will not be too revolted. The latter, however, involves, to be sure, shyness and awkwardness, but these can be overcome with time. What is left is the knowledge that "*x* knows my body and its ins and outs; knows in what ways my body is sensitive; knows what I like and what I dislike," and so on. These are all exposures that one-night standers simply do not have to deal with because they did not go through the time necessary to develop and have them.

What is important in the above discussion of one-night stands is the following point. Even if the talk is serious (and so not just chitchat), even if the venue is comparable to that used in affairs, and even if the two parties undergo feelings of vulnerability and trust similar to those undergone by parties in an affair, there is one crucial element found in casual sex and missing from affairs, an element which profoundly affects the phenomenological, ethical, and emotional dimensions of such sexual encounters. This is the fact that both parties in a one-night stand or a casual sex encounter *know* or *strongly believe* that what they are about to engage in is a one-shot sexual encounter, everything else equal (things might change: they might have sex only to find out that they have met the "right one"). The "know" might be too strong; and even if it is not too strong, it applies in *some* cases of one-night stands (many cases, surely, are ambiguous: at least one party might entertain doubts that this night is the first of many to come with this other person). Be that as it may, my point is conceptual and can be captured in a conditional: *if* the case is that of a one-night stand, and *if* the parties are clear (or know or strongly believe) on the fact that they are not after anything more serious, then their knowledge of this will deeply affect the above-mentioned similarities with affairs.

And now compare affairs to even quicker sexual escapades. Here I will draw on gay experiences since it is gay bars and venues that mostly offer the kind of atmosphere needed to facilitate such quick encounters (I do not mean to indicate that all or even most gay men engage in these sexual practices, of course). It is well known that in most major urban areas (especially those that are short on establishments advertised as gay), there will always be spots, such as particular parks, docks, and alleyways, where gay men cruise each other and often have sex right then and there. It is also well known that in most major urban centers there are a number of bathhouses where men can have sex with each other. It is also well known that many gay bars and discos often offer specifically designated areas (called "dark rooms" or "orgy rooms") in which men can have sex, and it is the orgiastic nature of it that often makes these a strong attraction. Add to these sex shops that contain "buddy booths" and one gets the general idea.

The conventions governing such sexual encounters and spaces are complicated. There are always ways for x to indicate to someone that x is interested in him, and ways to initiate the courtship. These ways differ from place to place in some subtle details. But one thing stands out: in almost all of them (the "almost" here indicates caution on my part to leave room for possible exceptions and future changes), speech plays a minimal role. Indeed, it virtually plays no role at all. If x tries to speak in an orgy room, then x would simply fail to grasp how one ought to conduct oneself in the room. And if x expresses emotion ("I really like you"), then x will be seen as, at best, joking or, at worst, demented. Speech plays no role, also, in cruising in parks and other public areas. It is eye contact and nonverbal behavioral expressions that carry the day.

I have dwelt on these comparisons to bring home an important point: the emotional and psychological involvement dwindles as one goes from affairs to one-night stands to anonymous sexual encounters. The idea is simply that depending on the type of sexual encounter, there could be a range of emotional and psychological involvement, going from full blown to nonexistent. Affairs, given that they are durable and given that they involve a good measure of intimacy, are fertile grounds for emotional and psychological involvement. Anonymous sex, given that it is quick, usually engaged in *only* for the sake of sex, and lacks verbal communication, is entirely inhospitable to emotional and psychological involvement. These do not, in general, exist in it. And in between there are cases and cases. One-night stands are less emotionally and psychologically involved than are affairs, but are more so than sexual encounters between sex workers and clients. And regarding the latter, even cases in which clients simply pour their hearts out to prostitutes, rather than have, or in addition to having, sex with them, these are just that; they are not cases in which the client falls in love with the prostitute.

The weakness in Steinbock's position should by now be obvious. By thinking of adultery mainly in terms of having affairs, Steinbock neglects a whole array of different types of adultery. And in doing so, she neglects types of adultery that involve minimal to nonexistent emotional and psychological aspects. This seriously weakens her argument by limiting its scope of application. Steinbock's argument will now be seen to plausibly apply only to types of adultery that are, more or less to a high degree, emotionally and psychologically invested. Steinbock's argument does not have the resources to address open relationships whose spouses engage only in anonymous sex with others; or only in one-night stands; or only with members of a swingers club; or only with sex workers. Steinbock cannot, given her bases, claim that such relationships deviate from the ideal. But if this is true, then she has, simply, failed to make a good case for her conclusion that sexual fidelity is the ideal in relationships.

Furthermore, even in those open relationships whose spouses engage in affairs, there is a limitation to Steinbock's argument. Steinbock is, of course, fully aware that sex does not necessarily lead to romantic love (1991, 190), and this has obvious implications for her argument. Perhaps the main one is that it will not be necessary that every adulterous *affair* is also a romantic love one or that it is one that will lead to romantic love. There could be cases of adulterous relationships that are purely sexual; both parties know this, both have no hopes for something "more," and both have no *desires* for something more. Such cases, moreover, are not hard to imagine. Let us say there are two couples: Joel and Cindy, and Janet and Don. Joel and Janet are having an affair with each other. Both of them are very happy with Cindy and Don. The only thing missing is exciting sex. This is *not* to say that the sex between them is nonexistent or that the couples shy away from it, but only that it is boring, or routine. And it may be that not much can be done about this. It may be that both Joel and Janet have lost sexual interest in their spouses, not in the sense that they find them ugly or repulsive, but simply in the sense that they do not find them sexually exciting any more. In seeking a sexual affair with each other, Joel and Janet may be seeking nothing more than that. Joel does not want affection from Janet. She does not want an ego boost. She does not want to spend time with Joel engaging in nonsexual activities. And she is not particularly interested in what Joel has to say and think about capital punishment, or any other topic for that matter (and vice versa in regard to all of these).

I have sketched this possibility in order to explain how Steinbock's conclusion, even when applied to affairs, is limited, and in order to supply a coherent picture of how an agent can rationally pursue a sexual affair (but more on this shortly). Let us then conclude that Steinbock's argument is weak because it neglects open relationships whose adulterous behavior is not emotionally and psychologically involved (or is involved to minimal degrees). And, though for less important reasons, it is weak because its conclusion does not give enough serious attention to the possibility that some adulterous affairs need be neither a sign of emotional betrayal of the spouse nor an indicator that the adulterous spouse is well on her way to falling in love with whomever she is having an affair with.

But now we can generalize a bit. If one wants to argue that open relationships are inimical to flourishing, one good way to do so is to argue that such relationships inhibit, or at least are not enhancing of, romantic love, a value that is both objectively important and subjectively desired by the agent. Here, we need to keep in mind that the agent is, under the second ideal, one who desires romantic love, as is evinced by the fact that she is in a relationship with another. And it seems to me that the Steinbock route is the only plausible one to take in offering such arguments. For how else is adulterous sex going to endanger the romantic love between the spouses other than by putting the adulterous spouse in a position to develop emotional ties to the one she is having sex with? And this almost always comes at the expense of the love for the spouse. True enough, the adulterous spouse might love both, but this is a rare enough phenomenon that we can safely set it aside.

Of course, one could argue that even too much anonymous sex can endanger the romantic love between two people if the spouses spend too much time seeking it, engaging in it, and planning their lives around it. This will surely have the consequence of neglecting their relationship that will, also usually, tend to make the romantic love between them wither away.[62] This is a plausible way to think about how even anonymous sex can endanger romantic love. But this is not a good case to make, because it can only be made in such a way that at least one spouse is portrayed as spending too much time and energy over sex, and *this* is surely a sign that the relationship is not going well to begin with. Steinbock's route, however, does not inevitably have to rely on such an assumption. Even if one is in a good relationship, the danger to romantic love comes through the general link between sex and the emotions of pleasure, trust, and affection.

But we have seen the difficulties that such a position will face. Not all adultery involves the kind of sex that is emotionally and psychologically invested. And once this is kept in mind, the danger to romantic love is considerably weakened. There could be, of course, conceptual ways other than the connection with romantic love by which adultery can put the flourishing of the agents at serious risk (by, that is, endangering another value that puts their love at risk). What these are, however, remain a mystery to me. So I will leave the burden of proving this on the shoulders of my opponents. (Indeed, even the connections that Steinbock adduces between sex, on the one hand, and romantic love, on the other hand, are not conceptual but contingent. I have elected to discuss them, however, because they are quite prevalent, and that is why Steinbock's argument is plausible. As to other contingent connections, I will discuss some of these below.)

What we can conclude, then, is that some forms of open relationships, namely, those that involve a good amount of intimacy and vulnerability between the spouse and his or her nonspousal lover, render likely the claim that the romantic love between the spouses is threatened. Because of this, such forms of open relationships render likely the claim that they are inimical to flourishing because both spouses consider their love for each other to be highly important. But we must also exercise caution. I have stated such open relationships "render likely" the claim the spouses' flourishing is endangered, but this is difficult to prove. The reason is that much will depend on each case. For example, much will depend on the reasons for the affair, much will depend on how resolute each spouse is in sticking with these reasons, and much will depend on the character of the person the spouse is having the affair with. What we should conclude, more cautiously, is that such types of open relationships are the ones that are most likely to endanger the romantic love between the spouses, and that whether they will do so will depend on each specific case.

As a corollary, we can also conclude from the above discussion that other forms of open relationships need not endanger the love between the spouses and, more importantly, are not likely to, if the spouses know what they are doing. Indeed, many such forms render the claims unlikely, given that these open relationships contain minimal to no psychological and emotional exposure, intimacy, and vulnerability.

The strong part of Steinbock's argument is the premise regarding the usual connections between sex and romantic love. I will address this strength as part of the discussion of the next issue, which is the direct compatibility of open relationships with temperance. I will sketch two ways in which a couple can be in love, pursue an open relationship, and yet be rational and virtuous (in that they are, at least, T1) in doing so. If my cases are plausible, then they will go quite a long way in showing that T1 does not require sexual monogamy. I will sketch two cases that occupy two extremes along a spectrum of open relationships. The treatment of what falls in between should, hopefully, be obvious.

Consider, first, the gay couple Marwan and Ziad.[63] At the time they met, they were both interested in sexual variety in their lives. When they met, they decided to keep their relationship sexually open, with both of them hooking up with other men every now and then. As their relationship progressed, they realized that they are truly in love with each other, and that theirs is not one of those yet-another-failed-attempt at being with someone. In order to foster the love between them but yet be able to maintain a sexually open life, they decide that they will no longer engage in any extramarital sex other than the anonymous type. They do so precisely because they want to minimize, if not altogether eliminate, the risk of getting emotionally attached to other third parties. In this way, they are able to have a sexually active and varied life, without also endangering the love between them.

It should be noted that neither Marwan nor Ziad are simpletons. They are not young and reckless men who are interested mainly in sex but who would also like to cultivate an image of themselves as being mature and so push themselves into being in a relationship. They can be as smart and as hard working as you want them to be. They can be extremely mature about issues surrounding romantic love and relationships, in the sense—minimally—that they both desire romantic love and commitment in their lives, but also in that neither will enter a relationship simply for the sake of being in one. When they enter one, they do so because they are convinced that this person is one that has a good chance of being an important and permanent part in the other's life (with as much guarantee as life often allows with these things).

In this vein, Ziad and Marwan's sexual escapades outside their relationship are neither obsessive nor the focus of their lives. They do not give them any more weight than they need to be given. They do not make it a point that they must have sex with outsiders at least once a week, or once a month. Indeed, they do not make it a point that a certain designated amount of "outside sex"—to (I think) coin a phrase—must be maintained within a designated time period. While doing so need not impugn the reasonableness of such a life, it could be that such insistence is an indicator that there is something troubling in the relationship. Rather, Ziad and Marwan accept this life as it comes: when the opportunity arises and not much else of more worth is at stake, then they welcome the outside sex. And this should indicate that being in an open relationship does not imply that outside sex will be engaged in every time an opportunity comes to the fore. Whether the opportunity is grabbed is an entirely circumstantial matter.

Moreover, when Ziad and Marwan decide to maintain a sexually open relationship, they do so not out of a sense that varied sex is as important as a relationship—if not even more important—and so they will never give it up. Rather, they do so out of the sense that sexual pleasure is one of the nicer pleasures that life has to offer, and unless there is a very good reason that they should give it up and become monogamous, then they will not. This is not to say that Ziad and Marwan believe that no couple should be monogamous; it is just that they realize that in *their* case, they are confident enough that sex with others is not a measuring stick for their love for each other. As Richard Mohr nicely puts it, "Gay men have realized that while sexual sacrifice may be part of the sacrifices that a couple choose to make in order to show their love for each other, it is not necessary for this purpose; there are many other ways to demonstrate mutual love. Monogamy is not an essential component of love and marriage" (1994, 50). Why go for outside sex to begin with? Because, as I mentioned above, sexual pleasure is an intense type of pleasure. When it is duly and appropriately pursued, there is no need to shun it. In this way, nonmonogamous relationships can, and do, enhance the life of couples, though of course they may not do so for every couple.

This case is at one end of the spectrum because, as part of its description, Marwan and Ziad end up settling for anonymous sex as the type of outside sex they are willing to engage in, and anonymous sex occupies one end of the spectrum of the connections between sex on the one hand, and romantic love and emotions on the other. But this is the only sense of "end of spectrum" that the first case exemplifies. In other senses, it is not so at all. For instance, it does not occupy one end of the spectrum in the sense that the openness of the relationship is permanent. Nothing is said about this, and Marwan and Ziad might very well decide to "close" their relationship later on in the future. Moreover, Marwan and Ziad could have begun their relationship in a monogamous way, and only later decided to open it, and perhaps in gradual ways. These different aspects can yield different ways in which we can construct the Marwan and Ziad case. Cutting across this variety, there are two aspects essential to the model. First, that the openness is intentionally part of a deliberate and rational way of leading one's life (this aspect is common to the next model also, and constitutes the main point of this section). Second, that the openness includes only anonymous sex (this aspect is what puts the Marwan-Ziad case at one end of the spectrum).

Consider now the heterosexual couple Makram and Hanan. Both are in their early to mid-forties. Both have been, and are, happily married, with two children away at college (let's make this case convenient by packing up and sending the children away!). However, after sexually experimenting with each other for a while, they have come to realize that their sex life is getting boring. They are confident enough in their love for each other and in their desire to be with each other that neither of them is threatened by the other having an extramarital affair. Neither Makram nor Hanan wants someone (other than Hanan and Makram, respectively) to dote over him or her, to cook with, to go traveling with, to watch movies with, and so on.[64] What they want is extra sexual spice to their lives, so they decide to sexually experiment further.

Suppose they know two people who are willing to have an affair with them (individually, that is). Hanan knows Khaled, an ambitious intern in his early thirties who works in her office. He is neither too young to be inexperienced and to brag, nor is he too old to be suspected of seeking affection under the guise of sex, so to speak. She knows that Khaled is sexually interested in her, she knows that he is not the romantic type, and she knows that he is single. Makram knows Samia, an old friend of his from college, a woman who has chosen an unmarried life because she has decided to make her career the focus of her life. Makram knows that Samia is sexually interested in him, and he knows that she is not the romantic type.

I have, of course, constructed these characters carefully. I have constructed them especially with an eye towards making sure that the sexual relations that ensue would not violate the dictates of other virtues. For example, Samia is not a minor; she is not Makram's student; and she is not his secretary. Neither Samia nor Khaled is married. And Makram and Hanan do not deceive each other in these things. Moreover, I have constructed these characters with an eye towards the idea that all of them can reasonably expect the relationships to be sexual and only sexual. Nevertheless, there is an element of fictitiousness to them that renders them implausible. This, I believe, stems from realistic rather than conceptual considerations. It is difficult to find a heterosexual couple that is willing to have such open *affairs* and, moreover, to make the case such that no difficulties will occur in the future. Do you mean to say, one might ask of me, that Makram does not feel jealous when Hanan leaves to meet the younger Khaled? Do you mean to say that Hanan never feels a tinge of sadness when she knows that her husband is "frolicking in bed with that tramp" Samia? How realistic are these cases? The point is not that heterosexual people in relationships have affairs only infrequently, or that heterosexual women have affairs only infrequently,[65] but that such *open, smooth* affairs are infrequent.

It is here, I think, where the strength of Steinbock's argument kicks in, and it does so most importantly at a practical level. The idea is that given the general conception that people (and not just Westerners) have that sexual activity indicates emotional intimacy between the sexual partners, it is, first, difficult to actually find that many couples who have such open affairs, and, second, it is difficult to find couples who are psychologically, emotionally, and morally able to bring themselves to actually engage in such open affairs, *even if* they themselves see no *theoretical* or conceptual difficulty in doing so. It is the second point that is of crucial importance (the first is merely a statistical one and requires evidential backing). And if we add a third *prescriptive* point, namely, that heterosexual couples *should not* engage in such open affairs, the force of this prescription can only ride on the possible damages that can ensue given the force of the second point (it cannot ride on the force of the conceptual connections between sex and emotions, because there are none).

The second point is not reducible simply to the practical difficulties of conducting open affairs; it is not the point expressed by one of John Updike's characters (Foxy) in *Couples*: "Adultery. It's so much *trouble*." The point rather illustrates the psychological, emotional, and moral inability of couples to bring themselves to accept and act upon the idea that *they* actually engage in open relationships. Sometimes, this can also illustrate the chasm between what we theoretically believe and what we can actually embark upon. A couple, for example, may have no difficulty claiming that sex, really, can be meaningless. But if they were to bring themselves to try to open their relationship, they would suffer acute emotional and psychological pains. Indeed, many couples would be even perfectly happy to accept boring sex in their lives rather than open up their relationship.

The causes and reasons for this attitude could be numerous. They can run the gamut from purely biological ones (we are inclined as a species to be incapable of such open nonmonogamy) to purely cultural ones (we have imbibed, deeply, cultural views to the effect that sex is always tied to emotions). But whatever the reasons, what is crucial here is what this tells us about the position I advocate: if open relationships are unrealistic, where does that leave us?

First, it does not affect the conceptual point, which is that open relationships can be perfectly virtuous and rational if given their proper place (I will briefly return to this issue in a moment). Second, it has a tremendous effect on the practical issue as to whether a couple should have an open relationship and of what type. A couple needs to be well informed about their reasons for wanting to have an open relationship; the spouses need to have minimal to nonexistent self-deception about their motives and about their ability to handle open relationships. For example, if they feel jealous, they need to know what its source is. Is it due to possessiveness? If so, then they might very well be unsuited for any type of open relationship. If their jealousy, however, is due to more benign sources, such as fear of losing their loved ones to another, then perhaps only open relationships that allow for emotionless sex are suitable for them.[66] The spouses should also think carefully about how they are to conduct their open relationships, when, with whom, when to give up the entire idea, and whom it is affecting (Do they have children, for example? Are the children young or old and leading their own independent lives? And, in either case, how will knowledge of their parents' open relationship affect them? Indeed, *should* the children, at any point in their lives, know about their parents' sex lives?). Furthermore, couples may very well differ in the range of their emotional and psychological capabilities. Some couples might have no difficulty in allowing for one-night stands in their open relationships. Others might find this difficult and opt for anonymous sex, or sex with sex workers. Still others might find even such types of sexual activity to be emotionally and psychologically taxing. But I will stop here as far as these issues are concerned so as to turn to more philosophical concerns.

I have sought in this section to make a case for the claim that open relationships need not be irrational, unvirtuous, and/or destructive, while also pitching the claim broadly enough so as to make room for contingent factors such as the emotional and psychological abilities of the spouses, their tastes, their ages, and other myriad factors that can come in assessing such issues. Both cases of Marwan and Ziad and of Makram and Hanan are meant to indicate how sexually open relationships can be rational and virtuous. The former case is more realistic, while the latter is less so, because gay couples have—for reasons we need not go into here—been able to some extent to escape societal expectations of relationships between the two genders. In both cases the spouses enjoy sexual activity and because of this are willing to open up their relationships. However, they do not do so out of an overvaluation of sex; nor do they do so at the expense of their relationship. Indeed, on the account I am offering, if the agents are in a relationship because they *highly* prize love and intimacy, and if they are incapable of handling an open relationship no matter how much they enjoy sex, then it would be irrational for them to open up their relationship. In all of this, the agents must decide how much they value romantic love and sexual variety. In the case of Firas, while Firas recognized the objective value of romantic love, he himself had no desire to have it in his life at that point in time. In this respect, he is able to rationally accommodate promiscuity in his life without overvaluing the general importance of sex. Someone, however, who values romantic love highly and yet who is willing to forgo meaningful romantic love relationships because he is simply unwilling to give up sexual variety and/or promiscuity smacks of incontinence: his desires rule his life even though he knows that they should not, simply because he knows that they are leading him to forgo a crucial good in his life. In this respect, his life is an irrational one.

Of course, there are cases and cases. A couple might decide to have an open relationship because their life together is, in general and not just sexually, getting tedious, boring, routine. While such open relationships could be justified, they are nonetheless a lesser of two evils: couples have them simply in order to avoid having to break up. On my account, such open relationships are, if not downright irrational, certainly less than rational. The spouses are looking in the wrong direction, so to speak. Rather than taking steps to scrutinize their relationship, they are engaging in patchwork remedies. They might not have much of a choice, of course; they might be in a situation in which breaking up is not an option. Nevertheless, such relationships are not rational, even if necessary sometimes; they are not conducive to a flourishing life.

We must also keep in mind that there are a number of variations in the cases between those of Marwan and Ziad, on the one hand, and Makram and Hanan, on the other. Makram and Hanan, for example, realizing that they are unable to handle open *affairs* in their marriage, might opt for a kind of sexual openness which leaves them less vulnerable. They might hire a sex worker. They might join a swinger's club. They might resort to one-night stands. Similar options exist for Marwan and Ziad. Whatever option a couple takes, what is crucial is that it be part of a deliberated upon, rational course of practice which does not threaten the love between the spouses by overvaluing sexual activity and sexual desires.

Let us get back briefly to T1. Couples that opt for an open relationship, as we have seen, need not believe that sex is more important than their love relationship; they need not believe that sexual activity may be pursued at the expense of other more worthwhile activities. They also need not engage in outside sex frequently, very often, or at regularly designated intervals. But T1 is specifically concerned with the issue of amounts in that a person whose life is driven by desire for sex is more than likely to make it the focal point of his life and so more than likely to spend too much time and energy seeking and engaging in sex. Since couples in open relationships need not be like this, and since they need not forfeit their romantic love because of their sexual lifestyles, we can safely conclude that open relationships are compatible with T1. As long as the sexual impulse that leads to them is part of a rational and virtuous life plan, then sexual activity is fully compatible with T1. The only notable exceptions are, as I stated, open relationshps involving a good amount of vulnerability and intimacy. These are the types of open relationships most likely to threaten the romantic love between the spouses, though whether they will do so will ultimately depend on each case.

6. The Third Ideal and T1

Does being a sex worker necessarily lead to having to forfeit some value essential to flourishing? Or does it make such forfeiture more likely? In this section, I will discuss four items—romantic love, a decent sex life, respect, and autonomy—that might be thought to be given up by sex workers due to the very nature of their work. If sex workers are likely to forfeit such goods, then there would be a good case to make that they cannot flourish or that they would have a hard time flourishing. However, I will argue that none of these goods are necessarily lost due to being a sex worker, and that they are not likely to. Moreover, I will discuss the reasons why many sex workers enter their profession, and use these reasons to argue how a life of sex work is perfectly compatible with virtue.

Does being a sex worker necessitate or make likely that the sex worker give up romantic love? Surely the answer to this is negative. A brief glance at the writings and experiences of sex workers confirms the fact that many of them have lovers and spouses with whom they are in love. Perhaps the thought is that, à la Kristjansson, the sex worker forfeits monogamy because of her active sex life; her sex life forces her, so to speak, to become unable to be monogamous. But of course this line of thinking is burdened with multiple mistakes.

First, not all sex workers engage in sex acts, narrowly construed in the way that the above line of thinking requires. Stripping and phone sex are not about actual sexual engagement in oral sex and intercourse; they do not require physical contact between the sex worker and the client (although some strippers are often willing to engage in lap dancing and other acts that require physical contact). Second, the best that the above reasoning establishes is that the sex work leads to forfeiting monogamy, not romantic love. And as we know by now, from the previous section, giving up the former does not entail giving up the latter, and it makes giving up romantic love likely only under certain forms of nonmonogamy, namely under those nonmonogamous encounters exemplified by extramarital affairs. But, of course, the kind of nonmonogamous sex acts that sex workers engage in are not of this sort.

Third, Kristjansson's argument derived much of its force from the very structure of the promiscuous person's sexual *desires*. That person was construed as someone who desires and who wants to have sex for the sake of having sex and with multiple partners to enhance the sexual experience. But the case with sex work is vastly different. Though almost all sex workers are certainly not prudish about sex, it is a myth and a false view to think of the sex worker as a woman who "can't get enough," who is driven by her lust to engage in "unspeakable" acts. The charged term "whore" carries precisely the connotations of someone who is base and driven by lust. But it is certain that this picture is extremely far from being accurate. As Peggy Morgan, a stripper, nicely puts it in referring to her work, "It's not sexual; it's *work*. Using our whole bodies to earn a living makes it clear how much sexual feelings really come from our minds: a lover may touch the same way a customer does, but produce an entirely different feeling" (1987, 25). The point is that while one can see how an argument based on the idea of a lustful person's desires can conclude that such a person is likely to forfeit monogamy, it is difficult to apply such an argument to sex work because sex workers are not accurately characterized by the basic idea of this argument.

Perhaps what is forfeited is not romantic love but something else. Perhaps what is forfeited is, paradoxically, a decent sex life. The thought could be that a sex worker cannot, or is not likely to, have a healthy, that is, pleasurable, sex life of her own because she engages in too much sex already. (The promiscuous person, no matter how promiscuous his behavior is, does not usually even come close to having as many sexual encounters as a sex worker has.) Too much of a good thing can lead to boredom with that thing. If a sex worker has to deal with sex all the time, then one would expect that she would lose her ability to enjoy a sex life of her own. This is a risk that comes with the trade; it is an "occupational hazard," as Primoratz calls it (1999, 92).

Again, however, not all sex workers engage in sexual acts of the kind that the above thought requires to be convincing. Engaging a client in a sexual conversation over the phone, for example, does not lead to a forfeiture of a sex life, let alone a decent one (skilled sex phone workers sometimes do all sorts of chores, such as ironing, while on the phone with a client). Furthermore, even for those types of sex work that do entail the kind of sex that this reasoning presupposes, there is no evidence that sex workers are less sexually fulfilled than other women, and, indeed, there is evidence that they are more sexually fulfilled.[67] Moreover, this reasoning makes the same crucial mistake as the one before it. One reason we are not tempted to believe that a heterosexual male (or a lesbian) gynecologist will not lose sexual interest in women's sexual organs even though he looks at these professionally on a regular basis is because we recognize an important and essential difference between his attitude towards women when they are his *patients* and when they are his *sexual partners*. Similarly, sex workers' basic attitude towards their work is not typically sexual or lustful. And this makes it perfectly easy to see how they can have a rich and healthy sex life outside their work.[68]

Is it respect that a sex worker forfeits? "Respect" refers to the *attitudes* of others towards the sex worker, and not necessarily to their behavior towards her. Furthermore, the lack of respect under consideration here is due to the sex worker's very status as a sex worker, rather than to the sloppiness of her work or her unprofessionalism. It is clear that such an attitude exists. Many religious people, for example, disrespect prostitutes (perhaps even condemn them). Perhaps many academics do so also. And perhaps also a good number of their male clients have disrespectful attitudes towards them. But then again, a large number of people do not disrespect sex workers and even downright respect them. In the case of male sex workers, being a male escort is even beginning to be considered a sign of prestige and glamour, as one recent magazine article has it.[69] In the case of women sex workers, their clients are made up of a variety of people, many of whom have a respectful attitude towards the sex workers and what they do. Many academics respect sex workers. And many other types of people have a respectful attitude towards them also.

It is because of such a mixed bag of results that this last reasoning is weak. What it needs to establish is the claim that there is an overwhelming attitude of disrespect for sex workers, across the board and from more or less all segments of the population. Otherwise, it is hard to see why a sex worker in Chicago cannot, or is not likely to, flourish just because the members of some Baptist Church in Montevallo, Alabama have an attitude of disrespect for sex workers in general. Indeed, some of those very same people who disrespect sex workers often also disrespect a host of other types of people, such as feminists and Democrats. Would this mean that feminists and Democrats cannot flourish because of this attitude of disrespect towards them? One hopes not.

More importantly, issues of lack of respect and of flourishing need to be handled with caution. Let us assume for the sake of the argument that the bag of attitudes is not so mixed, that it is mostly negative. While virtue ethics certainly emphasizes the concept of flourishing, virtue ethics admits of plenty of cases in which human beings find it difficult, and even do not, flourish due to contingent hazards to their lives. And it is often the case that part of such contingent hazards is the attitudes (and behavior) of others towards virtuous people. A just and humane white woman might very well expect to feel the ire of her fellow whites were she to fight and stand up for the rights of blacks in her racist country. An honest and virtuous Israeli citizen who stands up for the rights of the Palestinians to live in their land in dignity and freedom might very well invite the scorn and ill-treatment of many of his fellow citizens. But we do not, and neither would virtue ethics, counsel that they give up their political and moral stance. The reason is that virtue ethics is not a crass form of egoism; it does not invite its agents to calculate, as the moment warrants and demands, what sorts of behaviors and dispositions will lead them to be happy and live well. Nor can it conceptually do so, given the centrality of the virtues in its theoretical structure. For the virtues are deep and settled dispositions in the agent's character, and so if the agent has, say, the virtue of courage, she cannot just simply switch it off in a moment when she can benefit by acting cowardly (nor would she want to). Virtue ethics' claim regarding the connection between flourishing and being virtuous is that being the latter is one's best shot at the former because as rational and social entities the virtues are those traits that are most likely to allow us to live well. And this last claim is fully compatible with cases in which the agent does not lead a life as well as she could have, or even fails to flourish, due to contingent hazards external to her virtue and character.

The point of the two examples above about justice is not to make an analogy with sex work. After all, the work of sex workers is not like fighting for a just cause. The point, rather, is to dispel the impression—if it exists—that flourishing counts for everything within virtue ethics. With this point in mind, a virtuous woman might very well expect to deal with and to feel the disrespect of her society members, her community, and perhaps even her family members were she to opt to become a sex worker. But this does not show that she should—morally should—give up her profession. Indeed, we can strengthen the point about respect by adding to it other attitudes, such as scorn, hatred, and shunning. With such a gamut of attitudes, a sex worker might find it difficult to live a flourishing life. Consider, for example, the character of Sofia (or Sonia) Semionovna in Dostoyevsky's *Crime and Punishment*. Though she was forced into prostitution due to her poverty, and even though the people around her knew this, they nevertheless wanted to have nothing to do with her and treated her with scorn. With such attitudes, and in addition to her poverty, it was certainly difficult for her to lead a decent life. But if her reasons for becoming a sex worker are not vicious and do not go against virtue, then virtue ethics would not counsel, and rightly so, that she give up her profession. In the case of Sofia, her reasons (dire poverty) are indeed not vicious. (And she herself, as portrayed by Dostoyevsky, is morally decent.)

We should keep in mind the fact that others' attitudes towards one are, in a plausible sense, external goods. Depending on the attitudes, whether they are positive or not, one's chances for leading a decent life are certainly affected. In the case of sex work, such attitudes are ones that one can do without in order to lead a decent life. But such attitudes are also contingent, and more importantly, morally unjustified. If my argument has been on the right track, sex work does not justifiably elicit such attitudes. If this is so, and if the reasons why someone goes into sex work are not vicious, then we cannot simply claim that sex workers morally ought to give up their work. I will not conclude from this, however, that even though others' negative attitudes should not morally induce sex workers to give up their work, they nevertheless should prudentially do so because such attitudes do exist. And this is, after all, what matters for flourishing. I will not derive this conclusion because of the earlier considerations, namely, that such attitudes, though they do exist, are not widespread enough to seriously make a dent in a sex worker's life. They do not prevent her, for example, from having friends, a family, a lover, and a host of other things necessary for a well-lived life. Moreover, such negative attitudes are contingent and rest on what I take to be mistaken beliefs about sex work, about the role of sex in our lives, and about a number of other aspects connected to sex. And this further supports the conclusion that there is nothing about sex work, as such, that would require the forfeiture of respect or make such a forfeiture likely.

The fourth item one might think that a sex worker forfeits is autonomy. If sex work is a form of slavery, as some arguments have it, then the sex worker forfeits her autonomy. If she does so, then she cannot flourish. Carole Pateman, in a response (1983) to an article by Lars Ericsson (1980), argues that Ericsson misunderstands the feminist charge against prostitution, which is that prostitution (and so not all sex work, though Pateman is not explicit about this) is a form of slavery. If Pateman is right, then at least one form of sex work would be detrimental to flourishing. I will argue that Pateman's argument is far from compelling.

Pateman's argument seems to be as follows. In capitalist societies, labor power and services cannot be separated from the person offering them for sale (1983, 562). In the case of prostitution, the lack of separation of labor power and services from the laborer applies even more strongly because sexuality is connected to gender conceptions, and because sexual services are unlike other types of services. Pateman states,

> Sexual services, that is to say, sex and sexuality, are constitutive of the body in a way in which the counseling skills of the social worker are not. . . . Sexuality and the body are, further, integrally connected to conceptions of femininity and masculinity, and all these are constitutive of our individuality, our sense of self-identity. When sex becomes a commodity in the capitalist market so, *necessarily*, do bodies and selves. The prostitute *cannot* sell sexual services alone; what she sells is her body. (1983, 562; my emphasis)

This tells us that prostitution is a form of slavery—at least a temporary one that lasts for the duration of the sexual encounter between prostitute and client. Because of this, women would not consent to be prostitutes unless they have to, since—the assumption seems to be—no one would consent to slavery, temporary or not. Pateman states, "The difference between sex without love and prostitution is . . . that between the reciprocal expression of desire and unilateral subjection to sexual acts with the consolation of payment: it is the difference for women between freedom and subjection" (563). Therefore, prostitution is nothing but a form of men subjugating women, and this is what the feminist charge against prostitution is, according to Pateman: "Prostitution is the public recognition of men as sexual masters" (564).

In assessing Pateman's argument, Igor Primoratz offers the counterexamples of wet nurses and surrogate mothers: "Their bodies and gender are no less involved in what they do than the body and gender of the prostitute; and they charge a fee, just as the prostitute does" (1999, 104). Since wet nurses and surrogate mothers do not sell themselves just because of what they do, then Pateman's argument is not sound, because one might as well conclude the same thing about prostitutes. Primoratz concludes, "If what I have been saying is right, we still do not have an argument showing that prostitution is degrading *in itself*" (105; my emphasis).

I am not convinced, however, by Primoratz's response, for the simple reason that I think that Pateman can reply to him in convincing ways, given her argument. She can say that her argument is not meant to show that prostitution is wrong in itself, as Primoratz concludes, but only in capitalist societies. She can also reject the wet nurse and surrogate mother counterexamples on the grounds that the activities they engage in are not sexual activities, even though they necessarily involve sexual body parts. She might claim that the scope of her argument covers sexual body parts used sexually. Whether this would be a successful reply is questionable. In any case, it would be good to offer a more decisive response.

Since much of Pateman's argument hinges on the first premise—that in capitalist societies labor power and services cannot be separated from the person offering them for sale—a brief discussion of it is in order. (I will discuss it in such a way without needing to enter into larger issues regarding capitalism and its moral dimensions.) Pateman seems to think that the first premise is true because it is physically impossible to separate labor power from the body of the laborer. If, for example, I hire a plumber, *he*, and not some abstract "plumbing power," has to come and fix the problem at my home. This is obviously true. But it does not give Pateman what she wants, namely, that this is somehow a form of slavery because in hiring the labor power of the plumber I hire his body. Pateman states, "The employer appears to buy labor power; what he actually obtains is the right of command over workers, the right to put their capacities, their bodies, to use, as *he determines*" (562; my emphasis).[70] The pitfall is in the last three words: they are false. I, in hiring the plumber, cannot rightfully put his body to use as I determine; I cannot make him pose naked for me, for example, much as I would want him to. In other words, Pateman is too quick to infer from the fact that just because an employer has rights over the services of an employee, and just because these services come attached—so to speak—to the body of the employee, that the employer has full rights over the latter's body. This is an invalid inference.

Moreover, I do not even have the right to put the plumber's *plumbing capacities* to any use I want. I do not have the right, for example, to send him to my neighbor's house to fix her plumbing problem (not unless the plumber has agreed to this in advance or agrees to it upon request). It is important to mention this because of the following temptation. One might argue that even if what I say amounts to a good criticism of the first premise of Pateman's argument, it does nothing to criticize the second and third premises. After all, one might argue, the prostitute sells sexual services, and sex is connected to human bodies in intimate ways. I will grant this observation about sex and its intimacy to the body and to self-identities. But I will not grant that this yields the conclusion that prostitution is a form of slavery. For, in much the same ways that I do not have the right to send the plumber over to my neighbor's house, I do not have the right to use the prostitute's body in any way I determine. A client, for example, does not have the right to force the prostitute to engage in oral sex or in intercourse without the use of protection. Indeed, he does not have the right to perform sexual acts with her that she, for whatever reason, tells him—often in advance—that she will not do. That the prostitute uses her body is a given. But it will take much more to argue that this entails a form of slavery. The client, simply put, does not *own* the prostitute or her body, not even for the fifteen minutes or hour or whatever time duration that he pays for her services. Indeed, because the client is driven by his lust, whereas the prostitute usually is not, she is freer than the client in one crucial aspect: she is psychologically in charge of what they do together.

I am not denying, of course, that some clients force themselves on prostitutes in all sorts of ways and that the illegality of prostitution in many parts of the world makes it easier for the client to do so (since the prostitute cannot have legal recourse against him). Nor am I denying that in some types of prostitution such rights are lacking, such as many forms of streetwalking and child prostitution. Rather, my point is that even in capitalist societies, not all forms of prostitution are forms of slavery. This is both a descriptive and a normative point. It is descriptive, because as a matter of fact, many prostitutes and sex workers do successfully exercise such control over their bodies. It is a normative point, because morally speaking, just because a client pays for sexual services by the sex worker, it simply does not follow that the client owns her or her body—not even in capitalist societies—and it does not follow that both participants in the sex act view things this way, psychologically or phenomenologically.

My criticisms of Pateman's argument, if correct, indicate that it is not easy to argue that prostitution and sex work in general are forms of slavery, given the ability of sex workers to determine what clients are to do with their bodies. If so, then the burden of proof shifts to those who want to argue that prostitution is a form of slavery. Moreover, if my criticisms are correct, then the point of the fourth premise in Pateman's argument— that women would not consent to be prostitutes unless they had to— becomes moot. Since prostitution is *not* a form of slavery, then we are free to argue that oftentimes women do consent to be prostitutes and sex workers. Even if we grant that prostitution currently operates within patriarchy, women can still consent to it. Alan Soble puts the point well: "Whether women can consent to the sex acts of prostitution would seem to be as much a matter of their mental states, their particular needs and values, and the details of their lives as of their membership in a victimized class. The need to earn money can be a good reason to do something; it can also be coercive. Which it is in a given case cannot be established by sweeping claims about gender oppression" (1996, 36).

There are two points that at this juncture are important to make. First, the discussion of Pateman's argument indicates that sex work, as such, is not the type of work that leads its practitioners to give up their autonomy. That sex workers can, and often do, decide to enter this profession, and that they can, and often do, exercise control within it shows that they do not lose their autonomy. Of course, their freedom, broadly construed, would be limited. But this is the case with virtually every profession. Moreover, some types of sex work (streetwalking, for example) do result in large losses in the sex worker's autonomy. But this does not show, or make likely, that sex work as such leads to a forfeiture of autonomy. Second, this discussion, along with Soble's point quoted in the above paragraph, bring up the issue of why sex workers go into sex work. But before entering into it, a few important comments about the issue of the amounts of sex are needed as a preamble.

In my treatment of promiscuity, I argued that the issue of amounts is important as an indication as to how the promiscuous person is leading his life. When a man spends hours every day in pursuit of sex, he is no doubt engaging his sexual desires too *much*. And this *indicates* that his reason is the slave of his passions. If we now transfer this picture to sex work, and if we focus on the type of sex work that requires the obvious types of sexual acts (oral sex, intercourse), we might be misled into thinking that the sex worker is no doubt ruled by her sexual desires and that she is leading a slavish life. But it is worth repeating the point that this is not generally true because the sex worker typically does not approach her work as a way to satisfy her lust; she approaches it as work. And, with this point firmly in mind, we must give up the temptation to think of a sex worker as necessarily ruled by her sexual instincts and desires.

This leads head on to the issue of the reasons for going into sex work. Above, I stated that if the sex worker's reasons for becoming a sex worker do not stem from vices, then a sex worker is not morally required to give up her work. But what might the reasons for entering sex work be? And what are some differences between vicious and nonvicious ones? If sex workers are not generally in it to satisfy their lust, we are now in a position to speculate about the other possible reasons as to why they are in the sex work profession. According to Priscilla Alexander, "The specific reasons that prostitutes have given for choosing their work . . . have included money, excitement, independence, and flexibility, in roughly that order" (1987, 188). According to Vicky Funari, "There is no standard sex worker. Each woman has her own reasons for working. . . . The only safe thing to say is that we're all in it for the money" (1997, 28). What these remarks should do is to stifle another possible temptation, namely, that *all* sex workers are in sex work because they have no other options. While this is true with respect to some sex workers, it is by no means true of all of them or even of many of them. The fact that most of them are in it for the money should not indicate lack of options. If it did, then excitement, independence, and flexibility can hardly be cited as *reasons* for entering the profession. If sex workers are sex workers out of lack of other options, these items would be, at best, positive *byproducts* of being a sex worker, rather than reasons for entering this profession.

Nor should we think that, just because sex work has a social stigma attached to it, women who enter it do so out of *some* coercion, especially economic coercion.[71] The fact that sex work could yield quite a bit of monetary return should tell us, in no uncertain terms, that many women can and do choose it *precisely* because of this yield. People often choose all sorts of risky jobs, jobs which involve a lot of physical toil, or jobs which involve a lot of (physical) dirt and muck precisely because they can charge quite a bit of money. I do not wish to convey the idea that no women are coerced, economically or otherwise, into sex work; many are. But many are not, and we should not lose sight of this fact. Again, a cursory glance at the writings of sex workers should easily confirm this.

I have been engaging these well-worn points and arguments in order to make it clear that choosing to be, and being, a sex worker need not indicate irrationality on the part of the sex worker. They also need not indicate that the sex worker is leading an oppressed way of life, be it socially or economically. This can also be seen in the fact that even under decent economic and social conditions, a person, and more specifically a woman, can choose to become a sex worker and yet be as rational and as virtuous as one desires. For example, a woman might choose to become a sex worker so as to be able to have time to do what she really would like to do, such as write, or help the homeless, or travel. When the woman can do so without violating any other important obligations that she has, her reasons for entering the profession are perfectly permissible. Consider how many people (non–sex workers, that is) constantly express their wishes and desires to pursue some activity, hobby, or career that they cannot pursue given how hectic and demanding their jobs are. If sex work does indeed provide a good income, a good measure of independence, and time flexibility, then it makes perfect sense for someone to choose it as a job (and let's not forget that many academics choose their careers because of the independence and flexibility that being an academic gives them, though these—one hopes—are not the only reasons).

Notice that the success of the above example does not hinge on assuming that a situation of social inequality between men and women exists, or that a situation of gender oppression exists, or that the woman has no other economic options. For there is no reason to believe that in a society that has its genders on equal footing the sex profession will be any less lucrative, or that it will pay less money. As Pat Califia puts it, "While large and sweeping social change would probably alter the nature of sex work, the demographics for sex workers, and the wage scale, along with every other kind of human intimacy, I doubt very much that a just society would (or could) eliminate paying for pleasure" (1994, 242).[72] And if sex is such that people are always willing to pay for it (though so far it is mostly men who seem to do so), then even if one has other economic options, being a sex worker might very well be a better option economically. And if the stigma of being a sex worker is removed, then we might very well expect more people to enter the profession (though this might lead to lower incomes for sex workers due to competition).

The point is that money, flexibility, and independence are perfectly legitimate reasons for pursuing a profession. Moreover, because she is not driven by lust, they give the sex worker a measure of freedom as far as sex and sexual encounters are concerned: "The freedom to choose one's reasons for engaging in sex is an important part of sexual freedom" (Soble 2002b, 183). However, they do not, as such, give one a blank check to be used whenever the agent so desires. In the above example, these three features of sex work are used by the woman as reasons in a decent way because they do not violate any other obligations she has. In addition, she has not chosen sex work out of greed for money. She has not chosen sex work out of laziness. She has not chosen sex work out of fear of undertaking tasks that require a good amount of dependence. So she has not chosen her profession in a way that indicates her lack of proper measure of how to weigh the importance of instrumental goods such as money. She has not chosen her profession in a way to indicate that she lacks proper and reasonable ambition. And she has not chosen sex work in a way to indicate that she lacks courage. She has chosen sex work because it allows her, given her life, to pursue her writing career, for instance.

The reader can generate for herself numerous more examples in which being a sex worker might be part of a rational, flourishing life and contrary to no virtue, and so generate examples, along the lines of the above one, in which one's reasons for being a sex worker are ethically decent. This is not to claim that every person should be a sex worker. Even though one can have good reasons to be an academic, and even though being an academic need not be contrary to the virtues, it does not follow from this that everyone should be an academic. Similar reasoning applies to sex work. Moreover, the claim that sex work can be part of a virtuous, flourishing life is not the claim that all sex workers are leading flourishing lives (far from it). It is also not the claim that the decision to become a sex worker can be undertaken lightly, and it is not the claim that even when being a sex worker makes perfect sense, one does not have to sometimes give up on it in order to be virtuous. Here, we can cite some vicious reasons for being a sex worker. In this respect, they are no different essentially from vicious reasons for choosing any other profession. When one chooses a profession simply out of greed, out of laziness, or out of cowardice, out of stupidity, and/or at the expense of other important obligations in life, such as those from one's family, friends, sanity, and emotional health, then the reasons simply indicate a defective character. These need not preclude one from being good at what one does, but they do entail a defective character on the part of the agent. Moreover, when one is coerced to become a sex worker due to a lack of other options, this indicates that one's life is not going well, is not flourishing, and this is most obvious when one does not like one's career—to put the point somewhat mildly.

Given that sex work is primarily about *work* rather than sexual *desire*, its discussion under T1 is somewhat out of place. However, sex work does involve sexual behavior, from behavior that requires actual physical contact such as prostitution, acting in pornography, sadomasochism, and some forms of stripping, to behavior that requires no actual physical contact but that is nevertheless sexual, such as some forms of stripping, phone sex, and nude modeling. I have argued that sex work, much like any other profession, can be—and not in the logical weak sense of "can"—part of a rational, virtuous, and flourishing life. Of course, in a society in which sex work is associated with a good amount of stigma, being a sex worker might have a heavy price, and such a price can make the sex worker's life a difficult one to lead. Hopefully, we may look to a better future and to a better society.

7. The Gender Issue

Are there important differences between men and women that might be thought relevant to the discussion so far? In other words, is there a need to modify the above discussion in light of the thought that there are these differences between the genders? I will argue that the answer to this question is complicated, but that there does not, as of yet, seem to be a need to modify my conclusions in any conceptual or basic ways.

I have been conducting this entire discussion of sex without paying much attention to gender difference. I have for example discussed sexual promiscuity in a way that seems to forget that men tend to be more promiscuous than women. I have discussed open relationships in such a way that the only really convincing example of a relationship that contains partners who engage in outside anonymous sex is a *gay male* relationship. Perhaps my only nod to gender differences has been my more or less consistent use of the pronoun "she" when it comes to sex work and the pronoun "he" when it comes promiscuity under the realistic assumption that most sex workers are women and that most promiscuous people are men.[73]

But surely, one can complain, this obliviousness to gender issues assumes too much. Surely it is men who have been promiscuous, given that women, in most parts of the world, have always been required to be chaste or devout mothers and wives. And surely it is generally true that it is men who enjoy casual sex, not women. And when it comes to open relationships, we hardly have examples of these from among heterosexual couples and lesbian couples. Most of the examples come from gay male couples. Surely this issue needs to be addressed. Yes it does. But I am not sure what to say about it given the lack of crucial information from which to draw conclusions that are interesting, plausible, and general enough to apply to men and women. Let me explain.

The gender issue can be expressed in the claim that there are two possible ways in which my entire discussion is inapplicable to women. These two are that, first, women cannot be sexually active and experimental as men can be and are, and, that, second, women should not be sexually active in the ways I have been defending (the option that women *are* not sexually active in the above ways can be explained, ultimately, by either the "cannot" or the "should not"). For the sake of manageability, I will confine myself to discussing promiscuity, since promiscuity is the most salient fact that some sociobiologists and philosophers point to when it comes to the sexual behavioral discrepancy between men and women. It is my contention that the jury is still out with respect to these two ways in which my discussion is said to be inapplicable to women, and this is what I meant when I wrote in the above paragraph that we lack crucial information and plausible arguments. The topics in this area are vast and can take up a book on their own. I will then only indicate the direction of my arguments rather than engage in an exhaustive and an in-depth discussion.[74]

Consider first the "can" claim, namely, that women cannot be promiscuous. This "cannot" seems to indicate some type of impossibility, that, in some sense, it is impossible for women to be promiscuous. Given that women sex workers are promiscuous, the sense in question must be something along the lines of, "women cannot be promiscuous because they do not *desire* to be so. If they are, it is because they are either sex workers or are somehow forced into being promiscuous." But strictly speaking, this claim is false. There are, and have been, women who are quite promiscuous by choice. Furthermore, with the current changing times, one finds more and more women who are sexually promiscuous. However, some might argue that we should construe the "can" claim a bit more weakly to the effect that women find it *difficult*, though not impossible, because of their nature, to be promiscuous. But what nature is this?

Sociobiology, the view that "all aspects of human culture and behavior . . . are coded in the genes and have been molded by natural selection" (Lewontin, Rose, and Kamin 1984, 235–36), emerges. We are often told that during the early stages of humankind, it has been advantageous for women to be monogamous, and so with time their monogamy has become coded for in their genes. It is to the advantage of men, however, to be promiscuous, and with time promiscuity has been coded for in men. Such genetic predilections need not preclude acting contrary to them, but doing so does not come easy. If this hypothesis of sociobiology is true, it does not entail that when men, for example, are being promiscuous they are thinking such things as "This will help spread my semen around and so increase the chances of passing on my traits," or that they are promiscuous because of considerations such as passing on their traits. This is because sociobiological hypotheses are explanations of ultimate causes, and not of individual actions and the intentional behaviors of human beings (Sober 1993, 198).

However, the various hypotheses of sociobiology are still in weak shape. My main criticism here is not that sociobiology is merely crude biological determinism, and thus women can act contrary to their genetic dispositions (as far as sexual behavior, at least, is concerned). This criticism will not have much force in the face of the claim that it is *difficult* for women to act contrary to their genetic dispositions. My main criticism, rather, is that one can imagine a number of incompatible sociobiological hypotheses about what is advantageous to women, and that, at the present time, there is no plausible way of adjudicating between them. Consider promiscuity. One hypothesis is that it is advantageous for women to be sexually monogamous because in this way they can rely on the help and protection of the man in raising their children to sexual maturity. Since pregnancy lasts a long time, and since rearing children is time consuming and risky, it is to the advantage of women, according to this hypothesis, that they be monogamous, because then they can ensure the help of a spouse. But consider another hypothesis: it is advantageous for women to be promiscuous because in doing so they can elicit the help, support, and protection of a number of men in raising their children to maturity. The men will help because they are not sure which one of them is the father, and so it is to their advantage to chip in. If one dies, the mother has others to help out (Fisher 1992, ch. 4). These two hypotheses are at odds, and it is difficult to see which one can be confirmed to a good degree of probable certainty. In this sense, the jury is indeed out with respect to sociobiology.

I am not arguing that sociobiology is bankrupt science. My point is simply that as far as certain issues are concerned—in our case those of promiscuity—sociobiology does not seem to offer a definitive, or even a highly probable, answer. If this is correct, then it is hard to see how the "cannot" claim, understood to mean "biologically impossible or difficult," can be supported.

There is another way of understanding the "can" in a weak sense. This is the idea that cultural indoctrination (or gender ideology) makes it difficult for women to be promiscuous given that women typically grow up in cultures that tell them, in various forms and through diverse channels, that they should be sexually faithful and devout wives. It is even worse when such cultures have a negative attitude towards sex and are willing only to tolerate it, rather than (to use a recently fashionable though somewhat nauseating term) celebrate it. Women, in such social ambiances, simply grow up finding it difficult to be sexually active in the ways that men are. It is in this sense that they "cannot" be promiscuous.

But this reasoning is easy to dispose of. Cultures change. Due to political, moral, religious, and economic pressures, cultures often change their mores and beliefs. Western cultural mores, for example, have witnessed some deep changes with respect to women and women's sexuality. Were cultures to change to the point at which both men and women are treated in equal and similar ways at least as far as sexual behavior is concerned, women might very well find it in them, so to speak, to be promiscuous. Whether this will happen is too soon to tell. Attitudes towards women have changed, but not to the extent where women have achieved full social, cultural, legal, moral, religious, and cultural equality with men. And it is this full equality that is necessary for us to see whether women can be as sexually promiscuous as men. In this respect, we still have no final answers.[75]

But it is also important to keep in mind that the idea that cultures and social mores change is not simply a truth that we can confidently assert from our philosophic armchairs. There is, as far as sexual mores are concerned, evidence for it. Consider open relationships. In an interesting article on swingers, Dan Savage (2002), the sex advice columnist, reports on the large number of heterosexual swinger clubs that have cropped up all across the United States, and in areas where to all appearances the people who live there lead traditional, monogamous married lives, just in the ways that the most zealous advocate of the traditional family would like them to. More to the point, one of the crucial aspects of extramarital sex that swingers emphasize is the comfort level of women. According to Savage, "The swinging movement would collapse if women felt unsafe or threatened . . . so clubs have to create an environment where women feel safe and free to lose themselves in the moment," while men have to be on their best behavior all the time (2002, 16). Neither single men nor men suspected of bringing prostitutes with them are allowed in the swinger club. What is interesting about this sensitivity to women is that it tells us quite a bit about the notion that women are coerced into swinging by domineering husbands, a belief that many hold about swingers. Bridget, a woman (married to David) whom Savage interviewed for his article, hates this idea. While she acknowledged that most women go to their first "party" because their husbands want them to, it is the women who end up insisting on going to more and more parties. According to her, "Here's this place where you can be totally sexually free and open in public and completely safe at the same time. How many women get to experience that in their lives? And to share that experience with my husband is a joy" (2002, 21).

While our culture perhaps still expects women to be monogamous and sexually passive, the evidence from swingers, if one cares to look at it, seems to suggest a somewhat different picture. Perhaps women's supposed sexual disinclination towards open relationships and promiscuity is due not so much to their natures as women, but more to cultural expectations, including the potential social punishments that threaten sexually active women. However, it seems to be the case that once such obstacles are removed, and once women, or at least some of them, feel safe, they have no difficulty enjoying their ability to be in open relationships and to be promiscuous. In any case, the evidence we have from women swingers and other sexually active women seem to suggest that cultural mores do have a lot to do with women's inclination towards monogamous sex, and that once such mores are relaxed, there seems to be no barrier facing the idea that women can and do desire sexually active lives.

Let me turn now briefly to the "should" issue, namely, that women should not be promiscuous. The "should" could refer to a prudential advice or to a moral command. As far as the prudential advice goes, the idea is that women should not be promiscuous because it is not in their interest to do so. This is the type of argument, I believe, that Shulamith Firestone advanced in *The Dialectic of Sex* (1970, ch. 6). Firestone argues that the women who succumbed to the sexual revolution were duped, because they have given up on the only weapon—sex—that they could have used to ensure commitment from a man, given women's inequality and hence need for male support (Firestone is silent, however, on the point as to how much responsibility the women themselves share for being duped). Women who became promiscuous gave men what men wanted without the latter giving women something in return, namely support.

Though Firestone's 1970 argument applies to a time when social configurations were more stultifying than they are now, we can still benefit from Firestone's interesting description of the dynamics of sexism. Firestone warns that as long as sexism and gender inequality exist, women should think seriously about what it means for them to be sexually promiscuous and to behave in sexual ways that men can engage in without having to pay a social price. In this respect, and to quote Linda LeMoncheck, "Sexual liberation is women's liberation when women can define its terms and conditions. Is promiscuity consistent with women's sexual empowerment? Could a promiscuous lifestyle promote such empowerment?" (1997, 54). LeMoncheck continues to offer a conditional answer: much depends on the woman's awareness and knowledge of the relationships between sex, gender, and oppression. A woman who opts for a promiscuous lifestyle may very well know that she will incur the dismissal of society. But she may nevertheless be able to empower herself sexually and become her own sexual *subject* by deciding to give up on monogamy and marriage as they exist in an oppressive society.

The general idea behind LeMoncheck's claims is correct. Whether women are duped by becoming promiscuous or by adopting nontraditional sexual lifestyles depends on why the women are adopting these roles, on their political, moral, and social knowledge of their societies, and on their purposes. While there is room to quibble within these parameters, the idea is on the right track. Prudentially, and given the history of sexism and oppression, if women are to benefit and be empowered by living nontraditional sexual lives, they had, to put it simply, better know what they are getting themselves into. In this respect, we cannot make general claims that women should not be promiscuous or that it makes perfect sense for women to be promiscuous. Much depends on the circumstances.

The other general sense of "should" is the ethical one. In a way, of course, the ethical and the prudential senses can be closely related. Women who undertake promiscuous lifestyles in not-so-prudential ways put their very integrity, self-identity, and respect at risk. And these are ethical notions. In this respect, the remarks above are sufficient to deal with this sense of the ethical "should." But there is of course a more general sense of "should," captured by the idea that promiscuity should not be a undertaken because it is unvirtuous, inimical to flourishing, or leads to wrongdoing. And it is this sense of "should" that this book has been concerned to refute.

Notes

Introduction

1. This claim is found pervasively, for example, in R. Solomon's 1990 book on love.

2. What I say in this section is meant to be very rough and does not do justice to the actual history of philosophical thought on care, love, and sex.

3. For anthologies, see Chapman and Galston 1992, Crisp 1996, Crisp and Slote 1997, Flanagan and Rorty 1993, French, Uehling, and Wettstein 1988, Hursthouse, Lawrence, and Quinn 1995, Kruschwitz and Roberts 1987, Paul, Miller, Jr., and Paul 1998 and 1999, and Statman 1997. For nonanthology books, see Baron, Pettit, and Slote 1997, Broadie 1991, Dent 1984, Foot 1978 and 2001, Hursthouse 1999b, MacIntyre 1984 and 1999, McKinnon 1999, Miller 1995, Pincoffs 1986, A. Rorty 1980, Slote 1983, 1992, and 2001, Swanton 2003, R. Taylor 1991, Wallace 1978, and Zagzebski 1996. For articles not published in any of the above anthologies, see (and this is only a sample) Audi 1995, Clowney 1990, Elliot 1993, Foot 1994 and 1995, Garcia 1990, Gottlieb 2001, Hartz 1990, Hursthouse 1986, Kultgen 1998, McKerlie 2001, Oakley 1996, Prior 2001, Savarino 1993, Sherman 1989 and 1999, Slote 1995, Stohr and Wellman 2002, Swanton 1995 and 2001, Trianosky 1987 and 1988, and Waide 1988. For some examples of applying virtue ethics, see Bogen 1980, Foot 1978, Halwani 1998b and 2002, Hill 1983, Hursthouse 1995 and 1997b, Roberts 1988, and R. Solomon 1997.

4. This is similar to the distinction that J. Driver 1996 makes between virtue theory and virtue ethics. The latter is a moral theory independent of and possibly rivalling others, while the former is an account of what the virtues are.

5. I also do not intend to go into, anywhere in this book, how virtue ethics construes the notion of right action and how it construes the role of emotion in virtuous action. This has been ably done by Hursthouse (1999b, parts 1 and 2). See also Swanton 2001 and 2003, part 4, especially ch. 11, for a different view.

6. As I was doing the final revisions on this book, Swanton's 2003 book on virtue ethics appeared. Swanton offers a view of virtue ethics that is not entirely Aristotelian (see especially ch. 4), but that also does not have the serious defects that, in my opinion, Slote's has. Unfortunately, I did not have the time to incorporate Swanton's insights into the present book. But I do refer the reader every now and then to her views at some critical junctures.

7. Given that these elements are what makes a type of virtue ethics Aristotelian, I am not convinced by Susan Moller Okin's view that once we rid ourselves of Aristotle's sexist beliefs, there's not much of Aristotle left to render one's ethical position Aristotelian. See especially Okin 1996, but see also Okin 1979, ch. 4. See also note 10.

8. I am thus sympathetic to S. Buckle's claim that "Aristotle's focus on the virtues is not *instead of* a focus on law: law takes its place within his theory, and as something obligatory in the good life. His focus on the agent is not *instead of* a focus on actions" (2002, 568). I must note, however, that Buckle's attack on contemporary virtue ethics as being non-Aristotelian is highly uncharitable, as Buckle focuses on implausible versions of virtue ethics. This is especially puzzling since he cites Hursthouse's *On Virtue Ethics* (1999b) yet does not address the version of virtue ethics defended in that book.

9. The original definition goes as follows: "A virtue [is] a deep and acquired excellence of a person, involving a characteristic motivation to produce a certain desired end and reliable success in bringing about that end" (Zagzebski 1996, 137). I modified the definition by adding "worthwhile type" in order to make explicit the idea that virtues are concerned with what is moral, and so worthwhile, and by adding at the end "a characteristic disposition to emotionally react to one's situation" to highlight the idea that the emotional involvement in virtue is not only confined to *motivation* for action, but is also found in one's emotional *reaction* to the situation.

10. It is, of course, a debatable issue whether one can depart from Aristotle in these respects and yet be able to maintain that one's position is still Aristotelian. I think one can, but this debatable issue is not a proper part of the project of this book.

11. See Nussbaum 1988 for some suggestions as to how the content of a virtue can be specified differently according to cultural variations.

12. See Homiak 1993 for an excellent argument to the effect that we can accept Aristotle's ethics despite his remarks on women, manual labor, and slavery.

13. I should also add that this book is not an exegesis of other past philosophers' thought on the virtues, such as Plato, the Stoics, Aquinas, Hume, and Kant, or the ideas of those figures whose views are very much hospitable to a discussion of virtue, such as Marx, Hegel, and Nietzsche. There is much work that needs to be done by way of investigating how the thought of the last three can lend itself to virtue ethics or whether it can lead to forms of virtue ethics that are not neo-Aristotelian or neo-Greek in general. Swanton 2003 makes some headway in this respect, since much of her view of virtue ethics is inspired by some of Nietzsche's thoughts.

Chapter 1: Care

1. Gilligan certainly believed (i), and it is arguable that she held (ii), given her gestalt analogy; see "Moral Orientation and Moral Development" in Kittay and Meyers 1987. In *In A Different Voice* (1982) Gilligan states that the justice and care perspectives are not in conflict; see pages 33, 100, 105, 149, 156, 165–7, and 173–4.

2. Regarding conceptual criticisms, for example, Broughton 1993 accuses Gilligan of interpreting the responses of her interviewees to fit the results she desires. Moody-Adams 1991 criticizes Gilligan's choice of moral issues: while abortion might lend itself more easily to responses centered around care, sexual harassment, sexual abuse, and sexual discrimination do not. For empirical studies that yielded results different from Gilligan's, see the essays in part 3 of Larrabee 1993 and the book's bibliography.

3. The connections between care and oppression is a topic that Card 1995 takes up.

4. As Marilyn Friedman puts it, "The different voice hypothesis [care perspective is distinct from that of justice] has a significance for moral psychology and moral philosophy which would survive the demise of the gender difference hypothesis [women's reasoning is distinct from men's]" (1993, 121; 1995, 63).

5. This is the issue that Calhoun 1988 addresses, although her concern is not care ethics and virtue ethics, but care ethics and a justice perspective.

6. This is one of the concerns of McLaren's paper (2001). For another, more detailed elaboration of this issue, see Baier 1995, especially the first essay, and Friedman 1993, ch. 6. For an elaboration of the feminist desiderata for ethics, see Jaggar 1991 and Koehn 1998, 5–9.

7. I do not address Ruddick's (1989) views since these are more about conflict resolution than about building a moral theory around the notion of care. I also don't discuss Tronto's (1993) views since these use a notion of care that is broader in scope (applied to public policy issues) than the one I am interested in (see, however, notes 21 and 44).

8. I will return to these claims by Noddings in section 5 where I address the issue of Noddings's rejection of the claim that care is a virtue.

9. Noddings 1984, 5. Further page references in the body of this chapter are to this book.

10. By "persons" I do not exclude babies and children, but animals, plants, and inanimate objects. Noddings's reason for insisting on people as being the recipients of care is her requirement of completion and acknowledgement of caring by the cared-for. Such completion cannot be attained by animals, plants, and things. The discussion, however, is more complex because Noddings does allow for some completion in some types of animals (1984, ch. 7).

11. See Mayeroff 1971, especially 1–49.

12. One criticism of Noddings, worth briefly mentioning, is offered by Hoagland 1990. Hoagland argues that Noddings offers a dangerous unidirectional model of caring, such that one person can end up doing all the caring. In adult rela-

tionships, and especially within sexist societies, this is not morally praiseworthy. However, Hoagland's criticism of Noddings is uncharitable. For even though Noddings relies on models of caring that are unidirectional (e.g., mother and child, teacher and student) her account is not logically committed to this position. See p. 69 of Noddings (1984) for a logical statement of her account. See also Noddings 1990, p. 123 for an apt response to Hoagland's criticisms.

13. In *Nicomachean Ethics*, Aristotle recognizes something similar to this in his discussion of concord between friends: "Now concord also appears to be a feature of friendship. Hence it is not merely sharing a belief. . . . Nor are people said to be in concord when they agree just about anything. . . . Rather, a city is said to be in concord when its citizens agree about what is advantageous, make the same decision, and act on their common resolution" (1167a20–30). Aristotle's point here is that friendship involves concord because friends often have shared goals and act together to support these goals.

14. I owe this point to my student, Rebecca Franke. I should add that Mayeroff also emphasizes the necessity of knowledge of the cared-for to caring. See 1971, ch. 2.

15. Marianne Janack suggested this case to me.

16. Some, however, might find this to be controversial. Claudia Card, for example, wonders whether the friend has asked for advice to begin with. If the friend has not, then interfering in this way *would be* controversial. While I am sympathetic to this claim, it does not seem to me to rest on a picture of *friendship*; it seems to rest more on a picture of two people who are more like colleagues or acquaintances. In these types of relationships, interfering without being asked would certainly be controversial.

17. These features of acting from care are not of my own concoction, but are found in the literature on the subject. I include some references in the body of the text.

18. Blum 1980 offers an extended argument that acting out of altruistic emotions and friendship need not utilize principles but also need not be unthinking. See especially ch. 4.

19. One should also not equate care with moods, which usually lead to impulsiveness. It is perfectly possible for one not to be in the mood to, say, help a friend, but nevertheless help him out of care. Moods are not the same as altruistic emotions such as caring. See Blum 1980, ch. 2.

20. For an interesting and nontechnical account of these issues, see Greene 2000.

21. This suggestion has not gone unnoticed in the literature. In addition to McLaren (2001), Flanagan and Jackson make this suggestion: "But there is every reason to think that Gilligan's program would benefit from moving in a more virtue-theoretical direction, insofar as the conception of moral agency she describes is potentially so much thicker than Kohlberg's, embedded as it is in self-conception and social context" (1993, 74). In his remark that friendship is a virtue or "involves a virtue," Aristotle might be taken to make such a suggestion. But Aristotle, of course, did not frame the issues in contemporary terms. Tong 1998 makes the sug-

gestion that care ethics is a "species" of virtue ethics, and seems to defend it on the basis that both approaches give the emotions a central role. But Tong's view is not elaborated, and its concerns are mainly fleshed out along gender and historical lines (see also Tong 1997 for a defense of the idea that care should be thought of as a virtue in medical practice). Putman 1991a also argues for the thesis that putting caring in the context of virtue ethics allows us to distinguish between good and bad caring relationships. The thrust of his paper is aimed at arguing that care is—generally—a virtue, but his paper lacks a good discussion of the roles of emotion and reason in caring action. Curzer 2002 claims that care is a virtue, but he construes it so broadly that care loses its focus as a trait directed at those near and dear to us. (See section 5 in this chapter.) Blum 1993 claims that not all of the concerns of care ethics can be "encompassed within what currently goes by the name of 'virtue theory'" (58). But Blum does not explain this claim nor does he give examples, and without these it is difficult to assess it given that virtue ethics has been fleshed out differently by different philosophers. Swanton argues that caring must be construed in a thick way so that it can plausibly be construed as a virtue: "In [the agent's] (fully virtuous) caring, [the agent] must not display an unhealthy need for the cared-for to be dependent on her, . . . not display feelings of resentment or martyrdom, and so on" (1997, 501). I should add that a thin account of a virtue simply identifies the field of the virtue, whereas a thick account spells out what it is to be well-disposed with respect to the field of the virtue (on this distinction, see Nussbaum 1988). Finally, Tronto rejects construing care as a disposition and as a virtue. Against the former, she argues that thinking of care as a disposition allows it to be "sentimentalized and romanticized" (1993, 118). Against the latter, she argues that thinking of care as a virtue does not seem to be able to handle in a realistic way "the kinds of problems that caring will confront in the real world" (161). Neither argument is remotely plausible. That caring as a disposition can be sentimentalized is no argument against it if, indeed, caring is a disposition. And if caring is indeed a virtue, then it might not be plausible to require of it to handle the problems that Tronto wants to deal with.

22. On this, see especially Hursthouse 1986 and Nussbaum 1988.

23. Some might object that many advocates of care ethics caricature the claims of traditional moral theories, such as Kantian ethics and utilitarianism, by attributing to them exaggerated claims, such as construing our lives as being nothing but dealing with each other as "abstract" individuals following "abstract principles." No one, however, can deny that, for example, both Mill and Kant had very detailed things to say about the moral lives of individuals. But if so, then making it seem as if virtue ethics is the only theory that can accommodate care ethics would be implausible, for surely Kantian ethics and consequentialism might very well do so. For example, the latter theory might insist on the idea that human beings enter in caring relationships since this would best promote an overall desirable state of affairs. While I share the worry that Kantian and consequentialist claims have often been caricatured, and while I do not wish to deny the obvious possibility of Kantian and consequentialist theories being able to accommodate the desiderata of care ethics, my claim is simply that virtue ethics can also do so, and to argue for this

claim there is obviously no need to argue that the other theories fail in this respect. However, having said this much, there is also the issue of theoretical priority: Do Kantian ethics and consequentialism give theoretical priority to the desiderata of care ethics or do they think of them as instrumental to maintaining what these theories consider to be important? I will leave this question open, arguing only that virtue ethics does give the claims of care ethics theoretical priority.

24. For good discussions of virtue ethics and the emotions, see Annas 1993, especially pp. 53–66; Aristotle's *Rhetoric* (in addition, of course, to his two *Ethics*); Hursthouse 1997a and 1999b, part 2; Nussbaum 1986, especially ch. 10, and Nussbaum 1994; and Sherman 1989, especially ch. 5.

25. We should not confuse the claim that "X does so-and-so because it is just" with the claim that "X's intention *in* acting justly is to make sure that he is a just person." While it is important that a virtuous agent be concerned with his character, the latter claim smacks of undue attention to the repercussions of one's *specific* actions to one's character, and it is very different from the former claim. The former claim states that the reasons for X's actions are the deserts of others, not X's interests in how his action rebounds on his character. For a discussion of the closely related issue of the tension, in acting virtuously, between the virtuous person's concern for her virtue and her concern for others, see Annas 1993, pp. 249–62.

26. For similar arguments from a Kantian perspective regarding the regulative role of reason, see, for example, Baron 1995.

27. As Putman puts it, "Putting caring into the context of virtue theory gives the agent a perspective from which to judge the appropriateness of the virtue in particular situations" (1991a, 236). Putman defends a thesis very similar to mine, but his remarks are sketchy.

28. Unfortunately, in this essay Jeske criticizes an Aristotelian justification of friendship by criticizing *one way* in which an Aristotelian can offer such an account, thus neglecting other possible ones—such as the one hinted at in this chapter.

29. There are two points here to be kept in mind. First, merely saying that virtuous people are just says nothing about what laws and institutions a society ought to have. This is an issue, however, that is conceptually different from the one I am tackling. I am claiming that virtue ethics does recognize justice as an integral component of the ethical life. *Which* laws a society ends up having is a different matter altogether. Second, one might wonder about the ease with which I claim that Card's worry about justice to strangers is met under virtue ethics, since Aristotle did not have much to say about justice to strangers (see Annas 1993, 312–16). Aristotle's discussion is mostly centered on justice to other members of one's *polis*. But this is not a grave problem. For one thing, Aristotle did not deny that justice can be extended to people outside one's *polis*; he was simply silent on this issue. For another, there is nothing in Aristotle's account that would prevent such an extension.

30. The type of impartiality under discussion here is what is sometimes called "level 1" impartiality: impartiality at the level of day-to-day decisions regarding our actions. This is opposed to level 2 impartiality, which is a higher-order level concerned with which rules and principles to be adopted; see Baron 1991.

31. I borrow these three aspects of partiality from Archard 1995. I should note that Archard adds the fourth feature that there is an intrinsic morality of partiality, a morality exhibited in a number of ways, such as that different types of partiality (e.g., to friends and to lovers) have different moral features and expectations (see 136–38). I have left this feature out because its treatment requires discussion that goes beyond my aims, and because it is not necessary for my account.

32. Blum argues that "impartiality is a moral requirement only in certain restricted sorts of situations. It is not a morally incumbent perspective to take up in every situation. In particular, friendship does not typically involve us in situations in which impartiality between the interests of our friends and those of others is a moral requirement" (1980, 46).

33. I borrow this case from Baron 1995, 126.

34. I borrow this example from Blum 1993, 55.

35. For Aristotle's views, see *Nicomachean Ethics*, book 5. See also Aristotle's *Politics*. Aristotle's remarks about justice are scattered throughout this latter work, but a couple of important passages are 1282b15–1283a20 and 1332a8–1332a20.

36. It is also difficult to find or construct cases in which partiality can be plausibly said to morally override the valid claims of justice. Friedman, for instance, gives three cases ("stories") the point of which is to show that sometimes considerations of special relationships legitimately override those of justice and rights (1987, 195). The cases are those of Abraham's willingness to sacrifice Isaac, Socrates's indignation at Euthyphro's willingness to prosecute his own father, and a stranger's willingness to steal a drug to save a woman's life (a modification of the now famous Heinz dilemma). The point of the first case is that Abraham's special relationship with God may override Isaac's right to life. But it is obvious that such an answer is highly controversial and begs every question at hand (it is also not a suitable case to offer given the theological baggage it carries). Furthermore, the story need not be thought of as a conflict between maintaining a relationship (between Abraham and God) and not violating a right to life (Isaac's); it could be thought of as a conflict between maintaining two relationships (between Abraham and God, *and* between Abraham and Isaac). The point of the second case is to show that prosecuting one's father, even if one's father is a murderer, might be wrong, and so, in some cases, considerations of special relationships (duties to one's father?) override those of justice. But Friedman does not argue the case, making it appear as if the fact that Socrates's frowning upon Euthyphro's purported action is enough to convince us that the latter's action is wrong. Furthermore, there is an interpretation of the dialogue that makes Socrates's indignant response directed not at Euthyphro's action, but at the latter's *overconfidence* that he *should* prosecute his father (Socrates mocks Euthyphro's decision by saying, "you think you have such accurate knowledge of things divine" (Plato 1982, 172). Also, we often see on the media cases in which parents turn their children in to the law, and we do not usually react with indignation at such cases, nor do we usually think less of the parents for doing so. The last case given by Friedman is the story of a woman who steals a drug from a pharmacist (who overcharges for the drug) in order to save the life a person who

needs the drug. Since we are hesitant to approve of the theft, this is supposed to show that our initial, approving reaction to the original Heinz case derived from the fact that Heinz was the husband of the person who needed the drug. But again, Friedman is not convincing. She states that we would not say that a *personal risk* (via stealing) should be taken to save the person's life (198). However, this is to throw dust in our eyes, because the issue is not whether we would be willing to take a personal risk, but whether we would approve of the stranger's action of stealing the drug, and, I suspect, we would (the issue of risk shows only that people are often too cowardly to do what is morally right). In addition, the reason we would approve of stealing the drug in the original case is not simply because Heinz is the husband, but because we think of the pharmacist as also being quite vicious in refusing to give the drug to Heinz in return for an installment payment plan, *especially* since the drug is overpriced. It is not an issue of considerations of care overriding those of justice and rights, but one of recognizing the druggist to be a vicious person whose rights could morally be infringed given the urgency of the situation. (Friedman's points remain the same in her later work of 1993, 99–109.)

37. I borrow this case from McFall 1987.

38. For an excellent discussion of virtue ethics and irresolvable dilemmas, see Hursthouse 1999b, ch. 3.

39. See Hospers 1961, specifically the section on rule utilitarianism, for an argument along these lines.

40. Hursthouse 1997b offers an example involving abortion. The idea is that under some particular circumstances, having or not having an abortion is right.

41. I am very much indebted, in what follows, to Hursthouse 1999b, especially part 3, and MacIntyre 1999, especially ch. 7. I should also note that in what follows I will not go into the details of the ethical naturalism that underpin my remarks. For good accounts of it, see Hursthouse 1999b, part 3, and Foot 2001, especially chs. 2 and 3.

42. Card stated this worry in personal correspondence.

43. Slote also uses this notion of care in an essay (1998b), which drops the language of virtue entirely.

44. Compare Slote's understanding of "care" to the definition offered by Tronto: "On the most general level, we suggest that caring be viewed as a *species activity that includes everything that we do to maintain, continue, and repair our 'world' so that we can live in it as well as possible.* That world includes our bodies, our selves, and our environment, all of which we seek to interweave in a complex, life-sustaining web" (1993, 103; italics in original). Putting aside Tronto's desire to use a broad concept of care so as to effect positive changes in our conceptions of morality and politics, her definition of "care" is simply too broad; it includes too much and one is hard pressed to see what can be excluded from it. Tronto claims that some of the activities that are not caring include the pursuit of pleasure, creative activity, production, and destruction (104), but she never explains why these are excluded from her definition. And it seems easy to make a case that these can be viewed as caring activities, given the definition. Even destruction can be often

viewed as necessary in order to pave the way for a better world. Indeed, even wars can on Tronto's definition be caring activities (this idea is partially reflected in the saying "If you want peace, be prepared for war").

45. I owe this point to Flanagan and Jackson: "it is not impossible to see both the justice and care saliences in a moral problem and to integrate them in moral deliberation" (1993, 73).

46. One can also argue that people care about justice, and so care considerations enter into justice reasoning. However, the notion of care employed here does not have the emotive components (engrossment and displacement) which are part of the conception of care I am dealing with.

47. See Udovicki 1993 for some cautionary remarks against too much insistence on justice in intimate relationships. However, Udovicki wants to also argue that justice is not necessarily a primary virtue in intimate relationships. I think that she fails in making this claim, and at best argues for the conclusions that (i) always using justice to solve problems in relationships can yield the wrong moral results, and (ii) too much insistence on justice can ruin a relationship. Both of these conclusions are sensible, but they are a far cry from the claim that justice is not a primary virtue in relationships (on this, see Okin 1989, especially ch. 2).

48. Special thanks to Margaret McLaren who pointed out the need to discuss Aristotle's claim in this connection.

49. At the end of his essay, Sher states: "The oppositions of concrete and abstract, personal and impersonal, duty and care are not recent empirical discoveries, but generic determinants of the moral problematic. We have always known that a proper theory must assign each its proper place. What we have not known, and what Gilligan's findings bring us little closer to knowing, is what those places are" (1987, 187–88). This chapter should be construed as an attempt to supply such "proper places."

Chapter 2: Love

1. The philosophical literature on love has recently become quite rich. Alan Soble's works have been seminal in bringing this topic, after a long historical neglect, to the philosophical forefront. Here is a brief sample of some work it is worthwhile to consult: Lamb 1997; Martin 1996; Singer 1984, 1994, and 2001b; Soble 1989, 1990, 1997b, and 1998; Solomon 1990; Solomon and Higgins 1991; Verene 1995; White 2001; C. Williams 1995.

2. One controversial feature is that the romantic lovers desire union with each other (the union idea of love goes far back in time, of course; we find it, to give two examples, in Genesis in the Old Testament, and we find it in Aristophanes's speech in Plato's *Symposium*). It is a controversial feature because no one has been able to give a satisfactory account of what this desire really amounts to, let alone what the union notion amounts to. For some headway in this respect, see Nozick 1991. For criticisms of Nozick, see Soble 1997c.

3. There are two things to note. First, we should keep in mind that one and the same good could be both instrumentally *and* intrinsically good. Second, we should not make the mistake of thinking that just because something is intrinsically good then it is indispensable to a flourishing life. The pleasure of eating ice cream is an example of the former but not the latter. Donald Levy 1997, I think, makes this mistake, though demonstrating this would take me too far afield.

4. The reason, I think, why Thomas is misled into the belief that romantic love does not admit of rational justification is that he wants to account for popular beliefs about romantic love, namely, that it is something that happens to us, and so is a phenomenon that we have little to no control over. (It is usually said that people *fall in* love—in the nice words of Depeche Mode [the pop group], "We slip and slide as we fall in love.") But this does not entail that it is immune from rational assessment. Generally, emotions—including anger—can easily wash over us, but we are still required to give a story, rationally speaking, to account for their occurrence (with the exception, perhaps, of a few, such as depression and gloominess). On the rationality of love, see Soble 1990, ch. 7. See also Green 1997, who argues that romantic love can be rational even though it is not an emotion.

5. Of course, Ehman is not the only one to take such a position. For a historical figure, see, for example, Kierkegaard 1962. For a contemporary figure see B. Williams (Smart and Williams, 1973), who argues that utilitarianism is faulty on the grounds that it denies individuals the ability to have personal commitments, including commitments to individual people. This entails that utilitarianism is hostile to romantic love in so far as the latter entails a commitment to one person. See also Stocker 1976.

6. It is actually somewhat misleading to call the requirement of romantic love in Ehman's case "exclusivity," because exclusivity, in its weak form, is the claim that in romantic love one loves only one person at a time. But this claim is usually understood to rule out other *romantic* loves, not everybody else, *simpliciter*, as Ehman seems to require. For an excellent discussion of exclusivity, see Soble 1990, ch. 9.

7. In his discussion of friendship, Montaigne offers an arguably even stronger view than Ehman's: "In the friendship which I am talking about, souls are mingled and confounded in so universal a blending that they efface the seam which joins them together so that it cannot be found" (1987, 211–12). He adds, "Everything is genuinely common to [the friends] both: their wills, goods, wives, children, honour and lives" (214).

8. On consequentialism, see Pettit's "The Consequentialist Perspective," in Baron, Pettit, and Slote 1997. On Kantian ethics, see especially Baron 1995 and Herman 1993b. For an argument that love can be construed as a moral emotion in a specifically Kantian manner, see Velleman 1999. Central to Velleman's argument is that love need not involve desires to be with the loved one, to promote her welfare, and so on. To support this contention, Velleman gives counterexamples involving love in which such desires do not exist. But his examples are not convincing as examples of love. Moreover, even if they are, they are atypical, and hence do not affect the majority of cases of love.

9. We should not confuse moral justifications of romantic love with moral justifications of other, closely related phenomena. Soble, for example, justifies preferring, by the lover, one beloved over others in terms of the autonomy of the lovers and in terms of worthwhile objects (or properties): "The morality of the preferential choice flows from the value of autonomy, not only from the value of the object of that choice. The suggestion is that as long as lovers have some control over their preferences and over their ability to distinguish worthy from unworthy objects of love, the responsibility for making justifiable distinctions between the beloved and others is the lover's" (1990, 282). Yet though romantic love is not the same as the preferential choice for a particular beloved, the justification of the latter can also easily lend itself to the former. So one can argue that as long as one has some control over one's life, the morality of romantic love comes from one's responsibility and ability to plan one's life in such a way so as to make room for romantic love in it.

10. These points I owe to Soble, who has done an adequate job of sorting these issues out. See 1990, ch. 12.

11. This objection has its historical and contemporary philosophical defenders. An important historical defender is Kierkegaard 1962, and for a good discussion of his views, see Hannay 1991, ch. 7). One can also make a good case that Schopenhauer, in *The World as Will and Representation*, construes romantic love as a form of egoism. For contemporary advocates of this objection, see, for example, Nakhnikian 1978 and Nygren 1982.

12. How much sacrifice a lover must undertake in order to be a lover is controversial. There are probably no strict boundaries that can be plausibly defended. On this issue, see Soble 1990, ch. 12, especially section 4.

13. I have not, of course, examined all the positions. D. P. Verene, for example, claims that contemporary society has wrongly equated the erotic with the pleasurable, and ethical inquiry has become "an activity of discovering the limits that may or may not be set for the extension of [the quest for] the best techniques to induce pleasure in one's partner and in oneself" (1975, 113). We need to recover the experience of eros in order to experience the world as alive, because it is through the erotic that we human beings are connected to creativity (111). Morality, then, stifles the erotic, according to Verene, because it seeks to put limits on what sexual activities are or are not justified. Though it sounds interesting, Verene's position is somewhat difficult to come to terms with because of the vagueness of some of the claims. I am not sure how to understand the claims that the erotic is connected to creativity, and that it is the "feeling for the erotic that underlies the creation of ethical and aesthetic forms" (111). Nor is it clear why Verene asserts that our society has conflated the erotic with the pleasurable, and what the differences between them are.

14. Robert Solomon (1991) is one notable exception in his claim that romantic love is a virtue. I will examine his position below.

15. One can also offer a non-Aristotelian account of virtue and then argue, using differences in action, that love is not a virtue. This is a topic, however, beyond my scope.

16. For similar accounts, see also Pitcher 1965, G. Taylor 1979, and Hamlyn 1989. See also Soble's discussion of them (1990, ch. 7, section 5).

17. He discusses this issue specifically in light of Soble's defense of the possibility of deeply irrational emotions, emotions whose inner feel does not connect well with what their possessors believe about the object of their emotions. See Soble 1990, ch. 7, section 5.

18. On the view that emotions need only involve thoughts, see Carroll 1990, ch. 2; Greenspan 1980; and Stocker 1996, ch. 1, section 4.

19. It should be obvious that as a general account of emotions, beliefs and desires are not sufficient. What is also needed is some sort of feeling or affectivity; otherwise, why speak of *emotions?* But we need not worry about this issue as far as Green's argument against romantic love being an emotion is concerned.

20. I think, however, that Green is mistaken in the identity claim, because it is open to counterexamples: the desires might also characterize a sexual friendship, and a friendship that is not very intimate either. Green would be better off using Newton-Smith's (1989) notion of g-necessity and claiming that these desires generally characterize cases of love and that this *generality* is a necessary truth.

21. The claim that the virtues structure and are constitutive of romantic love is repeated on pp. 5, 10, and 15. It is defended against the objection that they merely enable romantic love on pp. 20–21.

22. He does, however, sometimes say that love is a virtue. On p. 121, for example, he states, "Rather than making honesty subordinate to love, it is possible to regard these virtues as equally valuable and in need of balancing." Notice how love is claimed to be a virtue, in need to be balanced with that of honesty.

23. Nor would Martin accept this consequence; he accepts many of the emotions on my list as emotions, and I would surmise that he would accept the rest also (he just does not list the rest).

24. We should also strike the word "beloved" from this rough understanding of how to view romantic love, otherwise we are in danger of circularity.

25. It is important to note that just because an emotion is dispositional, and just because virtues are dispositional, it does not follow that dispositional emotions are virtues. Being dispositional is a property that can characterize some emotions, the virtues, and a host of other traits that are neither emotions nor virtues. Indeed, a nonliving thing can have the property of being dispositional, with the classic example being that of sugar, which has the disposition of melting in water under the right conditions.

26. None of these claims deny that romantic love can be very enriching to human lives, of course.

27. Romantic love also seems to falter on the definition of "virtue" that Christine Swanton recently offered: "A *virtue* is a good quality of character, more specifically a disposition to respond to, or acknowledge, items within its field or fields in an excellent or good enough way" (2003, 19). Romantic love, on my view, is a dispositional emotion, and usually a longstanding one. But it need not necessarily respond to items within its field in excellent or good enough ways. If, how-

ever, we retain the assumption that romantic love is suffused with wisdom, then, on the face of it at least, it would fit Swanton's definition.

28. The claim that romantic love is not a virtue has support from some scholarship on Aristotle. For example, Nussbaum argues that "there is no trait of being loving or of being friendly that stands to love exactly as being courageous stands to courageous action, viz. as its mainspring and, impediments absent, its sufficient condition" (1986, 344). And Price also concludes that romantic love is not a virtue: "Put abstractly, the point is that love itself is not a virtue, and does not involve choice; it is not excluded that some choices may serve both love and virtue" (1997, 241).

29. Strictly speaking, Solomon should not have concluded that romantic love shows that we should not consider virtues to be traits. At best, he should have concluded that it shows that we should not consider *all* virtues to be traits.

30. The reader should compare Solomon's views on romantic love found in his essay discussed here with those found in his 1990 book. The views are basically similar, except that in the book Solomon claims that the goal of shared identity (or self) is an impossible goal to reach, though not impossible to strive for (147, 268). This is somewhat puzzling because Solomon understands shared identity as each self defining itself partly through the other (152), and this does not seem to be an impossible goal at all. In any case, for his views on shared identity and love, see chs. 11 and 12, and pp. 268–277.

31. In the last section of his paper, Solomon enumerates some of the "virtues of love." But these should not be thought of as yet other ways in which romantic love is a virtue. As the expression "virtues of love" indicates, and as Solomon's discussion does, these virtues are some benefits that result from being in love. Solomon, I should note, does not bother to explain to the reader how the following expressions, which he uses, are to be understood and how they differ from each other: "love is with virtue" (p. 510; by implication from his "love is without virtue"); "the virtues of love" (p. 511, 512), and "love is a virtue" (*passim*).

32. This claim does not contradict Stocker's plausible one that emotions reveal and are constituted by value (1996). When x gets angry at y, x reveals that x values being treated with dignity, for example. When y feels upset that his haircut has been botched up, this (perhaps) reveals that y cares (too much?) for outside appearances. But change x's and y's beliefs, and their emotions will be shed. So there is no incompatibility.

33. He is right only in that given the fighter's passions, we can trust that he will fight with gusto and that he will continue to do so; that is, he will not rationalize his way out of fighting. But what we cannot trust is that he is fighting for the right reasons.

34. Martin makes this claim about sexual fidelity also in his 1994 essay. As to open marriages, I will discuss these in more depth in the next chapter.

35. I have in mind here desires that constitute romantic love, as opposed to those that ground it or that result from it. See Soble 1990, 103–4 for these distinctions.

36. Soble argues that the view that genuine love is loving y in virtue of y's identity properties faces a dilemma: either x loves y for all of y's identity properties, in

which case the claim becomes the uninformative one that *x* loves *y* because *y* is *y*, or *x* loves *y* for a subset of *y*'s identity properties. The problem in the latter option is that if another subset of *y*'s identity properties changes, then *x*'s love will continue, but its object will now be *z*, a person other than *y*, given that a subset of *y*'s original identity properties has changed (1990, 225–26). However, I think that the second horn of the dilemma is not really a horn, not unless one assumes—as Soble seems to—that *each* of *y*'s identity properties is essential to *y* (and this assumes, in turn, that we understand "identity" to mean "essential"). But we can retain a robust meaning of "identity" without having to make these assumptions: an identity property is one that plays an important, though not essential, part in making *y* the person he is. This way, we can retain the main idea in the notion of "loving *y* for *y*'s identity properties," claim that *y* can lose some subset of his identity properties without ceasing to be *y*, and claim that *x* can continue to love *y* given that *x*'s love was based on a subset of *y*'s identity properties that did not change.

37. This is of course in contrast to Mill's position. Mill agreed that some pleasures are qualitatively better than others, but the decision as to which are which rests with those people who are experienced with both (1987, ch. 2). These experienced "judges" *may* be virtuous, but this would be a contingent issue, and Mill did not require that they be so.

38. Solomon argues that falling in love is a matter of choice. See 1990, ch. 17.

39. The distinction between infatuation and romantic love, especially the passionate phases of love, is hard to make. See Vannoy 1980, 181–86; Mendus 1989; and Soble 1989, 197, note 1; Kupfer 1993; and Martin 1996, 12–13. On the distinction between love and lust, see Stafford 1977 and 1988; and Lesser 1980.

40. For a good account of how the unity of the virtues doctrine construed as the claim that the virtues are identical has been understood by some of the ancients, see Annas 1993, 79–82, and Cooper 1998. For an argument that the virtues are incompatible, see Walker 1993.

41. B. Williams 1985, 36; Sherman 1989, 105; Badhwar 1996; and Hursthouse 1999b, 155–56 reject the entailment claim.

42. This is Becker's proposal (1990). One could also think of integrity as unifying the virtues in similar ways. Swanton makes the intriguing suggestion that objectivity as a virtue is structurally similar to that of practical wisdom in that it is inseparable from the moral virtues (2003, 179).

43. The first of these two accounts is Badhwar's (1996); the second is Watson's (1984).

44. Of course, to speak of people and their actual virtuousness is to depart from the ideal virtuous agent and to fall back on the idea that most people are virtuous to all sorts of degrees and extents. But this need not deny the insight that most people are not virtuous to high degrees and extents.

45. Of course, were people to be raised and morally trained in the right ways from infancy and yet end up being far from virtuous, then the Stoic claim becomes more plausible. But it is obvious that one reason why most people are far from being virtuous is the fact that their moral upbringing leaves much to be desired.

46. I am borrowing and adjusting, somewhat freely, from Joel Feinberg's *Harm to Others* (1984), especially chs. 1 and 5. See also Donald Levy 1980 for a slightly different account of basic human goods.

47. According to Paul Gregory, "Not everybody experiences love as an all-consuming passion, and, even for those who have experienced love in this way, such erotic passion . . . generally remains an exception" (1984, 265). Gregory might be mistaken in his claim that experiencing romantic love passionately is an exception, but he is right that not everybody has to go through the passion stage.

48. Whether such people intentionally do so or not is a different issue altogether. See Nozick 1991, 430 for examples—Jesus, Gandhi, Socrates, the Buddha, Beethoven—of people who somehow *define* themselves in such a way that their lives would not fit with a romantic *we*.

49. See Nussbaum 1986, ch. 7, especially pp. 215–16. Plato's account in the *Phaedrus* would be much closer to Socrates's speech in the *Symposium* if Socrates does not require that the lover dispense with the beloved as he climbs the ladder towards the Good. Price 1997, ch. 2, argues that Socrates does not have such a requirement.

50. On this, see Alexander Nehemas and Paul Woodruff's introduction to Plato (1995).

51. I will discuss in detail the compatibility of one-night stands and lack of a sexual monogamous relationship with a flourishing life in the next chapter.

52. On these issues, see Soble 1990, chs. 9–11; see also Soble 1997b, especially essays 36–39. A few philosophers have also argued that romantic love and friendship should be modeled on each other, with romantic love losing some of its traditional traits, such as exclusivity and jealousy, and friendship acquiring some new dimensions such as sexual activity. See Gregory 1984 and McMurty 1997.

53. See Nussbaum's (1986) discussion of it, ch. 12, pp. 357–58.

54. Thus, it seems to me that Richard White is just plain wrong in claiming that Aristotle's account of friendship is defective because it does not recognize differences between the friends. At the very least, White should have recognized that Aristotle's views do not necessarily imply that they have no room for difference. See White 2001, ch. 1, especially pp. 24, 29, and 44.

55. Juha Sihvola puts the point this way: "Aristotle . . . sees an emergence of the best kind of friendship, that based on virtue, from erotic love in which the partners have developed affinity and affection as well as reciprocal concern and respect between themselves" (2002, 213).

56. I should note that this view applies not only to heterosexual relationships, but also equally well to same-sex ones as well as to other types of relationships as long as none of these expresses or stems from vice or lack of virtue.

Chapter 3: Sex

1. For a similar position on the moral neutrality of sex, see Primoratz 1999, especially ch. 12: "Sex has no special moral significance; it is morally neutral. No

act is either morally good or bad, right or wrong, merely in virtue of being a sexual act" (173). On adultery, see Wasserstrom 1978, and the other references given in section 5 below.

2. I will, however, use "temperance" in this chapter to mean what Carr means by "chastity," that is, I will use "temperance" to refer to that aspect of it relevant to sexual desire, unless otherwise noted.

3. On this distinction, see Dent 1984, ch. 2. Indeed, my discussion of temperance owes much to this book, especially ch. 5. Young 1988 also attributes a similar distinction to Aristotle between common and peculiar appetites. Recently, Singer made the distinction between sex as an appetite and sex as involving interpersonal concerns (2001a, 59, and 72–78), though I think that the latter is broader than the notion of sex as desire and so Singer's distinction is not identical with mine and Dent's. For further discussion of these points and their connection to the social construction of sexual desire, see Nussbaum 1999, especially the essay "Constructing Love, Desire, and Care." On the construction of sexual desire and orientation, see Stein 1990 and Halwani 1998a.

4. See Dent 1984, 145. In "Free Agency," Gary Watson makes comparable remarks regarding valuing and desiring: "There seem to be two ways in which, in principle, a discrepancy may arise. First, it is possible that what one desires is not *to any degree* valued . . . ; one assigns *no* value whatever to the object of one's desire. Second, although one may indeed value what is desired, the strength of one's desire may not properly reflect the degree to which one values its object" (1975, 209–10). It seems to me that the first way is basically what I mean by "giving weight to" a desire. I have not discussed the second way because it involves giving different weights to different desires and so prioritizing them, depending on what the agent considers more important, and this second way does not really represent a difference in kind in how one responds to one's desires. (Watson, of course, wants to connect his remarks to the issues of freedom of the will and action; such connections are not part of my topic.) See also Wielenberg 2002 for a similar distinction between brute pleasures and value-based ones.

5. Hursthouse, during her discussion of a temperate person as one who either would not have certain sexual desires or one whose sexual desires would vanish as soon as one realizes what kind of sexual desires these are (e.g., desire for a child), states, "Perhaps . . . [the advocate of temperance] should not claim that they can be brought into complete harmony [with reason], but she can admit the possibility of a few twinges of lust and regret without losing a robust distinction between temperance and (mere) self-control" (1999b, 249). I agree with Hursthouse that we can maintain a distinction between temperance and self-control even if the temperate person can and does experience morally nasty sexual desires. However, Hursthouse prefaces this distinction with the remark that it should be made given the caveats made earlier about the idea that virtuous conduct gives pleasure to the agent. But I am unsure how this has much to do with the claim that temperate people can nevertheless feel ethically unhealthy sexual desires, because cases of attenuated pleasure in virtuous people involved circumstances external to the agent's character (war, poverty, etc.), whereas the

claim here is that temperate people, given the rootedness of sexual desire, can and sometimes do, feel these unhealthy desires. Consider the case of a poor virtuous agent who decides to return a wallet full of money to the right authorities but who feels attenuated pleasure in doing so. Such an agent does not have a generally occurring and recurrent desire to steal or to keep others' money and goods. The circumstance external to her character is her poverty, while stumbling across the wallet is the event that tested her virtue. Compare this to a case of a virtuous agent who was able to give no weight to his pedophiliac sexual desires, and so he does not have a generally occurring and recurrent desire to have sex with children. He stumbles across a beautiful preteen youth and comes to feel the twinge of sexual desire. What is the external circumstance here? There isn't one (or more than one). Stumbling across the youth is the counterpart to stumbling across the wallet. But there is no counterpart to poverty. The reason is simple: the agent's sexual desires are internal to him.

6. I also think that Aristotle's remarks on this issue are compatible with mine. He says, for example, that "someone is temperate because he does not feel pain at the absence of what is pleasant, or at refraining from it" (1985, 1118b35). This, of course, says nothing about whether the temperate person feels bad sexual desires; rather, Aristotle seems to be claiming that the temperate person is not pained because he is not indulging bad sexual desires, and whether such desires are present or not seems irrelevant here. Aristotle does believe of course that virtues are in a way natural to us (1985, 1144b3), and so temperance is in a sense natural to us. Again, however, this is silent on the point as to whether one can be temperate despite the presence of bad sexual desires. I cannot go into all of Aristotle's remarks, but I think that the point is clear.

7. For a brief but wonderful discussion of this issue, see Hursthouse 1999b, 245–47.

8. This is the main reason, I think, why Aristotle rejects the life of gratification (as being the happy life) by calling its proponent "slavish" (1985, 1095b19): such a person is the slave of his appetites and uses his reason simply to satisfy his desires. I use this point below to argue that promiscuity, nonmonogamy, and sex work are compatible with temperance.

9. Hursthouse 1999a gives such an interpretation, and my discussion here owes much to hers. She is also careful not to deny that temperance is *also* a matter of amounts (e.g., "But it is clear that Aristotle thinks licentiousness leads, *not merely* to ill health but to other vices," p. 111; my emphasis). What is not clear in Hursthouse's essay is how the two interpretations of Aristotle's views on temperance are connected. My position is that we have two conceptually independent (but perhaps causally connected) views of temperance.

10. Again, for this discussion of temperance and the conceptual ways the two types of temperance could part company, see Hursthouse 1999a.

11. I am not claiming, of course, that the wrongness of rape is exhausted by the violation of the victim's autonomy and rights.

12. See the discussion of the unity of the virtues in section 3.1 of the previous chapter. For some good literature on the issue of the unity of the virtues, see

Badhwar 1996; Becker 1990; Cooper 1998 and 1999, ch. 3; McKinnon 1999, 162–66; and Watson 1984.

13. I owe this point to Christopher Koch. It should be noted that the objection can also be raised about the example of honesty. But what I say in response to the one about rape applies equally well to the one about honesty.

14. For what I think is the best defense of this claim, see Hursthouse 1999b, part 1.

15. Of course one can do the action for both reasons, but I am separating these for the sake of keeping the analysis manageable.

16. We have to be careful, however, in our choice of examples. Had I used rape instead of adultery, the example would still illustrate the distinction but in a much more complicated way. Rape is wrong because, among other reasons, it is a *sexual* violation of the victim. However, saying this would not illustrate the distinction, because this sexual aspect belongs to those aspects of the action that are victim related. In other words, speaking of the sexual violation of the victim would not bring in the motives and reasons behind the action. Notice what would happen were we to do so: One can rape X because one desires to take revenge on X's parents, spouse, etc., and one can rape X because one wants to satisfy one's sexual desire. In *both* cases, the wrongness of rape is due, importantly, to its sexual nature. But only in the second case is it wrong because it is intemperate (in the first case it is wrong because it is, among other vices, vengeful).

17. There is a sense in which Goldman is correct, however. In a way, all of our moral rules for right and wrong action, ideals for good and bad characters, and reasons for claiming that such-and-such a life is flourishing whereas that one is not, can be reduced to a few concepts around which moral theories revolve and respond to, such as well-being (and harm, misery), pleasure (and pain, suffering), dignity (and servility, subservience), and autonomy (and slavishness, subservience). If Goldman's claim is that ultimately talk about the morality of sex must touch base with such concepts, then Goldman is correct. But this claim is correct at a deep level of this discussion, and would not impugn my remarks.

18. Please excuse the slant towards males in these examples, but these words of wisdom were told to me, and I am male.

19. Kant says something similar about drinking (which also applies to eating): "If I have drunk too much, I am incapable of using my freedom and my powers" (1963, 123). For a treatment of Kant's views on eating, drinking, and sexual activity, see Soble 2003.

20. For a good discussion of these issues, see Trianosky 1988.

21. One of the main problems with Wreen's (1991) otherwise fine essay is precisely its view of adultery as a *policy* that adulterers adopt. It seems to me that most adulterers do not commit adultery out of a policy.

22. The only explicit treatment of adultery from the point of view of virtue ethics that I know of is Halwani 1998b. Richard Taylor's (1982) and Mike Martin's (1994) treatment of the topic lend themselves to virtue ethics terms.

23. According to Carol Leigh, a.k.a. Scarlot Harlot (prostitute and feminist activist), it was she who coined the term "sex work." See "Inventing Sex Work" (1997).

24. See for example Belliotti 1993, Primoratz 1999, and Soble 1996.

25. For what I think is the best defense of ethical naturalism, see Hursthouse 1999b, part 3, and Foot 2001, especially chs. 2 and 3. See also MacIntyre 1999 and Nussbaum 1988 and 1995.

26. The gangster example was originally given, I believe, by Watson 1997. For an excellent discussion of this particular claim about how one goes about arguing that a type of human life is defective, see Hursthouse 1999b, especially ch. 10.

27. See, for example, the essays in Delacoste and Alexander 1987 and in Nagle 1997. The case of male sex workers, as far as this attitude towards the work is concerned, is basically the same, although male escorts (prostitutes) are often asked by their (predominantly) male clientele to have an orgasm at some point during the encounter. Still, this does not render the claim that male escorts see their work as *work* false. See Lawrence 2000.

28. One can argue that if sex work is illegal, and if a sex worker nevertheless engages in it, then she would in some sense be going against the virtue of justice. "In some sense" because one might propose that one way in which an agent can be just is to obey the laws of her society. This argument, however, should be taken very cautiously, because of the issue as to whether the laws themselves are just. If they are not, it is a stretch to argue that by violating them the agent is being unjust.

29. See for example Primoratz 1999, ch. 8, for a good discussion and further references. For a slightly less philosophical discussion, see the essays in Delacoste and Alexander 1987.

30. As a sample, see Lederer 1980; Bell 1987; Delacoste and Alexander 1987; Assiter and Carol 1993; Segal and McIntosh 1993; and Nagle 1997.

31. An argument along this line on pornography can be found in MacKinnon 1987 and 1993, and Dworkin 1989. Longino 1980 offers such an argument in regard to pornography also. In regard to prostitution, both Shrage 1994 and Satz 1995 give such an argument.

32. Many of the arguments against the sex industry have been premised on the idea that it *objectifies* women. But whatever the merits of such arguments, objectification is irrelevant to the one I am considering. For even if the women portrayed and/or partaking in the sex industry are portrayed and are doing so as *subjects*, they are nevertheless portrayed and are doing so—according to the argument I am investigating—as *sexual* subjects, as entities whose sexual desires are definitive of them. This is sufficient to reduce them to the status of bodies (since it is their bodies that lead their reason) and so lead to the oppression of women.

33. However, it is possible to argue—implausibly I believe—that sex work in our society is *essentially* characterized through oppressive sexist practices, and so once these practices are removed, what we have on our hands is no longer sex work, but something different altogether (sex therapy?). Shrage 1989 makes this type of claim. After saying that marriage can survive such societal changes because it is founded on nonoppressive principles, she states, "However, I am *unable to imagine* nonpernicious principles which would legitimate the commercial provision of sex and which would not substantially alter or eliminate the industry as it now exists" (p. 335 in Soble 1997a; my emphasis). Shrage, it seems, is unable to

imagine a principle, such as sex for money, which would keep the industry as a commercial sex industry throughout societal changes. Fortunately, this claim is not repeated in Shrage's later treatment of the subject (1994). Garry 1978, I should add, gives a couple of interesting examples of ways that pornography can be non-sexist in content, and she does so without assuming any major changes in society as far as sexism is concerned (although she does plausibly claim that the uptake among men for such hypothetical pornography movies might not be successful).

34. One need not be a certain type of feminist to offer reasoning similar to what is found here. Consider the following two sentences—offered in all serious-ness—by Roger Scruton: "[Fantasy] has a natural tendency to realise itself: to remake the world in its own image. The harmless wanker with the video-machine *can at any moment* turn into the desperate rapist with a gun" (1986, 346, my emphasis). Surely the "can at any moment" is true but means only "logically pos-sible"; surely the wanker's character (and remember: Scruton is an Aristotelian in his ethical views) has something to do with his becoming a rapist! There are lots of "wankers" who would never even think of raping someone, let alone actually doing it. What Scruton needs to do to support his point is to argue that the "can" refers to psychological likelihood.

35. I might be accused that in pitching the argument at such a general level, I turn it into a glaringly bad argument. However, the reason I have done so is because all of the other particularized versions of the argument—particularized in the sense that it is about one type of sex work rather than another, or in the sense that it sketches a more detailed way of how sex work oppresses all women, or both—that I have come across have failed. For instance, Shrage's 1989 and 1994 version has been aptly criticized by Primoratz 1993 and 1999. The criticisms of MacKinnon's and Dworkin's views are familiar: see, for example, Assiter and Carol 1993; Segal and McIntosh 1993; Soble 1996. Moreover, I wanted to give the basic idea behind the number of these similar arguments and to discuss it.

36. Among contemporary philosophers, variations of this argument can be found in Finnis 1994, and Finnis and Nussbaum 1993. Both Punzo 1969 and Scruton 1986 accept versions of this argument.

37. See Elliston 1975; Ellis 1986; Halwani 1995; Herman 1993a; Nussbaum 1995b; Soble 1996, ch. 1; Soble 1998, especially ch. 3; Soble 2002b, especially ch. 2; Primoratz 1999, especially ch. 8.

38. I must emphasize that this might not be a plausible conclusion, because when it comes to Kant's views on sex, things are much more complicated. The rea-son is that Kant sees something especially problematic in sexual desire. Regarding the workers example, Kant would rightly claim that the workers are not the object of a bodily appetite, in our case, the sexual appetite. Rather, it is their services that are targeted by the one who hires them, and they are targeted not out of an appetite, either (Kant, 1963, 162–68). This indicates that sexual activity might not easily satisfy the requirements of the categorical imperative. Moreover, Kant laid emphasis on the fact that sexual acts outside of marriage also debase the humanity in the agent, not just in the agent's sexual partner. But there is hope. Lara Denis (1999) convincingly argues that homosexual sex and masturbation need not vio-

late Kant's Categorical Imperative. Though Denis does not discuss promiscuity, sex work, and open relationships, one can make a good case that these need not violate the Categorical Imperative either. In any case, the discussion that follows on objectification is conceptually distinct from Kant's specific treatment of these issues. For another excellent treatment of Kant and sex, see Soble 2002a.

39. I wish to indicate that my use of Nussbaum's classification does not commit me to agreeing with her conclusion in that essay. Indeed, I disagree with it. Roughly put, Nussbaum concludes that objectification is morally in the clear only in the context of a healthy and respectful relationship. (I use the ambiguous "morally in the clear" on purpose, because Nussbaum actually concludes with two different claims, without evincing awareness that these are different. On the one hand, she claims that objectification is morally *permissible* in the context of a healthy and respectful relationship, but, on the other, that it is a morally *good* thing in that context.) I disagree with this conclusion because it entails that any form of sexual activity outside the context of such a relationship is wrong, an entailment I do not accept. For a good discussion of Nussbaum's essay, see Soble 2002a.

40. On the difficulty of defining "promiscuity," see LeMoncheck 1997, 30–41. On promiscuity and casual sex, see also Elliston 1975 and Ellis 1986.

41. The fact that a word has an inherently negative or immoral meaning does not entail that the phenomenon or phenomena the word refers to is not open to ethical debate, because word meanings most often reflect the way people use them at a point in time, and people's beliefs are, of course, open to ethical criticism.

42. Anscombe says this: "Those who try to make room for sex as casual enjoyment pay the penalty: they become shallow. They dishonor their own bodies; holding cheap what is naturally connected with the origination of human life" (1976, 148). Kristjansson often, though not always, refers to this as Anscombe's "argument." I would hardly call this an argument; nor does Anscombe give an argument for this claim elsewhere in her essay.

43. Kristjansson, in further describing this mushroom picker, states, "and he would dismiss any reference to the interests of 'the individual mushroom M' with understandable levity" (101). This remark, however, is dangerously misleading. What Kristjansson means by it—I think—is that the promiscuous person is not interested in the nonsexual aspects of his potential sexual partner, and this is true enough—we are speaking about casual sex, after all. But his remark nevertheless conjures in the mind of the reader an image of someone who gives not one jot of attention to the desires and wishes of his sexual partner and so makes the promiscuous person look as if he is a highly immoral person. This would be, of course, a false image of promiscuous people. At best, it would be true of only some of them.

44. For some powerful criticism of the view of love as union, see Soble 1997c.

45. See for instance Soble 1998, ch. 7; Goldman 1997, section 3; and, for the most comprehensive treatment, Vannoy 1980, ch. 1.

46. Steinbock 1991, 190–91.

47. The language of addiction is faithful to the position of Kristjansson; he uses it as an analogy as to why we should abstain from casual sex: it is too risky since it may lead to forfeiting real love.

48. An earlier argument to the effect that sexual practices not condoned by traditional morality can lead to the forfeiture of love is given by Scruton (1986, *passim*, but especially ch. 11). Scruton's account is explicitly Aristotelian, and Scruton treats the capacity for love as a virtue (337). His argument attempts to give a description of the "natural course" of sexual desire which, according to Scruton, culminates in (romantic) love (specifically, union with the beloved). One serious problem with his account is that the so-called description of the course of sexual desire turns out to be heavily normative and so question-begging against those who claim that casual, and other forms of, sex are not necessarily immoral. I have not dealt with Scruton's position because it has been adequately dealt with by others. See, for example, Primoratz 1999, 21–31 and *passim*; Soble 1996 and 1998, *passim*; and Stafford 1988.

49. Perhaps promiscuity leads to emptiness, a feeling that one's life is going nowhere and/or has no serious and significant dimensions, as some promiscuous people report. This, however, is surely not a necessary result of promiscuity. Furthermore, one can be promiscuous and yet lead as rich a life as is possible, and this richness in one's life may do a great deal to help prevent—or at least attenuate—the above feeling.

50. Of course, some philosophers, such as Kant and Augustine, thought that *all* sex does this. My concern is not with this extreme form of the argument. See Kant 1963 and selections from Augustine's *The Good of Marriage* in Rogers 2002.

51. I say "sketchy" because much has been written on issues of deliberation and planning in a virtuous life. Dent 1984; Sherman 1989, especially ch. 3; and Richardson 1997 are noteworthy landmarks. The discussion that follows has been informed by, and is certainly heavily indebted to, them.

52. None of these remarks entail that being a food critic, an athlete, a life guard, or having, in general, a vocation revolving around the activities mentioned, including sex, is a worthless or mistaken life. There is a world of difference between wanting to be a tennis champion, on the one hand, and claiming that deriving pleasure from playing tennis is, and should be, the overarching goal in one's life. Much as the food critic's reasons for being a food critic are not exhausted by the pleasures of eating, so are the tennis champion's reasons for wanting to be a champion exhausted by the pleasures of playing tennis. Similarly but more relevantly, consider someone who desires to be a sex expert. Perhaps he wants to refine the art of sex and seduction and write a book on it. Perhaps he wants to become a teacher in sex and sexual activity. My remarks do not entail that this would be a worthless life, or a life that revolves around a valuational mistake.

53. Thus, I need not be advocating what Michael Bayles has called "vulgar hedonism," a hedonism which he inveighs against and which he characterizes as being focused on sexual liberation with the result that sex is unduly emphasized ("out of all proportion to its significance for a eudaimonistic life—that is, a life worth living, including elements besides pleasure") (1984, 130). The examples of such sexual liberation that Bayles gives are premarital sex, gay liberation, no fault divorce, open marriages, polygamy, and orgies (notice how Bayles seems to assume in his essay that such forms of sexual liberation have no place in a *eudaimon* life).

I say that I "need not" be advocating vulgar hedonism because it is unclear on Bayles's account whether the "undue emphasis on sex" is necessary for characterizing vulgar hedonism. If it is, then I am certainly not advocating such a hedonism. If it is not, and if sexual liberation is sufficient to characterize it, then I am, under his construal, a defender of such hedonism (though I would take exception and not defend a few items on his list of examples of sexual liberation).

54. A number of other philosophers seem to hold this view also. Here's Nozick: "The most intense way we relate to another person is sexually" (1989, 61).

55. Elliston 1975 identifies three advantages to promiscuity: (i) it can contribute to the growth of human personality; (ii) it can help educate the agent in mastering the techniques of body language; and (iii) it can be a form of authentic sexuality and so help make us more open to others. But though Elliston gives a reasonable defense of promiscuity, he ultimately defends it as instrumentally good: "From this temporal perspective promiscuity has definite but limited value in the movement toward a sexual ideal. . . . The intentionally lifelong relationship is intrinsically more valuable. . . . The value of promiscuity is located in the pursuit of just such ideals" (1975, 240). My defense of the value of promiscuity is not just that it is instrumentally good.

56. Perhaps most of, if not all, couples feel monogamy to be a sacrifice, and with good justification, given that it requires them to give up on the satisfaction of a very natural impulse. But the adjective "serious" is meant to indicate the point that different couples might feel this sacrifice differently, especially in terms of the degree of its burdensomeness. Some couples barely mind it; others mind it more; still others mind it so much that they decide to be nonmonogamous. And some individuals have such strong sexual desires that they decide not to enter monogamous relationships to begin with (so as not to end up having to lie and to deceive their spouses).

57. I am, then, quite aware that there are interesting and serious conceptual issues regarding what constitutes sexual activity. However, I take it that certain paradigm cases, such as sexual intercourse, oral sex, and mutual masturbation, do constitute sexual activity, and it is these that I mainly have in mind in this discussion. I have these mainly in mind not only because I believe that these make up the majority of adulterous behavior, but also because this is a good way to set aside the conceptual issues regarding what constitutes sexual activity. On this, see Soble 1996, ch. 3, and 1998, ch. 1.

58. For some philosophical literature on adultery see Taylor 1982; Wasserstrom 1984; Steinbock 1991; Wreen 1991; Martin 1994; Halwani 1998b; Primoratz 1999, ch. 7.

59. For an excellent treatment of the importance of subjective and objective elements to happiness, see McFall 1989.

60. I have imagined this case and, I must confess, found no difficulty thinking of Romeo as loving both women. Steinbock's treatment of the issue of the exclusivity of love is the weakest in the essay. Steinbock gives no arguments against the idea that one can love more than one person at a time; she simply states that "our ideal" of romantic love has no room for it. However, the issue of the exclu-

sivity of love is not relevant to my concerns, and so I will not pursue these points further.

61. Examples of other philosophers who make this mistake are Daniel Putman (1991b), who on page 50 shuttles back and forth between "extra-marital sex" and "having an affair"; Cicovacki's (1993) examples of adultery are all of affairs; and Martin, who in addressing the issue of how sexual exclusivity expresses and protects love, states that the "affection, time, attention, and energy (not to mention money) given to an extramarital partner would lessen the resources they devote to sustaining their marriage" (1994, 80). This clearly indicates that Martin has affairs in mind. But surely one can be sexually nonexclusive in ways other than having an affair!

62. According to Dr. Patrick Carnes—an expert on sex addiction—"sexual addiction is defined as any sexually-related, compulsive behavior which interferes with normal living and causes severe stress on family, friends, loved ones, and one's work environment." Notice how the definition is inherently evaluative. Be that as it may, according to Carnes, "[s]exual addicts make sex a priority more important than family, friends, and work." Of course, the people I have in mind in my discussion are not sexual addicts. Moreover, according to Carnes, sexual addicts comprise three to six percent of the population and that most of them "come from severely dysfunctional families. Usually at least one other member of these families has another addiction." If this is true, then perhaps too much anonymous sex, as such, would not endanger a relationship. It would if it were a manifestation of sexual addiction. For the views of Carnes, see SexHelp.com.

63. For some interesting ways in which actual gay and lesbian couples have struggled with the issue of monogamy, see Marcus 1998, especially ch. 4.

64. This is overstated, of course. Either of them might very well seek the company of friends, relatives, and acquaintances to do these things with. What I mean is that neither of them wants to do these things with someone else *romantically*, or the way lovers do, or the way happily married people do. It is not crucial to my account, furthermore, that we have a precise grip on what these expressions mean.

65. In most studies of sexual behavior, men report having more sexual partners than women. This raises the problem of how this is possible when these men are having sexual encounters with women. Einon 1994 plausibly argues that prostitutes and "hypersexual" women cannot account for this discrepancy, and she tries to account for it by claiming that—and I state this roughly—men exaggerate their promiscuity. Another explanation, again roughly, could be that men and women rely on different definitions or understandings of "sexual encounter" or other related terms. For the studies and these explanations, see Einon 1994 and Soble 1998, 184–88.

66. Philosophers have often viewed jealousy as being a negative emotion. For example, R. Taylor 1982 takes jealousy to be possessiveness; Scruton 1986 argues that because jealousy is so destructive, we should strive to be sexually faithful; in her otherwise fine piece on the topic, G. Taylor takes the view that jealousy is a vice (1988). Primoratz recognizes that jealousy could take on good forms. His remarks on this, though brief, are to be commended (1999). For another view that does not take jealousy to be necessarily bad, see also Farrell 1989.

67. See Primoratz 1999, 93.

68. There is one important caveat to this. Male escorts are often asked by their clients to achieve orgasm, and this can cause a serious dent in the male escort's sex life, especially if he has a spouse who might get upset by the fact that his spouse is always "tired from work." As Lawrence puts it, "The escort becomes 'sexed-out' from working so often, and loses interest in having sex in his personal life. Alternatively, he may not orgasm at home to save his sexual energy for his work" (2000, 236). Lawrence goes on to offer a number of solutions to these difficulties, such as the escort taking vacations, and the escort raising his rates so as to decrease the number of clients while maintaining his income level (237). This should indicate to the reader that the problem of a sex worker getting to lose sexual interest in her own life due to her work is, at best, a contingent one.

69. See Weinstein 2001.

70. A number of feminists hold a similar view. For example, Dworkin states, "Prostitution: what is it? It is the use of a woman's body for sex by a man, he pays money, *he does what he wants*" (1997, 140; my emphasis).

71. This position is well known in the literature. See for example, MacKinnon 1987, especially ch. 14.

72. Califia correctly identifies a number of reasons as to why sex work will not cease in a just society. For example, some people do not want to be in monogamous or even any type of romantic relationship. Some people might be too busy to be involved in such relationships, even if they wanted to. There will still be people who are ugly, uncharming, disabled, elderly, and/or with terminal illnesses. There will still be fetishists with their own particular sexual requirements. All of these people would have very good reasons to seek sex workers to have their sexual needs met (Califia 1994, 244–46).

73. The latter claim, that men are more promiscuous than women, should be construed as a popular belief that might very well be false. If heterosexual men are promiscuous, *whom* are they sexually active with, if not women? On this, see note 65 above.

74. For a helpful survey of many of the points at issue and a good bibliography, see ch. 2 of LeMoncheck 1997; other chapters are also quite helpful.

75. There is a famous argument about gay people's happiness, with the same defective structure. In a 1984 article that has been widely anthologized, Michael Levin argues that the most plausible hypothesis to explain gay men's unhappiness is not homophobia, but homosexuality itself, since, according to Levin, there is evidence that gays are much more accepted in Western societies than they used to be. But Levin is mistaken in his reasoning because we must consider not just a few pockets of positive cultural change with respect to gay people, but a hypothetical situation in which gay people attain *full* equality in society in general. On this point, see Murphy 1987.

References

Adams, Robert M. 1976. "Motive Utilitarianism." *Journal of Philosophy* 73: 467–81.

Alexander, Priscilla. 1987. "Prostitution: A Difficult Issue for Feminists." In *Sex Work: Writings by Women in the Sex Industry*. See Delacoste and Alexander 1987.

Annas, Julia. 1980. "Aristotle on Pleasure and Goodness." In *Essays on Aristotle's Ethics*. See Rorty 1980.

———. 1993. *The Morality of Happiness*. New York: Oxford University Press.

Annis, David. 1987. "The Meaning, Value and Duties of Friendship." *American Philosophical Quarterly* 24: 349–56.

Anscombe, G. E. M. 1976. "Contraception and Chastity." In *Ethics and Population*, edited by M. D. Bayles. Cambridge, Mass.: Schenkman.

Archard, David. 1995. "Moral Partiality." In *Moral Concepts*, edited by P. French, T. Uehling, Jr., and H. Wettstein. Midwest Studies in Philosophy, vol. 20, pp. 129–41. Notre Dame: University of Notre Dame Press.

Aristotle. 1984. *Eudemian Ethics*. Translated by J. Solomon. In *The Complete Works of Aristotle*. See Barnes 1984.

———. 1984. *Politics*. Translated by B. Jowett. In *The Complete Works of Aristotle*. See Barnes 1984.

———. 1984. *Rhetoric*. Translated by W. Rhys Roberts. In *The Complete Works of Aristotle*. See Barnes 1984.

———. 1985. *Nicomachean Ethics*. Translated by Terence Irwin. Indianapolis: Hackett.

Assiter, Alison, and Avedon Carol, eds. 1993. *Bad Girls and Dirty Pictures: The Challenge to Reclaim Feminism*. London: Pluto Press.

Audi, Robert. 1995 "Acting from Virtue." *Mind* 104: 449–71.

Badhwar, Neera. 1993. "Altruism Versus Self-Interest: Sometimes a False Dichotomy." In *Altruism*, edited by E. F. Paul, F. D. Miller, Jr., and J. Paul. New York: Cambridge University Press.

———. 1996 "The Limited Unity of Virtue." *Nous* 30: 306–29.

Baier, Annette. 1995. *Moral Prejudices: Essays on Ethics.* Cambridge: Harvard University Press.

Baker, Robert, Kathleen Wininger, and Frederick Elliston, eds. 1998. *Philosophy and Sex.* 3d ed. Buffalo, N.Y.: Prometheus Books.

Barnes, J., ed. 1984. *The Complete Works of Aristotle.* Vol. 2. Princeton: Princeton University Press.

Baron, Marcia. 1991 "Impartiality and Friendship." *Ethics* 101: 836–57.

———. 1995. *Kantian Ethics Almost Without Apology.* Ithaca, N.Y.: Cornell University Press.

Baron, Marcia, Philip Pettit, and Michael Slote. 1997. *Three Methods of Ethics.* Oxford: Basil Blackwell Publishers.

Bayles, Michael. 1984. "Marriage, Love, and Procreation." In *Philosophy and Sex.* 2d ed., edited by R. Baker and F. Elliston. Buffalo, N.Y.: Prometheus Books.

Becker, Lawrence. 1990. "Unity, Coincidence, and Conflict in the Virtues." *Philosophia* 20: 127–43.

Bell, Laurie, ed. 1987. *Good Girls, Bad Girls: Feminists and Sex Trade Workers Face to Face.* Toronto: The Seal Press.

Belliotti, Raymond. 1993. *Good Sex: Perspectives on Sexual Ethics.* Lawrence, Kans.: University Press of Kansas.

Benhabib, Seyla. 1987. "The Generalized and The Concrete Other." In *Women and Moral Theory.* See Kittay and Meyers 1987.

Blum, Lawrence. 1980. *Friendship, Altruism, and Morality.* New York: Routledge.

———. 1993. "Gilligan and Kohlberg: Implications for Moral Theory." In *An Ethic of Care.* See Larrabee 1993.

Bogen, James. 1980. "Suicide and Virtue." In *Suicide: The Philosophical Issues,* edited by P. Battin and D. Mayo. New York: St. Martin's Press.

Broadie, Sarah. 1991. *Ethics with Aristotle.* New York: Oxford University Press.

Broughton, John. 1993. "Women's Rationality and Men's Virtues." In *An Ethic of Care.* See Larrabee 1993.

Buckle, Stephen. 2002. "Aristotle's *Republic* or, Why Aristotle's Ethics Is Not Virtue Ethics." *Philosophy* 77: 565–95.

Calhoun, Cheshire. 1988. "Justice, Care, Gender Bias." *Journal of Philosophy* 85: 451–63.

Califia, Pat. 1994. *Public Sex: The Culture of Radical Sex.* Pittsburgh: Cleis Press.

Card, Claudia. 1990. "Caring and Evil." *Hypatia* 5: 101–8.

———. 1995. "Gender and Moral Luck." In *Justice and Care: Essential Readings in Feminist Ethics,* edited by V. Held. Boulder, Colo.: Westview Press.

Carr, Brian. 1999. "Pity and Compassion as Social Virtues." *Philosophy* 74: 411–29.

Carr, David. 1986. "Chastity and Adultery." *American Philosophical Quarterly* 23: 363–71.

Carroll, Noël. 1990. *The Philosophy of Horror, or Paradoxes of the Heart.* New York: Routledge.

Carver, Raymond. 1989. *What We Talk About When We Talk About Love*. New York: Vintage Books.

Chapman, John, and William Galston, eds. 1992. *Virtue*. Nomos, vol. 34. New York: New York University Press.

Cicovacki, Predrag. 1993. "On Love and Fidelity in Marriage." *Journal of Social Philosophy* 24: 92–104.

Clowney, David. 1990. "Virtues, Rules, and the Foundations of Ethics." *Philosophia* 20: 49–67.

Cooper, John. 1998. "The Unity of Virtue." In *Virtue and Vice*. See Paul, Miller, Jr., and Paul 1998.

———. 1999. *Reason and Emotion: Essays on Ancient Moral Psychology and Ethical Theory*. Princeton: Princeton University Press.

Crisp, Roger, ed. 1996. *How Should One Live? Essays on the Virtues*. New York: Oxford University Press.

Crisp, Roger, and Michael Slote, eds. 1997. *Virtue Ethics*. New York: Oxford University Press.

Curzer, Howard. 2002. "Admirable Immorality, Dirty Hands, Care Ethics, Justice Ethics, and Child Sacrifice." *Ratio* 15: 227–44.

Davion, Victoria. 1993. "Autonomy, Integrity, and Care." *Social Theory and Practice* 19: 161–82.

De Bernieres, Louis. 1994. *Corelli's Mandolin*. New York: Vintage Books.

Delacoste, Frederique, and Priscilla Alexander, eds. 1987. *Sex Work: Writings by Women in the Sex Industry*. Pittsburgh and San Francisco: Cleis Press.

De Montaigne, Michel. 1987. "On Affectionate Relationships." In *The Complete Essays*. Translated by M. A. Screech. New York: Penguin Books.

Denis, Lara. 1999. "Kant on the Wrongness of 'Unnatural' Sex." *History of Philosophy Quarterly* 16: 225–48.

Dent, N. J. H. 1984. *The Moral Psychology of the Virtues*. New York: Cambridge University Press.

Driver, Julia. 1996. "The Virtues and Human Nature." In *How Should One Live? Essays on the Virtues*. See Crisp 1996.

Dworkin, Andrea. 1989. *Pornography: Men Possessing Women*. New York: Dutton.

———. 1997. *Life and Death*. New York: Free Press.

Ehman, Robert. 1989. "Personal Love." In *Eros, Agape, and Philia*. See Soble 1989.

Einon, Dorothy. 1994. "Are Men More Promiscuous Than Women?" *Ethology and Sociobiology* 15: 131–43.

Eliot, George. 1998. *The Mill on the Floss*. New York: Oxford University Press.

———. 2001. *Silas Marner*. New York: The Modern Library.

Elliot, David. 1993. "The Nature of Virtue and the Question of Its Primacy." *The Journal of Value Inquiry* 27: 317–30.

Ellis, A. 1986. "Casual Sex." *International Journal of Moral and Social Studies* 1: 157–69.

Elliston, Frederick. 1975. "In Defense of Promiscuity." In *Philosophy and Sex*, edited by R. Baker and F. Elliston. Buffalo, N.Y.: Prometheus Books, 1975.

Ericsson, Lars. 1980. "Charges Against Prostitution: An Attempt at a Philosophical Assessment." *Ethics* 90: 335–66.

Farrell, Daniel. 1989. "Of Jealousy and Envy." In *Person to Person*, edited by G. Graham and H. LaFollette. Philadelphia: Temple University Press.

Feinberg, Joel. 1984. *Harm to Others*. The Moral Limits of the Criminal Law, vol. 1. New York: Oxford University Press.

Finnis, John, and Martha Nussbaum. 1993. "Is Homosexual Conduct Wrong? A Philosophical Exchange." *New Republic* 15 November 1993, 12–13.

Finnis, John. 1994. "Law, Morality, and 'Sexual Orientation.'" *Notre Dame Law Review* 69 (5): 1049–76.

Firestone, Shulamith. 1970. *The Dialectic of Sex: The Case for Feminist Revolution*. New York: William Morrow & Co.

Fisher, Helen. 1992. *Anatomy of Love: The Mysteries of Mating, Marriage, and Why We Stray*. New York: Ballantine Books.

Flanagan, Owen, and Kathryn Jackson. 1993. "Justice, Care, and Gender: The Kohlberg-Gilligan Debate Revisited." In *An Ethic of Care*. See Larrabee 1993.

Flanagan, Owen, and Amelie Oksenberg Rorty, eds. 1993. *Identity, Character and Morality: Essays in Moral Psychology*. Cambridge, Mass.: MIT Press.

Foot, Philippa. 1978. *Virtues and Vices and Other Essays in Moral Philosophy*. Berkeley: University of California Press.

———. 1994. "Rationality and Virtue." In *Norms, Values, and Society*, edited by H. Pauer-Studer. Dordrecht, The Netherlands: Kluwer Academic Publishers, 1994.

———. 1995. "Does Moral Subjectivism Rest on a Mistake?" *Oxford Journal of Legal Studies* 15: 1–14.

———. 2001. *Natural Goodness*. Oxford: Oxford University Press.

French, Peter, Theodore Uehling, Jr., and Howard Wettstein, eds. 1988. *Ethical Theory: Character and Virtue*. Midwest Studies in Philosophy, vol. 13. Notre Dame: University of Notre Dame Press.

Fried, Charles. 1970. *An Anatomy of Values*. Cambridge: Harvard University Press.

———. 1978. *Right and Wrong*. Cambridge: Harvard University Press.

Friedman, Marilyn. 1987. "Care and Context in Moral Reasoning." In *Women and Moral Theory*. See Kittay and Meyers 1987.

———. 1993. *What Are Friends For? Feminist Perspectives on Personal Relationships and Moral Theory*. Ithaca, N.Y.: Cornell University Press.

———. 1995. "Beyond Caring: The Demoralization of Gender." In *Justice and Care: Essential Readings in Feminist Ethics*, edited by V. Held. Boulder, Colo.: Westview Press.

Funari, Vicky. 1997. "Naked, Naughty, Nasty: Peep Show Reflections." In *Whores and Other Feminists*. See Nagle 1997.

Garcia, J. L. A. 1990. "The Primacy of the Virtuous." *Philosophia* 20: 69–91.

Garry, Ann. 1978. "Pornography and Respect for Women." *Social Theory and Practice* 4: 395–421.

Gilligan, Carol. 1982. *In A Different Voice*. Cambridge, Mass.: Harvard University Press.

———. 1987. "Moral Orientation and Moral Development." In *Women and Moral Theory*. See Kittay and Meyers 1987.

Goldman, Alan. 1997. "Plain Sex." In *The Philosophy of Sex*. See Soble 1997a.

Gottlieb, Paula. 2001. "Are the Virtues Remedial?" *Journal of Value Inquiry* 35: 343–54.

Green, O. H. 1997. "Is Love an Emotion?" in *Love Analyzed*. See Lamb 1997.

Greene, Melissa Fay. 2000. "The Orphan Ranger." *The New Yorker*, 17 July, pp. 38–45.

Greenspan, Patricia. 1980. "A Case of Mixed Feelings: Ambivalence and the Logic of Emotion." In *Explaining Emotions*, edited by Amelie Rorty. Berkeley: University of California Press.

Gregory, Paul. 1984. "Against Couples." *Journal of Applied Philosophy* 1: 263–68.

Halwani, Raja. 1995. "Are One-Night Stands Morally Problematic?" *International Journal of Applied Philosophy* 10: 61–67.

———. 1998a. "Essentialism, Social Constructionism, and the History of Homosexuality." *Journal of Homosexuality* 35: 25–51.

———. 1998b. "Virtue Ethics and Adultery." *Journal of Social Philosophy* 29: 5–18.

———. 2002. "Outing and Virtue Ethics." *Journal of Applied Philosophy* 19: 141–54.

Hampton, Jean. 1993. "Selflessness and the Loss of Self." In *Altruism*, edited by E. F. Paul, F. D. Miller, Jr., and J. Paul. New York: Cambridge University Press.

Hannay, Alastair. 1991. *Kierkegaard*. London: Routledge.

Hartz, Glenn. 1990. "Desire and Emotion in the Virtue Tradition." *Philosophia* 20: 145–65.

Hamlyn, D. W. 1989. "The Phenomena of Love and Hate." In *Eros, Agape, and Philia*. See Soble 1989.

Held, Virginia. 1995. "Feminist Moral Inquiry and the Feminist Future." In *Justice and Care: Essential Readings in Feminist Ethics*, edited by V. Held. Boulder, Colo.: Westview Press.

Herman, Barbara. 1993a. "Could It Be Worth Thinking about Kant on Sex and Marriage?" In *A Mind of One's Own: Feminist Essays on Reason and Objectivity*, edited by L. Antony and C. Witt. Boulder, Colo.: Westview Press.

Herman, Barbara. 1993b. *The Practice of Moral Judgment*. Cambridge, Mass.: Harvard University Press.

Hill, Thomas E., Jr. 1980. "Humanity as an End in Itself." *Ethics* 91: 84–90.

———. 1983. "Ideals of Human Excellence and Preserving Natural Environment." *Environmental Ethics* 5: 211–24.

Hoagland, Sarah Lucia. 1990. "Some Concerns about Nel Noddings' *Caring*." *Hypatia* 5: 109–14.

Homiak, Marcia. 1993. "Feminism and Aristotle's Rational Ideal." In *A Mind of One's Own: Feminist Essays on Reason and Objectivity*, edited by L. Antony and C. Witt. Boulder, Colo.: Westview Press.

Hospers, John. 1961. *Human Conduct: An Introduction to the Problem of Ethics.* New York: Harcourt Brace and Company.

Hursthouse, Rosalind. 1986. "Aristotle, *Nicomachean Ethics.*" In *Philosophers Ancient and Modern*, edited by G. Vesey. London: Cambridge University Press.

————. 1995. "Applying Virtue Ethics." In *Virtues and Reasons.* See Hursthouse, Lawrence, and Quinn 1995.

————. 1997a. "Virtue Ethics and the Emotions." In *Virtue Ethics: A Critical Reader.* See Statman 1997.

————. 1997b. "Virtue Theory and Abortion." In *Virtue Ethics: A Critical Reader.* See Statman 1997.

————. 1999a. "A False Doctrine of the Mean." In *Aristotle's Ethics.* See Sherman 1999.

————. 1999b. *On Virtue Ethics.* New York: Oxford University Press.

Hursthouse, Rosalind, Gavin Lawrence, and Warren Quinn, eds. 1995. *Virtues and Reasons: Philippa Foot and Moral Theory.* Oxford: Clarendon Press.

Jacquette, Dale. 2001. "Aristotle on the Value of Friendship as a Motivation for Morality." *The Journal of Value Inquiry* 35: 371–89.

Jaggar, Alison. 1991. "Feminist Ethics: Projects, Problems, Prospects." In *Feminist Ethics,* edited by C. Card. Lawrence, Kans.: University Press of Kansas.

————. 1995. "Caring as a Feminist Practice of Moral Reason." In *Justice and Care: Essential Readings in Feminist Ethics,* edited by V. Held. Boulder, Colo.: Westview Press.

Jeske, Diane. 1997. "Friendship, Virtue, and Impartiality." *Philosophy and Phenomenological Research* 57: 51–72.

————. 2001. "Friendship and Reasons of Intimacy." *Philosophy and Phenomenological Research* 63: 329–46.

Kant, Immanuel. 1963. *Lectures on Ethics.* Translated by Louis Infield. Indianapolis: Hackett.

————. 1993. *Grounding for the Metaphysics of Morals.* Translated by James Ellington. Indianapolis: Hackett.

Kierkegaard, Søren. 1962. *Works of Love.* Translated by H. and E. Hong. New York: Harper and Row.

Kittay, E. F., and D. Meyers. 1987. *Women and Moral Theory.* Savage, Md.: Rowman and Littlefield.

Koehn, Daryl. 1998. *Rethinking Feminist Ethics: Care, Trust, and Empathy.* New York: Routledge.

Kraut, Richard. 1989. *Aristotle on the Human Good.* Princeton: Princeton University Press.

————. 1999. "Aristotle on the Human Good: An Overview." In *Aristotle's Ethics.* See Sherman 1999.

Kristjansson, Kristjan. 1998. "Casual Sex Revisited." *Journal of Social Philosophy* 29: 97–108.

Kruschwitz, Robert, and Robert Roberts, eds. 1987. *The Virtues: Contemporary Essays on Moral Character*. Belmont, Calif.: Wadsworth Publishing.

Kultgen, John. 1998 "The Vicissitudes of Common-Sense Virtue Ethics, Part I: From Aristotle to Slote" and "Part II: The Heuristic Use of Common Sense." *The Journal of Value Inquiry* 32: 325–41 and 465–78, respectively.

Kupfer, Joseph. 1993. "Romantic Love." *Journal of Social Philosophy* 24: 112–20.

Lamb, Roger, ed. 1997. *Love Analyzed*. Boulder, Colo.: Westview Press.

Larrabee, Mary Jeanne, ed. 1993. *An Ethic of Care: Feminist and Interdisciplinary Perspectives*. New York: Routledge.

Lawrence, Aaron. 2000. *The Male Escort's Handbook: Your Guide to Getting Rich the Hard Way*. Warren, N.J.: Late Night Press.

Lederer, Laura, ed. 1980. *Take Back the Night: Women on Pornography*. New York: William Morrow.

Leigh, Carol. 1997. "Inventing Sex Work." In *Whores and Other Feminists*. See Nagle 1997.

LeMoncheck, Linda. 1997. *Loose Women, Lecherous Men: A Feminist Philosophy of Sex*. New York: Oxford University Press.

Lesser, A. H. 1980. "Love and Lust." *Journal of Value Inquiry* 14: 51–54.

Levin, Michael. 1984. "Why Homosexuality Is Abnormal." *The Monist* 67: 251–83.

Levy, Donald. 1980. "Perversion and the Unnatural as Moral Categories." *Ethics* 90: 191–202.

———. 1997. "The Definition of Love in Plato's *Symposium*." In *Sex, Love, and Friendship*. See Soble 1997b.

Lewontin, R. C., Steven Rose, and Leon Kamin. 1984. *Not in Our Genes: Biology, Ideology, and Human Nature*. New York: Pantheon Books.

Longino, Helen. 1980. "Pornography, Oppression, and Freedom: A Closer Look." In *Take Back the Night*. See Lederer 1980.

Louden, Robert. 1997. "On Some Vices of Virtue Ethics." In *Virtue Ethics: A Critical Reader*. See Statman 1997.

MacIntyre, Alasdair. 1984. *After Virtue*. 2d ed. Notre Dame: University of Notre Dame Press.

———. 1999. *Dependent Rational Animals: Why Human Beings Need the Virtues*. Chicago and La Salle, Ill.: Open Court.

MacKinnon, Catharine. 1987. *Feminism Unmodified: Discourses on Life and Law*. Cambridge, Mass.: Harvard University Press.

———. 1993. *Only Words*. Cambridge, Mass.: Harvard University Press.

Marcus, Eric. 1998. *Together Forever: Gay and Lesbian Marriage*. New York: Doubleday, Anchor Books.

Martin, Mike. 1994. "Adultery and Fidelity." *Journal of Social Philosophy* 25: 76–91.

———. 1996. *Love's Virtues*. Lawrence, Kans.: University Press of Kansas.

Mayeroff, Milton. 1971. *On Caring*. New York: Harper Collins.

McFall, Lynne. 1987. "Integrity." *Ethics* 98: 5–20.

———. 1989. *Happiness*. New York: Peter Lang.

McKerlie, Dennis. 2001. "Aristotle's Theory of Justice." *The Southern Journal of Philosophy* 39: 119–41.

McKinnon, Christine. 1999. *Character, Virtue Theories, and the Vices.* Ontario: Broadview Press.

McLaren, Margaret. 2001. "Feminist Ethics: Care as a Virtue." In *Feminists Doing Ethics,* edited by J. Waugh and P. Desautels. Lanham, Md: Rowman and Littlefield.

McMurty, John. 1997. "Sex, Love, and Friendship." In *Sex, Love, and Friendship.* See Soble 1997b.

Mendus, Susan. 1989. "Marital Faithfulness." In *Eros, Agape, and Philia.* See Soble 1989.

Meyers, Diana. 1987. "The Socialized Individual and Individual Autonomy: An Intersection between Philosophy and Psychology." In *Women and Moral Theory.* See Kittay and Meyers 1987.

Mill, John Stuart. 1987. *Utilitarianism.* Buffalo, N.Y.: Prometheus Books.

Miller, Fred Jr., 1995. *Nature, Justice, and Rights in Aristotle's* Politics. Oxford: Clarendon Press.

Mohr, Richard. 1988. *Gays/Justice: A Study of Ethics, Society, and Law.* New York: Columbia University Press.

———. 1994. *A More Perfect Union: Why Straight America Must Stand Up for Gay Rights.* Boston: Beacon Press.

Moody-Adams, Michele. 1991. "Gender and the Complexity of Moral Voices." In *Feminist Ethics,* edited by C. Card. Lawrence, Kans.: University Press of Kansas.

Morgan, Peggy. 1987. "Living on the Edge." In *Sex Work.* See Delacoste and Alexander 1987.

Murphy, Timothy. 1987. "Homosexuality and Nature: Happiness and the Law at Stake." *Journal of Applied Philosophy* 4: 195–204.

Nagle, Jill, ed. 1997. *Whores and Other Feminists.* New York: Routledge.

Nakhnikian, George. 1978. "Love in Human Reason." In *Studies in Ethical Theory,* edited by P. French, T. Uehling, Jr., and H. Wettstein. Midwest Studies in Philosophy, vol. 3, pp. 286–317. Notre Dame: University of Notre Dame Press.

Newton-Smith, W. 1989. "A Conceptual Investigation of Love." In *Eros, Agape, and Philia.* See Soble 1989.

Noddings, Nel. 1984. *Caring: A Feminine Approach to Ethics and Moral Education.* Berkeley: University of California Press.

———. 1990. "A Response." *Hypatia* 5: 120–26.

Nozick, Robert. 1989. *The Examined Life: Philosophical Meditations.* New York: Simon and Schuster.

———. 1991. "Love's Bond." In *The Philosophy of (Erotic) Love.* See Solomon and Higgins 1991.

Nussbaum, Martha. 1986. *The Fragility of Goodness: Luck and Ethics in Greek Tragedy and Philosophy.* New York: Cambridge University Press.

———. 1988. "Non-Relative Virtues: An Aristotelian Approach." In *Ethical Theory*, pp. 32–53. See French, Uehling, and Wettstein 1988.

———. 1994. *The Therapy of Desire: Theory and Practice in Hellenistic Ethics.* Princeton: Princeton University Press.

———. 1995a. "Aristotle on Human Nature and the Foundations of Ethics." In *World, Mind, and Ethics: Essays on the Ethical Philosophy of Bernard Williams.*, edited by J. E. J. Altham and R. Harrison. New York: Cambridge University Press.

———. 1995b. "Objectification." *Philosophy and Public Affairs* 24: 249–91.

———. 1999. *Sex and Social Justice.* New York: Oxford University Press.

Nygren, Anders. 1982. *Agape and Eros.* Chicago: University of Chicago Press.

Oakley, Justin. 1996. "Varieties of Virtue Ethics." *Ratio* 9: 128–52.

Okin, Susan Moller. 1979. *Women in Western Political Thought.* Princeton: Princeton University Press.

———. 1989. *Justice, Gender, and the Family.* New York: Basic Books.

———. 1996. "Feminism, Moral Development, and the Virtues." In *How Should One Live?* See Crisp 1996.

Pateman, Carole. 1983. "Defending Prostitution: Charges Against Ericsson." *Ethics* 93: 561–65.

Paul, Ellen Frankel, Fred Miller, Jr., and Jeffrey Paul, eds. 1998. *Virtue and Vice.* New York: Cambridge University Press.

———. 1999. *Human Flourishing.* New York: Cambridge University Press.

Person, Ethel Spector. 1995. "The Value of Romantic Love." In *On Love and Friendship.* See Williams 1995.

Pettit, Philip. 1997. "Love and Its Place in Moral Discourse." In *Love Analyzed.* See Lamb 1997.

Pincoffs, Edmund. 1986. *Quandries and Virtues: Against Reductivism in Ethics.* Lawrence, Kans.: University Press of Kansas.

Pitcher, George. 1965. "Emotion." *Mind* 74: 326–46.

Plato. 1982. *Euthyphro.* Translated by Lane Cooper. In *Plato: The Collected Dialogues*, edited by E. Hamilton and H. Cairns. Princeton: Princeton University Press.

———. 1989. *Symposium.* Translated by A. Nehemas and P. Woodruff. Indianapolis: Hackett.

———. 1995. *Phaedrus.* Translated by A. Nehemas and P. Woodruff. Indianapolis: Hackett.

Price, A. W. 1997. *Love and Friendship in Plato and Aristotle.* New York: Oxford University Press.

Primoratz, Igor. 1993. "What's Wrong with Prostitution?" In *The Philosophy of Sex.* See Soble 1997a.

———. 1999. *Ethics and Sex.* New York: Routledge.

Prior, William. 2001. "*Eudaimonism* and Virtue." *Journal of Value Inquiry* 35: 325–42.

Punzo, Vincent. 1969. *Reflective Naturalism: An Introduction to Moral Philosophy.* New York: Macmillan Company.

Putman, Daniel. 1991a. "Relational Ethics and Virtue Theory." *Metaphilosophy* 22: 231–38.

———. 1991b. "Sex and Virtue." *International Journal of Moral and Social Studies* 6: 47–56.

Rachels, James. 1989. "Morality, Parents, and Children." In *Person to Person*, edited by G. Graham and H. LaFollette. Philadelphia: Temple University Press.

Richardson, Henry. 1997. *Practical Reasoning about Final Ends*. Cambridge: Cambridge University Press.

Roberts, Robert C. 1988. "Humor and the Virtues." *Inquiry* 31: 127–49.

Rogers, Eugene F., Jr., ed. 2002. *Theology and Sexuality: Classic and Contemporary Readings*. Oxford: Blackwell.

Rorty, Amelie Oksenberg. 1980. *Essays on Aristotle's Ethics*. Berkeley: University of California Press.

Ruddick, Sara. 1989. *Maternal Thinking: Towards a Politics of Peace*. Boston: Beacon Press.

Satz, Debra. 1995. "Markets in Women's Sexual Labor." *Ethics* 106: 63–85.

Savage, Dan. 2002. "Swingers: A Love Story." *The Chicago Reader*, October 18.

Savarino, Mary Ella. 1993. "Toward an Ontology of Virtue Ethics." *Journal of Philosophical Research* 18: 243–59.

Schopenhauer, Arthur. 1958. *The World as Will and Representation*. Translated by E. F. Payne. Vol. 2. New York: Dover Books.

Scoccia, Danny. 2000. "Moral Paternalism, Virtue, and Autonomy." *Australasian Journal of Philosophy* 78: 53–71.

Scruton, Roger. 1986. *Sexual Desire: A Moral Philosophy of the Erotic*. New York: Free Press.

Segal, Lynne, and Mary McIntosh, eds. 1993. *Sex Exposed: Sexuality and the Pornography Debate*. New Brunswick, N.J.: Rutgers University Press.

Sexhelp.com! Dr. Carnes' Resources for Sex Addiction and Recovery. 4 June, 2003. <http://www.sexhelp.com/>.

Sher, George. 1987. "Other Voices, Other Rooms? Women's Psychology and Moral Theory." In *Women and Moral Theory*. See Kittay and Meyers 1987.

Sherman, Nancy. 1989. *The Fabric of Character: Aristotle's Theory of Virtue*. Oxford: Clarendon Press.

———, ed. 1999. *Aristotle's Ethics: Critical Essays*. Lanham, Md.: Rowman and Littlefield.

Shrage, Laurie. 1989. "Should Feminists Oppose Prostitution?" In *The Philosophy of Sex*. See Soble 1997a.

———. 1994. *Moral Dilemmas of Feminism: Prostitution, Adultery, and Abortion*. New York: Routledge.

Sihvola, Juha. 2002. "Aristotle on Sex and Love." In *The Sleep of Reason: Erotic Experience and Sexual Ethics in Ancient Greece and Rome*, edited by M. Nussbaum and J. Sihvola. Chicago: University of Chicago Press.

Simpson, Peter. 1992. "Contemporary Virtue Ethics and Aristotle." *Review of Metaphysics* 45: 503–20.

Singer, Irving. 1984. *The Nature of Love.* Vol. 1. 2d ed. Also vols. 2–3. Chicago: University of Chicago Press.

———. 1994. *The Pursuit of Love.* Baltimore: Johns Hopkins Univesity Press.

———. 2001a. *Sex: A Philosophical Primer.* Lanham, Md.: Rowman and Littlefield.

———. 2001b. *Explorations in Love and Sex.* Lanham, Md.: Rowman and Littlefield.

Slote, Michael. 1983. *Goods and Virtues.* New York: Oxford University Press.

———. 1992. *From Morality to Virtue.* New York: Oxford University Press.

———. 1995. "Agent-Based Virtue Ethics." In *Moral Concepts,* edited by P. French, T. Uehling, Jr., and H. Wettstein. Midwest Studies in Philosophy, vol. 20, pp. 83–101. Notre Dame: University of Notre Dame Press.

———. 1998a. "The Justice of Caring." In *Virtue and Vice.* See Paul, Miller, Jr., and Paul 1998.

———. 1998b. "Caring in the Balance." In *Norms and Values: Essays on the Work of Virginia Held,* edited by J. Haber and M. Halfon. Lanham, Md.: Rowman and Littlefield.

———. 2001. *Morals from Motives.* New York: Oxford University Press.

Smart, J. J. C., and Bernard Williams. 1973. *Utilitarianism: For and Against.* Cambridge: Cambridge University Press.

Sober, Elliott. 1993. *Philosophy of Biology.* Boulder, Colo.: Westview Press.

Soble, Alan, ed. 1989. *Eros, Agape, and Philia: Readings in the Philosophy of Love.* New York: Paragon House. Reprinted 1999.

———. 1990. *The Structure of Love.* New Haven, Conn.: Yale University Press.

———. 1996. *Sexual Investigations.* New York: New York University Press.

———, ed. 1997a. *The Philosophy of Sex: Contemporary Readings.* 3d ed. Lanham, Md.: Rowman and Littlefield.

———, ed. 1997b. *Sex, Love, and Friendship: Studies of the Society for the Philosophy of Sex and Love, 1977–1992.* Amsterdam: Rodopi.

———. 1997c. "Union, Autonomy, and Concern." In *Love Analyzed.* See Lamb 1997.

———. 1998. *The Philosophy of Sex and Love.* St. Paul, Minn.: Paragon House.

———. 2002a. "Sexual Use and What to Do About It: Internalist and Externalist Sexual Ethics." In *The Philosophy of Sex: Contemporary Readings.* 4th ed., edited by Alan Soble. Lanham, Md.: Rowman and Littlefield.

———. 2002b. *Pornography, Sex, and Feminism.* Amherst, N.Y.: Prometheus Books.

———. 2003. "Kant and Sexual Perversion." *The Monist* 86: 55–89.

Solomon, David. 1997. "Internal Objections to Virtue Ethics." In *Virtue Ethics: A Critical Reader.* See Statman 1997.

Solomon, Robert. 1990. *Love: Emotion, Myth, and Metaphor.* Buffalo, N.Y.: Prometheus Books.

———. 1991. "The Virtue of (Erotic) Love." In *The Philosophy of (Erotic) Love.* See Solomon and Higgins 1991.

———. 1997. "Corporate Roles, Personal Virtues: An Aristotelian Approach to Business Ethics." In *Virtue Ethics: A Critical Reader.* See Statman 1997.

Solomon, Robert, and Kathleen Higgins, eds. 1991. *The Philosophy of (Erotic) Love*. Lawrence, Kans.: University Press of Kansas.

Stafford, Martin. 1977. "On Distinguishing Between Love and Lust." *Journal of Value Inquiry* 11: 292–303.

———. 1988. "Love and Lust Revisited: Intentionality, Homosexuality, and Moral Education." *Journal of Applied Philosophy* 5: 87–100.

Statman, Daniel, ed. 1997. *Virtue Ethics: A Critical Reader*. D.C.: Georgetown University Press.

Stein, Edward, ed. 1990. *Forms of Desire: Sexual Orientation and the Social Constructionist Controversy*. New York: Routledge.

Steinbock, Bonnie. 1991. "Adultery." In *The Philosophy of Sex: Contemporary Readings*. 2d ed., edited by A. Soble. Lanham, Md.: Rowman and Littlefield.

Stocker, Michael. 1976. "The Schizophrenia of Modern Ethical Theories." *Journal of Philosophy* 73: 453–66.

———. 1987. "Duty and Friendship: Toward a Synthesis of Gilligan's Contrastive Moral Concepts." In *Women and Moral Theory*. See Kittay and Meyers 1987.

Stocker, Michael, with Elizabeth Hegeman. 1996. *Valuing Emotions*. New York: Cambridge University Press.

Stohr, Karen, and Christopher Heath Wellman. 2002. "Recent Work on Virtue Ethics." *American Philosophical Quarterly* 39: 49–72.

Swanton, Christine. 1995. "Profiles of the Virtues." *Pacific Philosophical Quarterly* 76: 47–72.

———. 1997. "The Supposed Tension Between 'Strength' and 'Gentleness' Conceptions of the Virtues." *Australasian Journal of Philosophy* 75: 497–510.

———. 2001. "A Virtue Ethical Account of Right Action." *Ethics* 112: 32–52.

———. 2003. *Virtue Ethics: A Pluralistic View*. New York: Oxford University Press.

Taylor, Gabriele. 1979. "Love." In *Philosophy As It Is*, edited by T. Honderich and M. Burnyeat. London: Penguin Books.

———. 1988. "Envy and Jealousy: Emotions and Vices." In *Ethical Theory*, pp. 233–49. See French, Uehling, Jr., and Wettstein 1988.

Taylor, Richard. 1982. *Having Love Affairs*. Buffalo, N.Y.: Prometheus Books.

———. 1991. *Virtue Ethics*. Interlaken, N.Y.: Linden Books.

Thomas, Laurence. 1989. "Friends and Lovers." In *Person to Person*, edited by G. Graham and H. LaFollette. Philadelphia: Temple University Press.

———. 1991 "Reasons for Loving." In *The Philosophy of (Erotic) Love*. See Solomon and Higgins 1991.

Tong, Rosemarie. 1997. "Feminist Perspectives on Empathy as an Epistemic Skill and Caring as a Moral Virtue." *Journal of Medical Humanities* 18: 153–68.

———. 1998. "The Ethics of Care: A Feminist Virtue Ethics of Care for Healthcare Practitioners." *Journal of Medicine and Philosophy* 23: 131–52.

Trianosky, Gregory. 1987. "Virtue, Action, and the Good Life: Toward a Theory of the Virtues." *Pacific Philosophical Quarterly* 68: 124–47.

———. 1988. "Rightly Ordered Appetites: How to Live Morally and Live Well." *American Philosophical Quarterly* 25: 1–12.

Tronto, Joan. 1993. *Moral Boundaries: A Political Argument for the Ethics of Care.* New York: Routledge.

Udovicki, Jasminka. 1993. "Justice and Care in Close Relationships." *Hypatia* 8: 48–60.

Vannoy, Russell. 1980. *Sex Without Love: A Philosophical Exploration.* Buffalo, N.Y.: Prometheus Books.

Velleman, David. 1999. "Love as a Moral Emotion." *Ethics* 109: 338–74.

Verene, D. P. 1975. "Sexual Love and Moral Experience." In *Philosophy and Sex.* 1st. ed., edited by R. Baker and F. Elliston. Buffalo, N.Y.: Prometheus Books.

———, ed. 1995. *Sexual Love and Western Morality: A Philosophical Anthology.* 2d ed. Boston: Jones and Bartlett Publishers.

Waide, John. 1988. "Virtues and Principles." *Philosophy and Phenomenological Research* 48: 455–72.

Walker, A. D. M. 1993. "The Incompatibility of the Virtues." *Ratio* 6: 44–62.

Wallace, James. 1978. *Virtues and Vices.* Ithaca, N.Y.: Cornell University Press.

Wasserstrom, Richard. 1984. "Is Adultery Immoral?" In *Philosophy and Sex.* 2d ed., edited by R. Baker and F. Elliston. Buffalo, N.Y.: Prometheus Books.

Watson, Gary. 1975. "Free Agency." *The Journal of Philosophy* 72: 205–20.

———. 1984. "Virtues in Excess." *Philosophical Studies* 46: 57–74.

———. 1997. "On the Primacy of Character." In *Virtue Ethics: A Critical Reader.* See Statman 1997.

Weinstein, Steve. 2001. "Escort Report." *Out*, March, pp. 90–95.

West, Robin. 1997. "The Harms of Consensual Sex." In *The Philosophy of Sex.* See Soble 1997a.

Wharton, Edith. 1970. *Ethan Frome.* New York: Charles Scribner's Sons.

White, Richard. 2001. *Love's Philosophy.* Lanham, Md.: Rowman and Littlefield.

Wielenberg, Erik. 2002. "Pleasure, Pain, and Moral Character and Development." *Pacific Philosophical Quarterly* 83: 282–99.

Williams, Bernard. 1985. *Ethics and the Limits of Philosophy.* Cambridge, Mass.: Harvard University Press.

Williams, Clifford, ed. 1995. *On Love and Friendship: Philosophical Readings.* Boston: Jones and Bartlett Publishers.

Wreen, Michael. 1991. "What's Really Wrong with Adultery." In *The Philosophy of Sex: Contemporary Readings.* 2d ed., edited by A. Soble. Lanham, Md.: Rowman and Littlefield.

Young, Charles. 1988. "Aristotle on Temperance." *The Philosophical Review* 97: 521–42.

Zagzebski, Linda Trinkaus. 1996. *Virtues of the Mind: An Inquiry into the Nature of Virtue and the Ethical Foundations of Knowledge.* New York: Cambridge University Press.

Index

abortion, 78, 204, 268n40
Abraham (Bible), 267n36
abuse, 31, 95–96, 153, 200
actions. *See also* right action; virtuous
    action
    emotions in, 12, 13, 81–82,
        261n5
    erotic passion and bad, 153
    gap between virtues and, 185–86
    for justice, 121
    of kindness/love, 104–8, 121–22
    reason, emotion and caring,
        39–44
    rightness of, 15, 75
    without meditation of principles,
        33
activities. *See also* sexual activity
    in friendship/love, 166–67
    sex as, 189
    war as caring, 269n44
acts
    love and immoral, 152–58
    sexual, 250
    virtuous *v.* harmful, 153–55
admiration, 117
adult bookstores, 184
adultery, 171, 178, 184, 197
    affairs and, 231
    Aristotle on, 181
    emotions and, 233–35
    through temptation, 192

as wrong, 215, 226–27, 229
"Adultery" (Steinbock), 229
affairs, 7, 229
    one-night stands *v.*, 227, 231–34
    open, 239–40, 242
affections
    desires, beliefs and, 117
    intimacy and, 229–30
    love and, 88, 101, 103, 115, 167
Alexander, Priscilla, 251
anger, 116, 129, 153
    patience as disposition to exhibit
        for, 64
    romantic love *v.*, 90, 117
Annas, Julia, 140–41
Anscombe, G. E. M., 170, 211, 217
appetites, 179–80
    Aristotle on, 181–82, 276n3
    desires *v.*, 174–75
Aquinas, Thomas, 262n13
Archard, David, 267n31
Aristotle
    on adultery, 181
    on appetites, 181–82, 276n3
    on conditions for virtuous action,
        41–44, 61
    on eating, drinking, and sex, 188,
        189
    on emotions as virtues, 128–29
    on ethical naturalism, 11–12
    on external goods, 12–13

301

Euthyphro, 267n36
evil, 47–48, 65–66, 200–201
excellence, 35, 37
exclusivity, 229
  of romantic love/friendship, 85,
    94, 165, 270n6, 284n61
The Exorcist (film), 110

fairness, 93, 104–5, 133, 134
faithfulness, 133, 134, 136, 173
family, 39, 80, 194, 229
fantasy, 200, 207, 280n34
father-son relationships, 46–47
favoritism, 53, 80, 93
fear, 109–11, 116, 129
feminist ethics, 19, 25
feminists
  on prostitution, 247
  on sex work, 3, 9, 201, 280n34
  on sexism, 8
fidelity, 133–35, 165, 173, 229, 234
financial warfare, 153
fine, as notion, 181, 182, 221–22
Finnis, John, 170
Firas (man), sexual life of, 219–24,
  241
Firestone, Shulamith, 258
Flanagan, Owen, 264n21
flourishing, 6, 7
  with care, 67–71
  definitions of, 12–13, 15
  as ethically basic, 39–40
  excellence as part of, 37
  with open relationships, 226, 229,
    235
  with *philia*, 38
  with promiscuity, 197, 209, 211,
    213, 216–17
  with romantic love, 13, 19–20,
    85, 88–89, 96, 98, 121,
    158–68
  with sex, 169–70, 197
  with sex work, 192, 195, 200,
    242, 245–47, 253
  through relationships, 39–40, 55,
    81
  virtue ethics on, 245–46

  virtues for, 17, 35
food, drink, sex and, 171, 180,
    181–83, 187–89. *See also*
    peanut eating
Foot, Philippa, 12, 13
Franke, Rebecca, 264n14
Fried, Charles, 169
Friedman, Marilyn, 49–52, 263n4
friendliness, 71
friends
  as another self, 44–45
  goals of, 45–46, 123
  living together, 166
  relationships between, 65, 67
friendships, 37, 51–52, 61–62
  Aristotle on, 6, 7, 20, 37, 44–46,
    80–81, 94, 158, 166–67,
    264n13, 266n27
  Card on, 264n16
  in care ethics, 23, 29–30, 32,
    36–37
  care/concern in, 150
  integrity and, 32
  as love, 85, 88–89
  Montaigne on, 270n7
  romantic love *v.*, 2, 94–95,
    160–68
  sex and, 7, 94, 165
  values/beliefs of, 49–52
fun, 142–43
Funari, Vicky, 251
fungibility, 207–8

Gandhi, 275n48
gangsters, 195
Garry, Ann, 279n33
gay bars, 220, 232–33
gay(s), 2, 254, 285n75. *See also*
    homophobia; homosexuality
  in bars, 207
  cruisings, 227, 232–33
  in health club, 212
  /lesbian couples, 236–39,
    241–42, 284n63
  liberation, 282n53
  marriages, 78
  in military, 78

slavishness, 221, 277n8, 278n17
  of gratification, 189
  of pleasure, 217
Slote, Michael, 14, 24, 28, 71–72,
  74–79
Soble, Alan
  on emotions, 272n17
  on love, 86, 103, 104, 140, 143,
    144–45
  on lovers' autonomy, 271n9
  on prostitution, 250
  on sex, 169, 170, 225
social issues, caring for intimates *v.*,
  76–78
society
  erotic in, 271n13
  isolation from, 120
  laws in, 75–79, 266n29
  public *v.* private in, 126–27
sociobiology, 255–57
Socrates, 267n36, 275n48, 275n49
Solomon, Robert, 124–32, 149,
  271n14
spontaneity, 42, 54
spouse(s)
  relationships between, 80
  sex with, 180, 197, 215
  sex with friend's, 182, 184, 185
  sex with others than, 177, 178,
    196, 205, 226, 231
  of ship's captain dilemma, 58–60
  and stranger in car accident, 56,
    60, 80
stealing, 177, 178
Steinbock, Bonnie, 215, 229–36,
  239
Steve, restaurant revulsion and,
  110–11
Stocker, Michael, 273n32
the Stoics
  on extirpation of passions/
    emotions, 154–57
  on good life, 13
  romantic love/virtues, 8, 137,
    151–58, 262n13
strangers
  compassion to, 100

justice to, 65, 266n29
kindness toward, 148–50
partiality/impartiality and, 55–58,
  60
relationships with, 126–27, 147
saving drowning, 100
and spouse in car accident, 56, 60,
  80
streetwalking, 194, 249
strippers, 169, 199, 243–44
stripping, 3, 192, 195, 243, 254
student testimonials, 213–14
subjectivity, denial of, 208
subservience, 278n17
suffering, 148, 278n17
Swanton, Christine, 262n6, 265n21,
  272n27, 274n42
The Swimming-Pool Library
  (Hollinghurst), 212
sympathy, 26, 33, 116
Symposium (Plato), 95, 161, 269n2
syphilis, 217

T1 (moderation), 187–88
  compatibility of promiscuity with,
    209–25
  first ideal and, 209–25
  second ideal and, 226–42
  T2 and, 182–84, 190–91, 195
  third ideal and, 242–54
T2 (not wronging others)
  T1 and, 182–84, 190–91, 195
  three ideals and, 196–209
"Taking Money For Bodily Services"
  (Nussbaum), 193
Taylor, Gabriele, 137–38, 158
teenagers, male, 202–3
temperance, 11, 13, 17, 171–90. *See
  also* intemperance
  Aristotle on, 5, 180–82, 188, 221,
    277n6
  continence *v.*, 170–71, 177–80,
    190–91
  promiscuity and, 12, 20–21
  sex and, 6, 64
temptation, 48–49, 192
tenderness, 64

whores, 243
wife-husband relationship, 36, 46
Williams, Bernard, 57, 270n5
wisdom, 47, 82–83. *See also* reason(s)
 in action, 13
 in love, 124, 139, 161
 moral, 148–49
 practical, 61, 68, 70, 102, 119,
  120, 132, 274n42
 regulative role of, 15, 52
 as virtue, 11, 74, 133, 148
wittiness, 71
women
 Aristotle on elitism, slavery and,
  17–18
 v. men and reason, 24–25
 v. men in romantic love, 163

v. men on morality, 7–8
oppression/objectification of,
 201–3, 205–8, 279n32,
 281n39
in sex industry, 201–3
sexual behavior of men *v.*, 221,
 254–59, 284n65
The World as Will and Representation
 (Schopenhauer), 271n11
Wreen, Michael, 278n21

Yasser (man in forties), life of,
 162–64, 168
Young, Charles, 188, 189

Zagzebski, Linda, 16, 70, 122, 124